BARRON'S

TEAS®

PRACTICE TESTS

Sandra S. Swick, B.S.N., M.S.N., Ed.D.

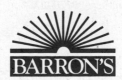

BARRON'S

Now Available!

Go to
barronsbooks.com/tp/TEAS/
to take a free sample
TEAS complete with
answer explanations and
automated scoring.

*Online tests can be accessed on most mobile devices, including tablets and smartphones.

All inquiries should be addressed to:
Barron's Educational Series, Inc.
250 Wireless Boulevard
Hauppauge, New York 11788
www.barronseduc.com

Library of Congress Control Number: 2017942757

ISBN: 978-1-4380-1028-1

PRINTED IN THE UNITED STATES OF AMERICA

9 8 7 6 5 4 3 2 1

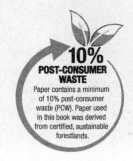

10%
POST-CONSUMER
WASTE
Paper contains a minimum
of 10% post-consumer
waste (PCW). Paper used
in this book was derived
from certified, sustainable
forestlands.

Contents

Introduction

━━━

If you purchased this TEAS book of practice tests, there's a good chance you have a nursing entrance exam in your future. If it's the TEAS, then this is the book you need to help you in your preparation. *TEAS Practice Tests* will give you information about: (1) why nursing entrance exams are important and necessary, (2) the format of the TEAS test, (3) study strategies and suggestions, including alternative options to consider if you are not offered admission to a nursing program, and (4) five TEAS practice tests with rationales for each question. There is also an additional sixth practice test online that can be accessed at *barronsbooks.com/tp/TEAS/*.

WHY DO I NEED TO TAKE A NURSING ENTRANCE EXAM?

Life is full of instances in which if you want something, you must show your worthiness by meeting specific criteria. You passed a written test and successfully drove for an examiner to receive your driver's license. You had to meet certain state criteria to graduate from high school, and you had to meet specific criteria for admission to a college or university. You also had to meet specific criteria to pass certain college courses. Nursing programs are no different. It's not uncommon for a nursing program to require a nursing entrance exam as part of its admission process. There are numerous entrance exams on the market, and nursing programs select an exam that best meets their needs. Nursing programs determine your probability of success based on your exam scores. Academic skills are one of the areas of interest in nursing programs. They include such factors as

- Critical and analytical thinking
- Problem solving
- Reading competency
- Mathematical ability
- Study habits
- Time management
- Written/oral communication

Your critical and analytical thinking skills, problem solving ability, reading competency, mathematical ability, and time management skills can all be measured by entrance exams. Registered nursing programs are competitive. Nursing programs rarely admit all applicants. A nursing program may have 200 applicants who meet or exceed all admission criteria but may only offer admission to 50 of them. Given the competitiveness of nursing programs, it may be a good idea to apply to more than one program.

Course work in a nursing program is the most difficult you'll ever attempt. Nursing courses build on previous courses. Prerequisite courses serve as groundwork for nursing courses, and courses become more difficult as you progress. What you learn in an introductory nursing course will serve as the foundation for other nursing courses.

THE TEAS TEST

Developed by Assessment Technologies Institute (ATI) the Test of Essential Academic Skills, better known as TEAS, is a standardized multiple-choice test that examines basic academic preparation in the areas of Reading, Mathematics, Science, and English and Language Usage. The TEAS is used by many nursing and other health science programs as one component of the admission process. As of this writing, the TEAS is offered in both paper and pencil and computer formats. A simple four-function calculator is embedded in the computerized format.

Visit *barronsbooks.com/tp/TEAS/* for access to a free online sample test!

Content Area	Number of Test Items	Time Allowed
Reading	53	64 min.
Mathematics	36	54 min.
Science	53	63 min.
English and Language Usage	28	28 min.
Total	170	209 min. (3.5 hr.)

STRATEGIES FOR SUCCESS

The key to doing well on any test is preparation and accurate application of testing strategies and knowledge. It's also important to examine how you prepare for a test and how you actually take a test. Do not completely rearrange your method of preparation if it consistently produces above-average grades and meets your goals. If your preparation is average or below average, and this is demonstrated in your past grades, you will need to reassess your study strategy in order to succeed on the TEAS.

Your performance on the TEAS test has the potential to positively or negatively impact your future. It is paramount that you have a course of study that will prepare you to do your very best. Having a goal to obtain the minimal required TEAS score is not acceptable because there are students whose goal is to obtain the highest score possible, and they will score higher than you. Plan on giving your best effort!

Your attitude can have a positive or negative impact on your preparation and performance on the TEAS. It can be overwhelming when you consider the amount of information the TEAS test encompasses. Do not let this mountain of material overwhelm you! This should not be new information. The TEAS addresses information to which you should have already been exposed. Your preparation for the TEAS actually started the day you started school many years ago. In all likelihood, you know much more than you think you do.

PAST PERFORMANCE

Do not delude yourself with the opinion that since you made As and Bs in your previous courses, you know the content and will be able to apply it when taking the TEAS. Test preparation is more than spending a number of hours in the presence of a book and your class notes. It is also much more than expecting admission to a nursing program when your study participation and preparation has been minimal. Developing and successfully implementing a realistic study plan or schedule can only enhance your TEAS scores. You can do this!

TESTING ACCOMMODATION

The U.S. Department of Justice's Americans with Disabilities Act (ADA) "ensures that individuals with disabilities have the opportunity to fairly compete for and pursue such opportunities by requiring testing entities to offer exams in a manner accessible to persons with disabilities. When needed testing accommodations are provided, test-takers can demonstrate their true aptitude."

> Do not assume that prior accommodation guarantees accommodation for the TEAS or that checking a box on the admissions papers guarantees accommodation.

If you require reasonable accommodation when taking the TEAS test, you should contact the nursing program as soon as possible to ensure that there is time to certify that accommodation is needed and it is adequately provided.

Student Services in the nursing program or at the educational institution can provide you with needed information, but it is your responsibility to take care of what needs to be done in a timely fashion.

MULTIPLE-CHOICE TESTS

The TEAS is in a multiple-choice format. You should already be familiar with this form of testing. Multiple-choice testing, such as in the TEAS, is adaptable and capable of measuring many types of learning outcomes at the knowledge and comprehension levels. These outcomes are measurable and observable. Words such as *identify, interpret, compare and contrast, apply, calculate, explain, formulate, solve,* and *evaluate* are frequently used when measuring students' learning outcomes and apply to testing as well.

Among the knowledge outcomes measured by multiple-choice tests are

- Knowledge of

  - Specific information
  - Terminology
  - Specific facts
  - Principles
  - Methods/procedures

- Ability to

  - Interpret cause-and-effect relationships
  - Compare and contrast material or objects
  - Justify methods/procedures
  - Read comprehensively and interpret what has been read
  - Perform mathematical and scientific functions
  - Think critically

The majority of standardized tests use multiple-choice formats. Examples are the GED, ACT, SAT, GRE, LSAT, HESI, NET, NLN PAX-RN, and NCLEX-RN. Multiple-choice items (questions) are composed of a stem and options. Items have one stem and typically three, four, or five options.

The stem presents the problem that needs to be solved. It typically asks a question, but it can also be fill-in-the-blank. There is no single type of stem. The following is an example of a question stem.

The United States President who delivered the Gettysburg Address is:

Options consist of the correct answer and distractors (incorrect answers). The correct answer is obvious to the individual who knows and understands the content of the question. Distractors are plausible options that distract from the correct answer. Distractors appear reasonable and are most often selected by individuals who do not know or understand the content being tested. Appropriate options for the above stem are:

(A) Abraham Lincoln (correct response)
(B) Andrew Johnson
(C) George Washington
(D) James Buchanan

You will notice as you take the practice tests in this book that the options are presented in alphabetical order. This was purposefully done to reduce using illogical methods of determining a correct answer when the actual correct answer cannot be determined. Selecting option C or the longest answer if the actual answer is not known will not work.

A STUDY PLAN FOR THE TEAS

Study plans are organized schedules or plans that delineate your learning objectives/goals and specific times of study for a period of time. Study plans serve three basic purposes: (1) You become more organized because your studying is not hit or miss, (2) you become accountable or responsible for your learning and obtaining of goals, and (3) guilt for not taking the time and effort to learn is basically eliminated because you have a workable plan to follow. Self-discipline and willpower are keys to reaching your goals.

Where to Start

It's always best to start at the beginning. The first thing you need to do is develop a realistic, organized study plan. Sacrifice is often a component of any serious planning, and you will most likely have to sacrifice some of your social time when preparing for the TEAS. You are the only person who can determine how much study time you need to prepare. You lessen your chances of gaining admission to a nursing program if you are not honest with yourself.

There is no correct or incorrect study plan. You may want to use the first practice test in this book as a diagnostic tool to give yourself an idea of your strengths and weaknesses. Do not time yourself if you do this—the purpose of doing this is to identify areas needing improvement, not to set a speed record.

Again, you are the expert when considering the amount of time to spend on each content area of the TEAS. Forget about your grades at this point and honestly assess how well you know, understand, and can apply information in each content area. If you have been a strong math student, you may not need as much time with math preparation. If you are weak in science, you'll need to devote more time to this area. It's important to remember that you are reviewing to take the TEAS. Preparatory time is not meant to teach you what you do not know.

TEAS CONTENT AREAS

The following pages address the content areas of Reading, Mathematics, Science, and English and Language Usage. The list of Test Elements included in each content area is not all-inclusive—it would be virtually impossible to list every element that has the potential to appear on the TEAS.

As you begin perusing the testing elements of each content area, you will see that vocabulary is essential. You need to understand what the words mean and be able to apply these meanings to specific problems or circumstances. Consider the following randomly selected items from the Test Elements of each content area:

- What is a *topic sentence* in a passage or paragraph?
- What are *inferences* of a passage or paragraph?
- What is a *bias*, a *stereotype*, or *tone* in an author's writing?
- What are the *differences* among the various writing types?
- How do you define a word or phrase from its *context*?
- What is *alliteration, slang,* or *allusion*?
- What is meant by *compare and contrast*?
- What is the *order of operations* in mathematics? Can you correctly apply them?
- What are key words that indicate specific *mathematical functions*?
- What is the *Pythagorean theorem* or *theory*? Do you know when and how to apply it?
- Do you know *geometry formulas* for such things as volume, surface area, and perimeter?
- How do you determine age, distance, and percentage change, and read charts and tables in word problems?
- Can you *convert* from one *measurement system* to another?
- What is the *purpose* of each body system? How does each work, and how does each system *affect* or *influence* other body systems? What anatomical structures comprise a system? Are these structures used by more than one system?
- What is a *Punnett square*, how do you set one up, and what do its results suggest?
- Can you read the *Periodic Table of Elements*?
- What is *atomic structure*? How do you determine it?
- What are *substances* and what are their unique characteristics?
- What are *acids* and *bases*? How does *pH* play into acids and bases?
- What is *scientific inquiry*, and can you define each of its components? What is the *scientific method*?
- Can you differentiate between types of sentences?
- What is the difference between *formal* and *informal writing*? Can you select examples of each?
- How well do you spell? Do you know *rules for spelling*?
- When do you use a *colon* as opposed to using a *semicolon*?

Can you define and discuss the italicized words in the above bulleted list? You should be able to. A strong vocabulary is necessary for performing well on the TEAS. Without an adequate vocabulary, you will not be able to understand and successfully apply the various test elements that may appear on the TEAS.

CONTENT AREA: READING

Number of Questions: 53   Time Allotment: 64 minutes

Test Elements*

- **Information Sources**
  - Primary
  - Secondary
  - Tertiary
- **Passage/Paragraph**
  - Summarize
  - Topic sentence
  - What are
    - Conclusions
    - Implications
    - Inferences
    - Predictions
- **Author**
  - Assumptions
  - Biases
  - Fact vs. opinion
  - Intent of writing
  - Point of view
  - Stereotypes
  - Tone
- **Writing Type**
  - Argument
  - Cause/effect
  - Compare/contrast
  - Exposition
  - Narrative
  - Persuasive
  - Poetry
  - Problem solve
  - Technical/scientific
- **Vocabulary**
  - Denotative vs. connotative meaning of words/passages
  - Phrase meaning
  - Word meaning
  - Word/phrase defined by context
- **Figures of Speech**
  - Alliteration
  - Allusion
  - Assonance
  - Cliché
  - Idiom
  - Jargon
  - Metaphor
  - Neologisms
  - Onomatopoeia
  - Personification
  - Simile
  - Slang
  - Synecdoche
- **Text Structure**
  - Chronology
  - Formal vs. informal writing
  - List
  - Problem/solution
  - Sequence
- **Type of Communication**
  - Announcement
  - Blog
  - Classified
  - Directions
  - Forum
  - Invitation
  - Memorandum
  - Newsletter
  - Newspaper
  - Recipe
  - Speech
  - Television/radio
- **Graphic Information**
  - Maps
  - Measurement
  - Tables/charts
  - Visual instruction
- **Information Resources**
  - Almanac
  - Anthology
  - Atlas
  - Bibliography
  - Biography
  - Concordance
  - Dictionary
  - Encyclopedia
  - Handbook
  - Index
  - Journals
  - Labels
  - Newspaper
  - Periodical
  - Thesaurus
  - Valid Internet sites

*List is not all-inclusive

CONTENT AREA: MATHEMATICS

Number of Questions: 36   Time Allotment: 54 minutes

Test Elements*

- *Arithmetic*
  - Addition, subtraction, multiplication, division
  - Arithmetic terms
  - Decimals
  - Exponents and powers
  - Fractions
  - Mathematical symbols
  - Measures of central tendency
  - Order of operations (KNOW THIS, AND BE ABLE TO APPLY IT)
  - Percentage
  - Place value
  - Rational numbers
  - Rounding numbers
  - Signed numbers
  - Square roots and cube roots
- *Algebra*
  - Absolute value
  - Algebraic fractions
  - Algebraic terms/symbols
  - Analytical geometry
  - Evaluating expressions
  - Factoring
  - Inequalities
  - Keys words indicating addition, subtraction, multiplication, division
  - Monomials
  - Ratio and proportion
  - Roots and radicals
  - Solving equations
- *Geometry*
  - Angles
  - Circles
  - Cube
  - Cylinder
  - Lines
  - Perimeter
  - Polygons
  - Pythagorean theorem
  - Quadrilaterals
    - Rectangle
    - Right triangle
  - Surface area of solid figures
  - Triangles
  - Volume of solid figures
- *Word Problems*
  - Key words/phrases
  - Age
  - Charts and tables
  - Distance
  - Geometry
  - Numbers
  - Percent
  - Percent change
  - Ratio and proportion
  - Simple and compound interest
  - Work/Time
- *Changing Phrases/Sentences into Equations*
- *Conversion from One Measurement System to Another*

*List is not all-inclusive

CONTENT AREA: SCIENCE

Number of Questions: 53   Time Allotment: 63 minutes

Test Elements*

- **Human Anatomy and Physiology**
  - A&P in general terms
  - Cardiovascular system
    - Blood
      - Formation
      - Hemostasis
      - Groups
  - Endocrine system
  - Gastrointestinal system
  - Immune system
  - Integumentary system
  - Muscular system
  - Neurological system
  - Renal system
  - Reproductive system
  - Respiratory system
  - Skeletal system
  - Vision/hearing
- **Life Sciences**
  - Biology
    - Adaptation
    - Anatomical positions and directional terms
    - Body tissues
    - Cell and cell membranes
    - Cell division
    - Cell metabolism
    - Classification systems
    - Genetics
      - Mendel
      - Punnett squares
    - Movement of substances
    - Parts and functions of cells
    - Organic molecules
      - Metabolism and cellular respiration
        - Carbohydrates
        - Fat and protein metabolism

- Nucleic acid
- Steroids
- Organs
- **Chemistry**
  - Acids and bases
  - Atomic mass
  - Atomic number
  - Atomic structure
  - Bonds/bonding
  - Characteristics of substances
  - Chemical reactions
  - Compounds
  - Electrons
  - Ions
  - Isotopes
  - Periodic Table of Elements
  - pH
- **Scientific Reasoning**
  - Laboratory glassware
  - Measurement tools
  - Metric system
  - Scientific inquiry
    - Controls
    - Design
    - Event
    - Object relationships
    - Process
    - Variables
  - Scientific method
    - Analysis
    - Conclusion
    - Experimentation
    - Hypothesis
    - Investigation
    - Problem identification

*List is not all-inclusive

CONTENT AREA: ENGLISH AND LANGUAGE USAGE

Number of Questions: 28

Time Allotment: 28 minutes

Test Elements*
(Based on Standard United States English)

- *Sentence Components*
  - Complement
  - Direct object
  - Indirect object
  - Predicate
  - Subject
- *Parts of Speech*
  - Adjective
  - Adverb
  - Conjunction
  - Interjection
  - Noun
  - Pronoun
  - Preposition
  - Verb
- *Types of Sentences*
  - Simple
  - Compound
  - Complex
  - Compound-Complex
- *Punctuation*
  - Brackets
  - Colon
  - Dash
  - Conjunction
  - Comma
  - Exclamation point
  - Hyphen
  - Parentheses
  - Period
  - Question mark
  - Quotation marks
  - Semicolon
  - Solidus
- *Spelling*
  - Plurals
  - Possessives
  - Contractions
  - Compound verbs
  - Technical terms
  - Slang
  - Prefixes
  - Root words
  - Suffixes
- *Vocabulary*
  - Commonly misspelled words
  - Commonly misused words
  - Formal use of words
  - Informal use of words
  - Word phrases
- *Writing*
  - Sentence formation
  - Sentence structure
  - Paragraphs
  - Formal vs. informal writing
- *Capitalization*
- *Abbreviations*
- *Quotations*

*List is not all-inclusive

DEVELOPING YOUR STUDY PLAN

Once you have thoroughly and realistically examined your strong and weak areas, your test preparation methods, and your ability to follow through on a task, you are ready to develop and implement your study schedule/plan.

This is your study plan, and it should meet your needs. Your plan should be realistic, honest, and achievable. Most of all, your plan should be something you want to do, not something you have to do. Remember, your goal is admission to a nursing program. Take the following questions into consideration as you develop your plan.

WHAT LENGTH OF TIME SHOULD I PREPARE/REVIEW FOR THE TEAS TEST. Considering the amount of material that could be covered on the TEAS, a minimum of four to five weeks is most likely needed. More time may be needed if you identify several areas of weakness. Keep in mind this time of preparation is not a permanent change in your life. It is temporary and has a specific goal.

ARE YOU A DAY OR NIGHT PERSON? When possible, schedule study times when you are at your best.

DO YOU STUDY BEST ALONE, IN A GROUP, OR BOTH? Your best method of study is what is most effective for you. Think long and hard before changing what works, and if you change your method, make sure it benefits you.

Study groups can sometimes be problematic. Ideally, a study group is a small group of individuals (no more than three or four) who come together to discuss previously identified topics for a specified amount of time. It's a time for sharing and clarifying information, not learning new information. Each member of a study group should come prepared to discuss a specific, previously decided topic. A member should not come to the group unprepared. If one group member rarely contributes, or if you are the only one talking, then the group is teaching the member who rarely contributes, or you are teaching the group what it does not know. In this case, you're helping them but you are not enhancing your learning. There should be no cell phones, texting or messaging, noise, or other distractions. Problems arise when study groups spend more time socializing than on focusing on the designated topic. The study group should have rules for what is acceptable and unacceptable, and individuals who cannot abide by the rules should leave the group.

HOW DO OTHERS FIT INTO MY STUDY PLAN? Are others supportive of your goals? Are they willing to give you uninterrupted time to review and study for the TEAS? If not, why not?

WHERE WILL YOU STUDY? The area should be well lit, comfortable, quiet, and have minimal distraction. The study area should have everything you will need readily available. Your cell phone should be turned off during study time—your focus needs to be on your preparation for the TEAS, not your social life. Leave your phone in another room, if necessary. Disruptions from others should be avoided. Find an appropriate study location if you cannot study at home.

WHAT WILL YOU STUDY? All of the content areas need to be addressed a number of times each week. Schedule to study more than one content area a day and all content areas each week. Make sure you include the elements included in the content area tables, as well as elements you have identified that may not appear in the content tables. Strong areas should not require as much study time as weak areas.

HOW LONG SHOULD I STUDY? Study time should be no more than 50 minutes per hour with 10 minutes away from the study area. Use an alarm clock if you need to. This 50/10 method will allow for an extended period of concentrated study with time to get away to stretch your legs and clear your mind. Using this method will allow for longer periods of study without a gradual decrease in performance.

ALLOW FOR SOME "MY TIME" IN YOUR STUDY PLAN. "My time" time is yours to do whatever you want. If you exercise or run on a regular basis, use "my time." If there is a favorite television program you enjoy, use "my time." This is your time; use it wisely.

WHAT IF SOMETHING COMES UP THAT I NEED OR WANT TO DO? Good study plans allow for some flexibility. Forgoing study time for something else does not relieve you of your study responsibility.

For example, let's say Saturday is a big study day, and a friend asks you to go out to dinner and see a movie on Saturday evening. Dinner and a movie will take six hours or more of your scheduled study time. Dinner and a movie will not be problematic provided you reschedule the hours taken away from studying. You can reschedule these hours by giving up some "my time" or waking up earlier or staying up later on a number of days to make up the time.

WHERE DO I START WHEN DEVELOPING MY PLAN? Things you must do, such as work, school, or other obligations, should be added first, and then add your study times. For each study period, you should include the content area plus a specific topic or element to review. For example, a time identified as English and Language Usage may specifically address the components of a sentence and parts of speech. It could also address an area in this category that you have identified as an area of weakness.

Below is a blank study schedule to help you organize your time. Use this schedule as a template to develop a study plan that meets your needs.

	Sunday	Monday	Tuesday	Wednesday	Thursday	Friday	Saturday
0700							
0800							
0900							
1000							
1100							
1200							
1300							
1400							
1500							
1600							
1700							
1800							
1900							
2000							
2100							
2200							
2300							
2400							

Study Time = 50 minutes with 10-minute break each hour.

Developing a realistic and workable study plan/schedule and following it will require honesty and discipline. Sound preparation for the TEAS can enhance your score(s) on the test and increase your potential for admission to a nursing program.

Prep/Study Time

You've completed your study schedule, and now it's time to implement it. Consider giving a copy of your finalized study schedule to family and friends, so they will know when you will be studying and unavailable. These individuals should understand and support your need to have an organized plan to prepare for the TEAS. Just as you are giving up personal time to prepare, supportive friends and family should be willing to give you this time to prepare.

Have everything you might need available for each specific time—collect these things prior to the study time. For example, if you have designated a certain time for anatomy and physiology, have your A&P book, notes, handouts, and other pertinent materials readily available.

A study schedule is a waste of time if there is no way to determine if your time has been unproductive or worthwhile. Plan some test time at the end of each study session to quiz yourself to see what you have accomplished. For example, if you have reviewed the cardiovascular system, write down everything you can think of regarding the system—define vocabulary specific to this system, the purpose of the system, what comprises the system, how does the system interact with other systems. Then check and see how accurate you have been. If you have reviewed fractions and decimals, work on problems that will demonstrate your understanding. You are the only person who can determine if a session has been worthwhile. Be honest with yourself, and restudy if you haven't accomplished what you had hoped to.

What Do I Do After I've Taken a Practice Test?

Use each practice test to help you determine your areas of strength and weakness. Take a practice test at strategic points in your study plan and take the test within the given time limits—use an alarm clock to time yourself. The rationales for each test are not simply for incorrect answers; they are also for correct answers. Read the rationale for each question to strengthen what you already know and to help you determine/understand why you incorrectly answered a question. For example, if you consistently miss geometry problems, you need to increase your review time on geometry.

TAKING THE TEAS

You've prepared for the TEAS, and now it's time to actually take the test. Consider the following:

- Arrive early to the testing site and maintain a realistic and optimistic attitude.
- Know where you're going and where you will park. Do a test run.
- Follow the directions for testing.
- The test is multiple choice, and you have to select the most correct or correct answer from four options.
- Know the amount of time for each content area and gauge your time accordingly. English and Language Usage allows one minute per question. Reading, Mathematics, and Science each allow more than one minute, but less than one and one-half minutes per question.
- Know before the test begins if you can leave an answer blank and return to it at a later time.
- Carefully read each question and each answer option before selecting an answer. Consider each option separately—you may find cases where each option is basically correct. In this case, your job is to select the most correct answer. Treating each option as either true or false

is helpful in some instances. Reducing the number of options by eliminating obviously incorrect options may also help.

DO NOT ARGUE WITH A TEST QUESTION OR THE OPTIONS! Focus on the information you are given. The question and its options will tell you everything you need to select the correct answer. Trust your ability to apply your knowledge and critical thinking skills.

DO NOT CHANGE AN ANSWER UNLESS YOU ARE 100% SURE YOU SELECTED AN INCORRECT ANSWER. Trust your first impression. The majority of test takers who change answers usually change correct answers to incorrect answers.

DO NOT GUESS UNLESS THERE IS NO OTHER OPTION! If you must guess, make it an educated guess based upon your knowledge and critical-thinking abilities. There are numerous illogical methods used to guess a correct answer to a question such as, if you don't know the correct answer, select option C or the option with the longest answer. Remember, if students are aware of these illogical methods, the writers of tests are also aware of these methods.

WHAT CAN I DO IF I'M NOT ADMITTED TO A NURSING PROGRAM?

There are instances in which individuals meet or exceed the minimal TEAS criteria and are still not offered admission. In this case, the first thing you should do is contact your advisor or the director of the nursing program and meet with him or her to discuss the reasons you were not admitted and develop a plan for moving forward. You should also consider why you want to be a nurse. Is nursing a family tradition, and the expectation is for you to also become a nurse? If this is the case, you need to stop and decide if you want to become a nurse to satisfy tradition or yourself. Tradition will not make a satisfying career. Nursing is not what you see on television in reality shows or soap operas. Nursing is demanding work that can be hard on your spirit, mind, and body. Becoming a nurse is time consuming and challenging, and may be the most difficult thing you've ever attempted. Nursing may also prove to be the most rewarding thing you'll ever do.

It is virtually unimaginable for a nursing program to offer admission to everyone who applies for a particular semester or academic year. The applicant pool for a specific admission time influences admission. A high applicant pool may mean not all qualified candidates will be offered admission.

Admission to a nursing program is highly competitive, and only those who demonstrate the highest probability of success will be offered admission. Meeting or exceeding a nursing program's admission criteria does not guarantee admission to the program. It means you qualify to seek admission.

Nursing programs rarely admit all candidates for admission because of many factors, and only the best of candidates for a particular semester or class will be offered admission.

The following is a partial list of factors that may influence admission criteria:

- The number of teaching faculty in the nursing program and their level of educational preparation is guided by the board of nurse examiners of each state.
- Policies of the institution or nursing program.
- State board of nursing rules and regulations that apply to the nursing programs. Limits are set on the number of students one faculty member can supervise in a clinical setting. This also includes students with past/present legal problems.
- The number and size of health care institutions in a town, city, or area. These institutions determine the number of nursing students that come to their facilities for clinical instruction. They also determine the availability of nursing units and numbers of students that can be on

a unit. If an area has more than one nursing program, it may give preference to one program over another.

- Nursing programs typically have admission criteria, and only those individuals who meet or exceed the criteria will be considered for admission. For example, imagine that a program has six criteria for admission and will offer admission to 50 individuals in the upcoming fall semester. Each criterion is scored from one to four points, and the score from each criterion is totaled. Individuals seeking admission are ranked according to their total criteria score (highest to lowest), and the top 50 individuals will be offered admission. If 185 individuals meet or exceed admission criteria and you are ranked 53, it is doubtful you will receive an offer of admission—there were too many other individuals with higher overall scores.

If you find yourself in this predicament, contact the nursing program to talk with the person who works with admissions. Consider the following questions for your discussion:

- Why was I not offered admission if I met the criteria?
- Were there specific criteria that contributed to my not receiving an offer for admission?
- Are there suggestions that can be given to increase my chances for admission?

LET'S GET STARTED!

Hopefully this section has helped explain what the TEAS is all about and has addressed your questions regarding the exam. The rest of this book consists of five complete practice tests each followed by detailed answer explanations. There also is a sixth test that you can access on your computer, tablet, and smartphone for additional practice. To access the test, go to *barronsbooks.com/tp/TEAS/* or scan the QR code on pages ii, 2, and 304.

Now let's get to work!

> ### Comments? Questions? Suggestions?
>
> E-mail: *picket31644@mypacks.net*
>
> Don't forget to include your e-mail address and a good description of why you're writing.

Practice Test 1

ANSWER SHEET
Practice Test 1

Reading

1. Ⓐ Ⓑ Ⓒ Ⓓ
2. Ⓐ Ⓑ Ⓒ Ⓓ
3. Ⓐ Ⓑ Ⓒ Ⓓ
4. Ⓐ Ⓑ Ⓒ Ⓓ
5. Ⓐ Ⓑ Ⓒ Ⓓ
6. Ⓐ Ⓑ Ⓒ Ⓓ
7. Ⓐ Ⓑ Ⓒ Ⓓ
8. Ⓐ Ⓑ Ⓒ Ⓓ
9. Ⓐ Ⓑ Ⓒ Ⓓ
10. Ⓐ Ⓑ Ⓒ Ⓓ
11. Ⓐ Ⓑ Ⓒ Ⓓ
12. Ⓐ Ⓑ Ⓒ Ⓓ
13. Ⓐ Ⓑ Ⓒ Ⓓ
14. Ⓐ Ⓑ Ⓒ Ⓓ

15. Ⓐ Ⓑ Ⓒ Ⓓ
16. Ⓐ Ⓑ Ⓒ Ⓓ
17. Ⓐ Ⓑ Ⓒ Ⓓ
18. Ⓐ Ⓑ Ⓒ Ⓓ
19. Ⓐ Ⓑ Ⓒ Ⓓ
20. Ⓐ Ⓑ Ⓒ Ⓓ
21. Ⓐ Ⓑ Ⓒ Ⓓ
22. Ⓐ Ⓑ Ⓒ Ⓓ
23. Ⓐ Ⓑ Ⓒ Ⓓ
24. Ⓐ Ⓑ Ⓒ Ⓓ
25. Ⓐ Ⓑ Ⓒ Ⓓ
26. Ⓐ Ⓑ Ⓒ Ⓓ
27. Ⓐ Ⓑ Ⓒ Ⓓ
28. Ⓐ Ⓑ Ⓒ Ⓓ

29. Ⓐ Ⓑ Ⓒ Ⓓ
30. Ⓐ Ⓑ Ⓒ Ⓓ
31. Ⓐ Ⓑ Ⓒ Ⓓ
32. Ⓐ Ⓑ Ⓒ Ⓓ
33. Ⓐ Ⓑ Ⓒ Ⓓ
34. Ⓐ Ⓑ Ⓒ Ⓓ
35. Ⓐ Ⓑ Ⓒ Ⓓ
36. Ⓐ Ⓑ Ⓒ Ⓓ
37. Ⓐ Ⓑ Ⓒ Ⓓ
38. Ⓐ Ⓑ Ⓒ Ⓓ
39. Ⓐ Ⓑ Ⓒ Ⓓ
40. Ⓐ Ⓑ Ⓒ Ⓓ
41. Ⓐ Ⓑ Ⓒ Ⓓ
42. Ⓐ Ⓑ Ⓒ Ⓓ

43. Ⓐ Ⓑ Ⓒ Ⓓ
44. Ⓐ Ⓑ Ⓒ Ⓓ
45. Ⓐ Ⓑ Ⓒ Ⓓ
46. Ⓐ Ⓑ Ⓒ Ⓓ
47. Ⓐ Ⓑ Ⓒ Ⓓ
48. Ⓐ Ⓑ Ⓒ Ⓓ
49. Ⓐ Ⓑ Ⓒ Ⓓ
50. Ⓐ Ⓑ Ⓒ Ⓓ
51. Ⓐ Ⓑ Ⓒ Ⓓ
52. Ⓐ Ⓑ Ⓒ Ⓓ
53. Ⓐ Ⓑ Ⓒ Ⓓ

Mathematics

1. Ⓐ Ⓑ Ⓒ Ⓓ
2. Ⓐ Ⓑ Ⓒ Ⓓ
3. Ⓐ Ⓑ Ⓒ Ⓓ
4. Ⓐ Ⓑ Ⓒ Ⓓ
5. Ⓐ Ⓑ Ⓒ Ⓓ
6. Ⓐ Ⓑ Ⓒ Ⓓ
7. Ⓐ Ⓑ Ⓒ Ⓓ
8. Ⓐ Ⓑ Ⓒ Ⓓ
9. Ⓐ Ⓑ Ⓒ Ⓓ

10. Ⓐ Ⓑ Ⓒ Ⓓ
11. Ⓐ Ⓑ Ⓒ Ⓓ
12. Ⓐ Ⓑ Ⓒ Ⓓ
13. Ⓐ Ⓑ Ⓒ Ⓓ
14. Ⓐ Ⓑ Ⓒ Ⓓ
15. Ⓐ Ⓑ Ⓒ Ⓓ
16. Ⓐ Ⓑ Ⓒ Ⓓ
17. Ⓐ Ⓑ Ⓒ Ⓓ
18. Ⓐ Ⓑ Ⓒ Ⓓ

19. Ⓐ Ⓑ Ⓒ Ⓓ
20. Ⓐ Ⓑ Ⓒ Ⓓ
21. Ⓐ Ⓑ Ⓒ Ⓓ
22. Ⓐ Ⓑ Ⓒ Ⓓ
23. Ⓐ Ⓑ Ⓒ Ⓓ
24. Ⓐ Ⓑ Ⓒ Ⓓ
25. Ⓐ Ⓑ Ⓒ Ⓓ
26. Ⓐ Ⓑ Ⓒ Ⓓ
27. Ⓐ Ⓑ Ⓒ Ⓓ

28. Ⓐ Ⓑ Ⓒ Ⓓ
29. Ⓐ Ⓑ Ⓒ Ⓓ
30. Ⓐ Ⓑ Ⓒ Ⓓ
31. Ⓐ Ⓑ Ⓒ Ⓓ
32. Ⓐ Ⓑ Ⓒ Ⓓ
33. Ⓐ Ⓑ Ⓒ Ⓓ
34. Ⓐ Ⓑ Ⓒ Ⓓ
35. Ⓐ Ⓑ Ⓒ Ⓓ
36. Ⓐ Ⓑ Ⓒ Ⓓ

ANSWER SHEET
Practice Test 1

Science

1. Ⓐ Ⓑ Ⓒ Ⓓ	15. Ⓐ Ⓑ Ⓒ Ⓓ	29. Ⓐ Ⓑ Ⓒ Ⓓ	43. Ⓐ Ⓑ Ⓒ Ⓓ
2. Ⓐ Ⓑ Ⓒ Ⓓ	16. Ⓐ Ⓑ Ⓒ Ⓓ	30. Ⓐ Ⓑ Ⓒ Ⓓ	44. Ⓐ Ⓑ Ⓒ Ⓓ
3. Ⓐ Ⓑ Ⓒ Ⓓ	17. Ⓐ Ⓑ Ⓒ Ⓓ	31. Ⓐ Ⓑ Ⓒ Ⓓ	45. Ⓐ Ⓑ Ⓒ Ⓓ
4. Ⓐ Ⓑ Ⓒ Ⓓ	18. Ⓐ Ⓑ Ⓒ Ⓓ	32. Ⓐ Ⓑ Ⓒ Ⓓ	46. Ⓐ Ⓑ Ⓒ Ⓓ
5. Ⓐ Ⓑ Ⓒ Ⓓ	19. Ⓐ Ⓑ Ⓒ Ⓓ	33. Ⓐ Ⓑ Ⓒ Ⓓ	47. Ⓐ Ⓑ Ⓒ Ⓓ
6. Ⓐ Ⓑ Ⓒ Ⓓ	20. Ⓐ Ⓑ Ⓒ Ⓓ	34. Ⓐ Ⓑ Ⓒ Ⓓ	48. Ⓐ Ⓑ Ⓒ Ⓓ
7. Ⓐ Ⓑ Ⓒ Ⓓ	21. Ⓐ Ⓑ Ⓒ Ⓓ	35. Ⓐ Ⓑ Ⓒ Ⓓ	49. Ⓐ Ⓑ Ⓒ Ⓓ
8. Ⓐ Ⓑ Ⓒ Ⓓ	22. Ⓐ Ⓑ Ⓒ Ⓓ	36. Ⓐ Ⓑ Ⓒ Ⓓ	50. Ⓐ Ⓑ Ⓒ Ⓓ
9. Ⓐ Ⓑ Ⓒ Ⓓ	23. Ⓐ Ⓑ Ⓒ Ⓓ	37. Ⓐ Ⓑ Ⓒ Ⓓ	51. Ⓐ Ⓑ Ⓒ Ⓓ
10. Ⓐ Ⓑ Ⓒ Ⓓ	24. Ⓐ Ⓑ Ⓒ Ⓓ	38. Ⓐ Ⓑ Ⓒ Ⓓ	52. Ⓐ Ⓑ Ⓒ Ⓓ
11. Ⓐ Ⓑ Ⓒ Ⓓ	25. Ⓐ Ⓑ Ⓒ Ⓓ	39. Ⓐ Ⓑ Ⓒ Ⓓ	53. Ⓐ Ⓑ Ⓒ Ⓓ
12. Ⓐ Ⓑ Ⓒ Ⓓ	26. Ⓐ Ⓑ Ⓒ Ⓓ	40. Ⓐ Ⓑ Ⓒ Ⓓ	
13. Ⓐ Ⓑ Ⓒ Ⓓ	27. Ⓐ Ⓑ Ⓒ Ⓓ	41. Ⓐ Ⓑ Ⓒ Ⓓ	
14. Ⓐ Ⓑ Ⓒ Ⓓ	28. Ⓐ Ⓑ Ⓒ Ⓓ	42. Ⓐ Ⓑ Ⓒ Ⓓ	

English and Language Usage

1. Ⓐ Ⓑ Ⓒ Ⓓ	8. Ⓐ Ⓑ Ⓒ Ⓓ	15. Ⓐ Ⓑ Ⓒ Ⓓ	22. Ⓐ Ⓑ Ⓒ Ⓓ
2. Ⓐ Ⓑ Ⓒ Ⓓ	9. Ⓐ Ⓑ Ⓒ Ⓓ	16. Ⓐ Ⓑ Ⓒ Ⓓ	23. Ⓐ Ⓑ Ⓒ Ⓓ
3. Ⓐ Ⓑ Ⓒ Ⓓ	10. Ⓐ Ⓑ Ⓒ Ⓓ	17. Ⓐ Ⓑ Ⓒ Ⓓ	24. Ⓐ Ⓑ Ⓒ Ⓓ
4. Ⓐ Ⓑ Ⓒ Ⓓ	11. Ⓐ Ⓑ Ⓒ Ⓓ	18. Ⓐ Ⓑ Ⓒ Ⓓ	25. Ⓐ Ⓑ Ⓒ Ⓓ
5. Ⓐ Ⓑ Ⓒ Ⓓ	12. Ⓐ Ⓑ Ⓒ Ⓓ	19. Ⓐ Ⓑ Ⓒ Ⓓ	26. Ⓐ Ⓑ Ⓒ Ⓓ
6. Ⓐ Ⓑ Ⓒ Ⓓ	13. Ⓐ Ⓑ Ⓒ Ⓓ	20. Ⓐ Ⓑ Ⓒ Ⓓ	27. Ⓐ Ⓑ Ⓒ Ⓓ
7. Ⓐ Ⓑ Ⓒ Ⓓ	14. Ⓐ Ⓑ Ⓒ Ⓓ	21. Ⓐ Ⓑ Ⓒ Ⓓ	28. Ⓐ Ⓑ Ⓒ Ⓓ

READING

NUMBER OF QUESTIONS: 53

TIME LIMIT: 64 MINUTES

> **Instructions:** Read each question thoroughly. Select the single best answer. Mark your answer (A, B, C, or D) on the answer sheet provided for Practice Test 1.

Questions 1–3 are based on the following passage. The passage is from the local newspaper.

A pick-up truck was found at the foot of a deep ravine in Rabbit Creek Canyon following one of the worst winter storms to hit Anderson County in the past 100 years. Road crews clearing snow from SR 328 discovered the vehicle shortly after dawn this morning. Investigators *surmise* the car slid on the icy road and went through the guardrail, plunging into the ravine below. One set of partially snow-dusted boot tracks led from the demolished pick-up truck into the woods. Anderson County Search and Rescue is currently searching the woods for the driver of the vehicle.

1. Which of the following is a synonym for *surmise*?

   (A) Calculate
   (B) Hypothesize
   (C) Inform
   (D) Measure

2. The passage states *a pick-up truck was found at the foot of a deep ravine . . . .* What does this phrase imply?

   (A) When looking into the ravine from above, it has a foot-like profile.
   (B) The depth of the ravine was not measured and supports the use of the word "deep."
   (C) The pick-up truck was found at the bottom of the ravine providing a more precise location.
   (D) The road crews had trouble locating the pick-up truck because of the depth of the ravine.

3. The passage was written to

   (A) demonstrate county employees are doing their jobs.
   (B) encourage residents to avoid driving during winter storms.
   (C) provide information of a happening in the county.
   (D) suggest the accident may not have happened if roads were sanded/salted.

Questions 4–5 are based on the following passage and chart.

The developers of full-service truck stops are including updated shower facilities in their newest constructions. Their goals are to provide truckers with the latest in shower facilities, while getting the truckers in and out of these facilities as quickly as possible. Shower facilities at 18 current locations were repainted using the following color themes, with data collected by color and average time spent in the shower area.

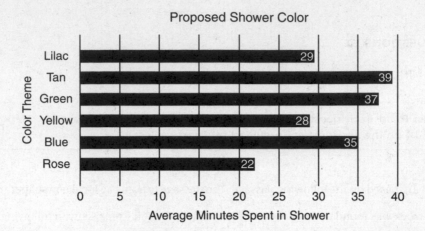

Proposed Shower Color

4. The graphic uses a _____ to present data.

(A) bar chart
(B) column chart
(C) pie chart
(D) line chart

5. What color theme meets one goal of the truck-stop developers?

(A) Green
(B) Rose
(C) Tan
(D) Yellow

Question 6 is based on the following passage.

Jenet, a university freshman, has wanted to be a member of the women's softball team since she saw them play six years ago while in public school. The softball team is consistently in the top three each season and has taken the championship title five years in a row. The team also has the highest grade point average and graduation rate of any university sport in the conference. Jenet tried out for the team and had an interview with the women's coach. At the interview the coach discussed the following items with Jenet:

- Performance in the classroom is as important, or more important, than performance on the field.
- A grade of "B" in each course attempted must be maintained to be a member of the team. Students unable to meet this criterion for any semester will be dismissed from the team, but may retry for team membership. There are no guarantees of readmission, and if a student is readmitted, she will play the position assigned, serve as a substitute for at least one semester, and will be ineligible for all away games and post-season games for one semester.
- A stringent code of conduct is enforced. Disciplinary action may lead to dismissal from the team.
- She has excellent softball skills and understanding of the game. Great experience.
- She is now considered a member of the softball team. She has strong potential to enhance the team.
- She may apply for full softball scholarship prior to the beginning of her second year. Over two-thirds of the team currently receive the full scholarship.

■ Her transcript grades are a mix of barely passing with a "C" average to a low "B" average. There is an expectation that she will adapt her behavior to meet the criterion to maintain membership on the team.

6. Based on the information in the passage, what is Jenet's best plan of action to maintain membership on the softball team?

(A) Develop a realistic plan of study that she can follow.

(B) Hire a tutor for all of her courses.

(C) Talk with her professors about being a member of the softball team and her need to maintain at least a "B" average in her courses.

(D) Work harder on her grades since she has finally reached her goal of being a member of the university softball team.

Questions 7–8 are based on the following passage.

Gettysburg Address by Abraham Lincoln

Four score and seven years ago our fathers brought forth on this continent, a new nation, conceived in Liberty, and dedicated to the *proposition* that all men are created equal.

Now we are engaged in a great civil war, testing whether that nation, or any nation so conceived and so dedicated, can long endure. We are met on a great battle-field of that war. We have come to dedicate a portion of that field, as a final resting place for those who here gave their lives that that nation might live. It is altogether fitting and proper that we should do this.

But, in a larger sense, we cannot dedicate—we cannot consecrate—we cannot hallow—this ground. The brave men, living and dead, who struggled here, have consecrated it, far above our poor power to add or detract. The world will little note, nor long remember what we say here, but it can never forget what they did here. It is for us the living, rather, to be dedicated here to the unfinished work which they who fought here have thus far so nobly advanced. It is rather for us to be here dedicated to the great task remaining before us—that from these honored dead we take increased devotion to that cause for which they gave the last full measure of devotion—that we here highly resolve that these dead shall not have died in vain—that this nation, under God, shall have a new birth of freedom—and that government of the people, by the people, for the people, shall not perish from the earth.

7. Select a synonym for the word *proposition* in the first paragraph.

(A) Assurance

(B) Knowledge

(C) Opposition

(D) Premise

8. The primary purpose of the Gettysburg Address was to

(A) acknowledge Union and Confederate survivors of the Battle of Gettysburg.

(B) propose a plan of action for postwar reconstruction.

(C) recognize Robert E. Lee's victory at the Battle of Gettysburg.

(D) set apart a cemetery for Union soldiers who died during the Battle of Gettysburg.

Questions 9–11 are based on the following passage.

The White Indian Boy is a novel written by Elijah Nicholas Wilson and was published in 1910. The novel is a compilation of stories of his adventurous life in the 1800s in what is now Wyoming. He was the son of Mormon pioneers. In the novel, Wilson writes of his adventures as a runaway and living with the Shoshone; his adoption as a brother of Chief Washakie; his experience as a stagecoach driver for the Overland Stage and a Pony Express rider. He was also a trapper and trader, and he treated diphtheria and small pox on the frontier. The town of Wilson, Wyoming, is named after him.

9. Based on information presented in the passage, what style of writing is used in *The White Indian Boy*?

   (A) Expository
   (B) Narrative
   (C) Persuasive
   (D) Technical

10. Based upon the passage, *The White Indian Boy* is an example of a(n)

    (A) autobiographical novel.
    (B) biographical novel.
    (C) secondary source novel.
    (D) third-person novel.

11. In which of the following sections in a library would you find a hard copy of *The White Indian Boy*?

    (A) Fiction
    (B) Reference
    (C) Serials
    (D) True-life

Questions 12–13 are based on the following passage.

Brenda was having a wonderful summer day playing in the fields with her dog, Bibi, until the ground shook. She thought she had imagined the shaking until she saw Bibi barking at something unseen. Frightened, she ran home as fast as she could, shadowed by an excited and still barking, Bibi. Upon rushing into the kitchen, she found her parents calmly sitting at the breakfast table drinking coffee and reading the morning newspaper. She screamed, "Mom, Dad, it's the end! We've got to get away! Hurry!"

Brenda's mom glanced up from reading the paper and smiled at Brenda's dad who looked at Brenda and calmly said, "Girl, when are you going to start listening to me? I told you at breakfast that the quarry would start blasting again today."

Brenda felt like such a fool. She vaguely remembered her dad telling her about the blasting at the quarry, but she wasn't paying attention because she was in a hurry to get outside and play.

12. What is the writing style of the passage?

    (A) Expository
    (B) Narrative
    (C) Persuasive/argumentative
    (D) Problem/solution

13. What is the *most* logical conclusion from reading this passage?

(A) Brenda is a child and doesn't fully understand the importance of listening to her parents.

(B) Brenda is a fool.

(C) Brenda's parents are good parents.

(D) Brenda probably remembered her dad telling her about the blasting and forgot about it when she started to play.

Questions 14–16 are based on the following e-mail.

Dear Valued Customer,

Are you tired of the inflated rates you are paying for repairs? What did you pay for your last home or motor home repair? Prices keep going up, and there's no relief in sight. As a valued customer of *locally owned* Hawkins Hardware, we are pleased to announce a new service to ease the burden on your wallet. Beginning September 1, we will be offering a warranty service for home and motor home repair. This fantastic offer is yours for the *paltry* sum of $50 a month, with a $55 service charge for each call—no additional charges will be assessed. This offer is being made to our credit account holders only. Give us a call at 555-555-5555 or go to *hawkinshardware.com* to find out more about this exciting offer you cannot afford to live without.

14. What mode of writing is the e-mail?

(A) Argumentative

(B) Expository

(C) Narrative

(D) Persuasive

15. What is an antonym for the word *paltry*?

(A) Beggarly

(B) Picayune

(C) Unimportant

(D) Valuable

16. What does *locally owned* imply?

(A) Decision-making regarding the hardware store is determined by the city fathers who understand what's best for the community.

(B) The hardware store is not owned by a large corporation with a chain of hardware stores. Theoretically, money spent in the community stays in the community.

(C) Chain-owned businesses tend to pay higher taxes than small "mom and pop" businesses in the community. This provides for economic growth.

(D) Locally owned suggests diversification within the community with the hardware store purchasing from local businesses.

Question 17 is based on the following passage.

You'll need this if you're coming to the summer sheep camp for the celebration. Take SH 42 west out of Wardsburg and proceed to the west end of Harris Corners. Turn left onto FM 2398, going toward Muleshoe, and proceed about 8 miles. Turn right onto the paved road just before the large sign advertising the Polk Leather and Boot Company. The paved road will turn into a dirt road after around 15 miles. The dirt road will take you to the summer sheep camp around 12 miles down the road. There is a telephone in a wooden box attached to a telephone pole where the pavement turns to dirt. Call 8733 if it has been raining, or you do not want to take your vehicle on a bumpy dirt road. Someone from the ranch in a four-wheel-drive vehicle will come, pick you up, take you to the sheep camp for the celebration, and then take you back to your car when you're ready to leave. There is a graveled parking area on the left. Make sure you lock your car. We've never had any problems, but one never knows. See ya soon!

17. The passage is an example of which type of writing?

(A) Entertaining
(B) Expressive
(C) Technical
(D) Informative

Questions 18–21 are based on the following passage and map.

Welcome to Pacific Mountains State Park. Located in the Cascade Range, running through the beautiful state of Oregon, Pacific Mountains State Park offers the ultimate camping and trail experiences for thrill-seeking nature enthusiasts. Situated at an elevation of 7,000 feet, the park's climate has the ability to change from hour to hour. Well-defined trails connect nine destinations within the park, and primitive trails abound in the area. Pacific Mountains State Park is handicap accessible, with two trails suitable for all ages and abilities.

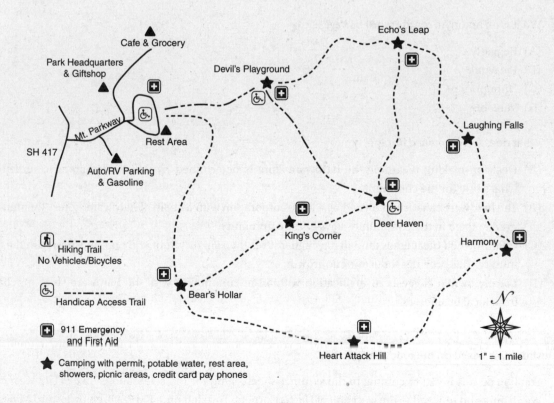

18. Greg is setting up camp at Deer Haven and discovers he has forgotten to bring matches. Based on the trail map, what is the shortest, most direct route from Deer Haven to the grocery?

    (A) Deer Haven to Devil's Playground to the grocery
    (B) Deer Haven to Echo's Leap to Devil's Playground to the grocery
    (C) Deer Haven to King's Corner to Bear's Hollar to the grocery
    (D) There is no direct route.

19. Based on the map, an estimated distance, in miles, of the perimeter hiking trails is

    (A) 6 to 8 miles.
    (B) 8 to 13 miles.
    (C) 15 to 21 miles.
    (D) 23 to 26 miles.

20. Each of the nine park destinations, as well as the entrance area, has designated 911 emergency and first aid facilities. What does this suggest?

    (A) Park visitors are frequently far from nonmountainous areas and are more prone to accidental injury.
    (B) The park administrators are health conscious.
    (C) Audacious individuals are more likely to sustain accidental injuries.
    (D) The state park system wants to decrease the chances of litigation from injuries occurring within the park.

21. While individuals of all ages and abilities are welcome at Pacific Mountains State Park, the official brochure is written to appeal to which of the following types of individuals?

    (A) Average individuals looking for a challenging and adventurous environment
    (B) Families, with young children, wanting a child-friendly environment
    (C) Super athletes wanting a structured environment
    (D) Retired individuals contemplating a peaceful environment

---

Questions 22–25 are based on the following passage.

Heart Failure

Heart failure is a chronic, progressive disorder frequently seen in older adults although it can occur at any age. Heart failure does not strike suddenly like a heart attack, but progresses quietly until symptoms appear. Individuals usually do not seek medical attention until symptoms begin to interfere with their activities of daily living. Without treatment, the heart continues to fail.

A diagnosis of heart failure does not mean the heart has quit working. It means the heart does not work as effectively as it once did. The diagnosis is also not a death sentence—with health-care provider prescribed management, an individual can live a fairly normal life within limitations. Management includes medications, lifestyle changes, and exercise to control or reduce symptoms.

Heart failure has numerous etiologies. They include coronary artery disease, heart valve disease, high blood pressure, heart attack, disorders that damage the heart muscle, and other conditions such as diabetes, thyroid, and kidney disease. Drug and alcohol misuse can also lead to heart failure. In heart failure, the heart gradually loses its ability to work effectively. This results in the heart not being able to pump enough blood to meet the body's metabolic needs.

Signs and symptoms of heart failure include: (1) congested lungs and/or shortness of breath with activity or when lying down caused by fluid backing up into the pulmonary veins; (2) swelling in the feet, ankles, lower legs, and/or abdomen and/or sudden weight gain caused by fluid buildup in body tissues; (3) rapid heart rate and increased respiratory rate caused by the heart trying to play "catch up" to meet the body's metabolic requirements; (4) nausea and anorexia caused by the gastrointestinal system receiving less blood; (5) tiredness and/or fatigue that affects the ability to complete everyday tasks (shopping, cleaning house, cooking, dressing, bathing) in a timely fashion; (6) troublesome cough or wheezing with or without bringing up white or blood-tinged sputum brought about by fluid backup into the lungs; and (7) changes in amount of urination, a decrease in the day and increase at night after going to bed.

There are a number of laboratory and diagnostic studies that can be performed to verify a diagnosis of heart failure. Among these are (1) an electrocardiogram (EKG) to look at the electrical activity and beating of the heart; (2) a chest X-ray to determine the size of the heart and to show fluid buildup around the heart, if present, and fluid buildup and congestion in the lungs; (3) pulse oximeter readings to determine oxygen saturation of the blood; (4) blood tests to determine kidney and thyroid function, the presence or absence of *anemia*, and a BNP that increases when heart failure exists or symptoms worsen and decreases when the condition is stable.

Your health-care provider should be consulted if you have reason to believe you have heart problems. He or she is your best source of information.

22. The passage is appropriate for

(A) a brochure.
(B) a journal for health-care professionals.
(C) the editorial section of a newspaper.
(D) a new age publication.

23. A simple, concise definition of heart failure is

(A) cardiovascular failure.
(B) heart disease of old age.
(C) pump failure.
(D) cardiopulmonary congestion.

24. A 70-year-old man is diagnosed with heart failure. When teaching him about his disease, the most important point for him to understand is heart failure

(A) can be treated but not cured.
(B) is a death sentence.
(C) is expensive to treat.
(D) will put unreasonable demands on his life.

25. Which of the following words is a synonym for *anemia*?

(A) Flushed
(B) Pallid
(C) Thin
(D) Uninteresting

Question 26 is based on the following partial table of contents from a gardening book.

26. What is incorrect in the table of contents?

   (A) Freezing temperatures should be included in Chapter 2.
   (B) Gardening tools should be included.
   (C) The list of vegetables should be more inclusive.
   (D) Tomatoes are fruits, not vegetables.

Questions 27–29 are based on the following passage.

The forest was darker and eerier than he remembered. He could have sworn he was being followed. He was certain he heard footsteps behind him, but when he stopped walking, the sound behind him stopped, too— he was sure of it. He turned and looked behind him and saw nothing but shadows in the quiet darkness. Nothing was moving. He started walking again, this time faster and with a sense of urgency. The sound behind him started again, too, and matched his pace. *Unnerved*, he broke into a run and ran like a man possessed.

27. What is the mood of this passage?

   (A) Controlled
   (B) Fearful
   (C) Melancholy
   (D) Regretful

28. Which of the following words is a synonym for *unnerved*?

   (A) Excited
   (B) Panic-stricken
   (C) Soothed
   (D) Worried

29. A reader would *most* likely expect to find the passage in which of the following?

   (A) A comedy novel
   (B) A mystery novel
   (C) A science fiction novel
   (D) A spiritual novel

Questions 30–31 are based on the following recipe.

PINEAPPLE NUT COOKIES

1/2 C. softened butter (do not use margarine)

1 C. packed brown sugar

3/4 C. cane sugar

2 large eggs

1 t. imitation vanilla (do not use pure vanilla extract)

3 C. all-purpose flour

1/2 t. baking powder

1 t. baking soda

1 1/2 C. crushed pineapple (drained well)

1 C. chopped nuts (pecan and walnut work best)

Preheat oven to 325°F. Liberally grease cookie sheet.

Mix moist/wet ingredients in large bowl; beat until smooth.

Add dry ingredients; mix until well creamed.

Place 2–3 t. dollops of dough about 3 inches apart onto cookie sheet.

Bake for 15 to 18 minutes or until golden brown around the edges.

Makes 4 dozen cookies.

---

30. Based on the recipe, what is the first action to be taken in preparing the cookies?

   (A) Allow the butter to soften.
   (B) Bake for 15 to 18 minutes.
   (C) Liberally grease the cookie sheet.
   (D) Preheat the oven to 325°F.

31. An individual with cocoa allergies would be concerned about which of the following ingredients?

   (A) Brown sugar
   (B) Imitation vanilla
   (C) Nuts
   (D) Pineapple

32. The order of operations states: When multiplication, division, parentheses, exponents, addition, subtraction, and square roots are contained in one problem, the order of operations is as follows:

1. Parentheses
2. Exponents and square roots
3. Multiplication and division, whichever comes first working from left to right
4. Addition and subtraction, whichever comes first working from left to right

In the problem below, what is the first action to be performed based on the order of operations?

$$40 - 29 + \frac{30}{5} + 44 \div (12 \cdot 3) =$$

(A) Add 5 and 44.
(B) Divide 30 into 5.
(C) Multiply 12 and 3.
(D) Subtract 29 from 40.

Questions 33–34 are based on the following chart.

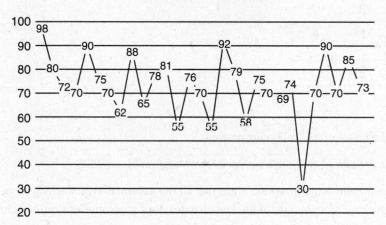

Midterm Grades

33. The above is a

(A) bar chart.
(B) cosmo graph.
(C) flow chart.
(D) line graph.

34. Twenty-nine students took the midterm examination. If a passing grade is 75 or above, how many students passed the exam?

(A) 11
(B) 13
(C) 15
(D) 20

35. Using the shape below, follow the directions to construct a new shape.

A	B	C
D	E	F

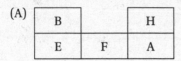 **STEP 1** Fold box C under box B.

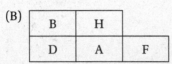 **STEP 2** Erase box D.

STEP 3 Attach box A to the right of box F.

STEP 4 Add a new box H above box A.

What does the new shape look like?

(A)

B		H
E	F	A

(B)

B	H	
D	A	F

(C)

A	B	
H	F	E

(D)

C	B	H
F		A

Questions 36–40 are based on the following passage.

Coming of Age in Samoa (chapter 2, pp. 26–27) by Margaret Mead, 1928.

By the time a child is six or seven, a girl has all the essential avoidances well enough by heart to be trusted with the care of a younger child. She also develops a number of simple techniques. She learns to weave firm square balls, to make pinwheels of palm leaves . . . , to climb a coconut tree by walking with flexible little feet, to break open a coconut . . . , to play a number of group games and sing the songs that go with them, to tidy the house . . . , and bring water from the sea, to spread out the copra to dry and to help gather it in when rain threatens, to roll the pandanus leaves for weaving, to bring a lighted faggot for the chief's pipe or the cook-house fire, and to exercise tact in begging slight favours from relatives.

But in the case of the little girls, all of these tasks are merely supplementary to the main business of baby tending. Very small boys also care for the younger children, but at eight or nine years of age they are usually relieved of the duty. Whatever rough edges have not been smoothed off by this responsibility for younger children are worn off by their contact with older boys. For little boys are admitted to interesting and important activities only as long as their behavior is circumspect and helpful. Where small girls are abruptly pushed aside, small boys will be patiently tolerated and they become adept at making themselves useful. The four or five little boys who all wish to assist at the important business of helping a grown youth lasso reef eels, organize themselves into a highly working team; one boy holds the bait, another holds an extra lasso, others poke eagerly about in holes in the reef looking for prey, while still another tucks the captured eels into his lavalava. The small girls, burdened with heavy babies or the care of little staggerers who are too small to adventure on the reef, discouraged by the hostility of the small boys and the scorn of the older ones, have little opportunity for learning the more adventurous forms of work and play. So while the little boys first undergo the chastening effects of baby-tending and then have many opportunities to learn effective cooperation under the supervision of older boys, the girls' education is less comprehensive. They have a high standard of individual responsibility, but the community provides them with no lessons in cooperation with one another. This is particularly apparent in the activities of young people; the boys organize quickly; the girls waste hours in bickering, innocent of any technique for quick and efficient cooperation.

36. The writing style in the above passage is

   (A) cause and effect.
   (B) compare and contrast.
   (C) expository.
   (D) narrative.

37. What is implied in the first line of the passage, *by the time a child is six or seven, a girl has all the essential avoidances well enough by heart to be trusted with the care of a younger child*?

   (A) A child of six or seven years is old enough to care for younger children in any society or culture.
   (B) Both girls and boys lack the adeptness to care for younger children.
   (C) Girls six or seven years of age understand the importance of staying away from danger.
   (D) All children can be trusted to care for younger children.

38. The passage contains numerous instances of young girls and boys being exposed to unwritten rules on how to behave in Samoan society. What exactly is the passage referencing?

   (A) Cognitive sociology
   (B) Community control
   (C) Social contract
   (D) Social norms

39. Which of the following best describes the relationship between the Samoan villagers and the author?

   (A) Communal enjoinment
   (B) Cynicism
   (C) Intolerance
   (D) Familiarity

40. *Coming of Age in Samoa* is a

   (A) primary source.
   (B) quaternary source.
   (C) secondary source.
   (D) tertiary source.

Questions 41–44 are based on the following passage and chart.

Puff-n-Stuff Bakery recently opened in the village and is planning on participating in the regional Harvest Fair. Their goal is not only to participate in the fair but to increase their sales after the fair. The following chart represents their sales in the week before the fair, the week of the fair, and the week after the fair.

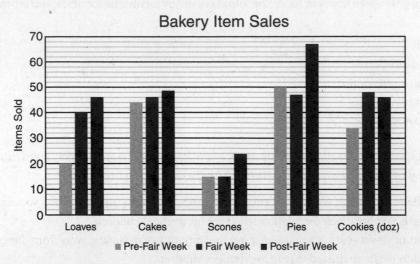

41. The chart is an example of a

(A) column chart.

(B) horizontal chart.

(C) stacked chart.

(D) vertical chart.

42. The total number of items sold in the week before and the week after the fair is approximately

(A) 350.

(B) 375.

(C) 400.

(D) 425.

43. Based on the chart, which of the following items should the Puff-n-Stuff bakers reevaluate?

(A) Cakes

(B) Cookies

(C) Pies

(D) Scones

44. Which of the following weeks had the highest average of sales?

(A) Fair week

(B) Number of sales are not provided; the answer cannot be determined.

(C) Post fair

(D) Pre-fair

Questions 45–49 are based on the following passage.

Remembrance

Evie, as an adult, often reflected on growing up in Wyoming. She lived with her parents and younger brother, Will, in Washakie County. Their home was in an oil camp three miles off of Highway 20 and several miles north of Worland, the county seat. Oil was big in Wyoming in the 1950s.

Evie became a well-known writer of historical Wyoming literature as an adult. She kept a daily diary from an early age until she died in 2014. The following is an excerpt written from when she was about ten years old.

Dear Diary. This is Friday, November 14, 1958. I'm going to bed in a little while. I haven't been to school for four whole days because of the biggest blizzard that came up Monday night and shut everything down. The road from the camp to the highway is blocked with lots of snow and really big drifts. The sun came out yesterday afternoon for the first time in four whole days and Mother let me and Will play outside until Daddy came home from work. She wouldn't let us go and play in the canal because she said the weather wasn't good enough. This morning the sun was out and we got to go play in the canal. Mother told us to come in if we started to get cold because the temperature was 20°. You remember, Diary, that they drain the canal water in the fall and it won't have water again until the spring. The blizzard made great big drifts that went from the canal road down into the canal. Me and Will had fun sliding into the canal. We took our shovels and threw them into the canal so we could dig hand holds in the snow so we could climb out. It was so much fun. We made two snow forts and had a snowball fight. I don't know who won because Mother called us in to have hot tea and crackers with butter and to potty, and then we played outside again until Daddy came home for lunch. Daddy says that if the men get the sidewalk cleared today, I can walk down to the office with him tomorrow and walk back home all by myself. After lunch, me and Will tried to make a snowman, but the snow was too deep and we couldn't roll the ball through the snow. Will got in big trouble because he was throwing snowballs at Sammy's horse. Mom made him come in the house to stay. Daddy had a snowball fight with me when he got home from work. It was so much fun. I hit Daddy with three snowballs, and he never did hit me. I got to stay up and watch the *Cisco Kid* on TV because I was good and took my bath and didn't mess up the floor with water. Will fell asleep and Daddy carried him to bed. I don't know why Will's so tired because he's not old enough to go to school yet. Daddy just said it's time to turn off the light, so goodnight, Diary. I hope the sidewalks get cleared soon! See you later, alligator!

45. The passage is an example of which source of information?

    (A) Primary
    (B) Quaternary
    (C) Secondary
    (D) Tertiary

46. The diary entry represents a young girl's

    (A) chronology of one day.
    (B) hidden secrets no one else knows about.
    (C) need to express herself.
    (D) venture into creativity.

47. What can you infer about Evie and her father's relationship?

    (A) Evie and her father have a better relationship than Evie has with her mother.
    (B) Evie and her father have a relationship that was typical of parent-child relationships in the fifties.
    (C) Evie and her father have a wholesome parent-child relationship.
    (D) Evie's father prefers her company to Will's.

48. What is Evie looking forward to?

(A) Another snowball fight with her father
(B) Going back to school on the bus
(C) Her brother, Will, getting into trouble again and being punished
(D) Walking home by herself from her father's office after the snow is cleared

49. Select the most logical summarization of Evie's diary entry.

(A) A diary entry written by a ten-year-old in Wyoming in the winter of 1950
(B) A grammatically poor diary entry of a ten-year-old child over 50 years ago during the winter of 1958
(C) A one-day diary entry by a ten-year-old girl living in Wyoming in the 1950s. The entry recounts a horrendous blizzard and winter activities with her brother, Will and their parents.
(D) A preposterous one-day diary entry made by a young girl in the 1950s. In all likelihood, the entry contains fabrications of the events she claims to have experienced.

Questions 50–51 are based on the following diagram.

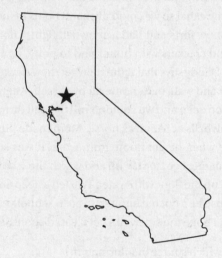

50. The above graphic represents which of the following states?

(A) Alabama
(B) Arizona
(C) California
(D) Oregon

51. Which of the following earthquake fault lines is found in the above state?

(A) Saddle Mountain
(B) San Andreas
(C) San Diego
(D) Southern Whidbey Island

Questions 52–53 are based on the following table.

Rank	Title	Local Jobs	Local Mean Salary	Typical Local Salary	National Growth % 2006–2016	National % with College Degree
1	Registered nurses	31,530	$65,390	$46,290–84,880	24%	56%
2	Sales representatives, wholesale and manufacturing, except technical and scientific products	31,260	$61,510	$26,240–106,270	8%	51%
3	Accountants and auditors	24,690	$67,270	$37,000–107,320	18%	79%
4	Elementary school teachers, except special education	23,740	$47,320	$36,470–60,760	14%	95%
5	Secondary school teachers, except special and vocational education	17,310	$46,020	$22,180–63,700	6%	96%
6	Computer systems analysts	14,900	$80,960	$44,320–122,490	29%	68%
7	Computer software engineers, systems software	13,960	$90,990	$57,390–129,390	28%	85%
8	Computer programmers	12,950	$80,400	$46,680–117,490	–4%	73%
9	Computer software engineers, applications	12,550	$91,800	$61,200–127,250	45%	85%
10	Middle school teachers, except special and vocational education	10,690	$48,860	$37,750–62,910	–11%	95%

52. Which of the following job titles has the lowest national growth percentage?

(A) Computer programmers
(B) Middle school teachers
(C) Registered nurses
(D) Sales representatives

53. Which column provides information on the average salary for a job?

(A) First column
(B) Fourth column
(C) Sixth column
(D) Third column

MATHEMATICS

NUMBER OF QUESTIONS: 36

TIME LIMIT: 54 MINUTES

Instructions: Read each question thoroughly. Select the single best answer. Mark your answer (A, B, C, or D) on the answer sheet provided for Practice Test 1.

1. Simplify the equation.

   $$4 \cdot 3(7 \div 2) + 75 =$$

   (A) 42
   (B) 89
   (C) 100
   (D) 117

2. Simplify the expression.

   $$a^8 \div a^6 =$$

   (A) $a^{0.02}$
   (B) $a^{1.3}$
   (C) a^2
   (D) a^{14}

3. Marcus is 20 years older than his youngest sister Cindy. The sum of their years is 66. How old is Cindy?

   (A) 12
   (B) 23
   (C) 46
   (D) 52

4. Add the following numbers.

   $$8,576 + 80.67 =$$

   (A) 8,495.67
   (B) 8,656.67
   (C) 8,681.67
   (D) 8,691.67

5. Mark is buying mulch for his garden plot which measures 10 yards by 8 yards. How many bags of mulch does he need to buy if one bag of mulch covers 25 square meters?

   (A) One bag
   (B) Two bags
   (C) Three bags
   (D) Five bags

6. Simplify the expression.

$$14 \div 5(\sqrt{36}) =$$

(A) 2.13
(B) 14
(C) 16.8
(D) 36

7. Two sisters are 15 years apart in age. In what year was the younger sister born if the older sister was born in 1988?

(A) 1973
(B) 1983
(C) 1993
(D) 2003

8. Simplify the equation. Round your answer to the nearest tenth.

$$15x - 30 \cdot 0 + 40 = 89$$

(A) –3.3
(B) 0.0
(C) 0.7
(D) 3.3

9. A contractor is planning to fence a yard that will join with the back of the house on three sides (see diagram below). The width of the house is 40 feet, and the length of the yard is 50 feet.

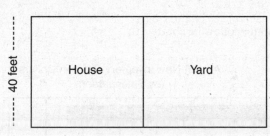

How many feet of fencing will the contractor need in order to fence the yard?

(A) 140 ft
(B) 160 ft
(C) 180 ft
(D) 200 ft

10. In $\triangle ABC$, $\angle A = 90°$ and $\angle B = 45°$. How many degrees are in $\angle C$?

(A) 45°
(B) 90°
(C) 225°
(D) 299°

11. Simplify the expression.

$$\frac{2}{9} \cdot \frac{5}{6} =$$

(A) $\frac{7}{15}$

(B) $\frac{4}{7}$

(C) $\frac{5}{27}$

(D) $\frac{4}{5}$

12. $2^4 \cdot 3^2 =$

(A) 48

(B) 68

(C) 36

(D) 144

13. Simplify the expression. Round your answer to the nearest hundredth.

$$69 \div 16 =$$

(A) 4.00

(B) 4.30

(C) 4.31

(D) 4.40

Questions 14–15 are based on the following chart.

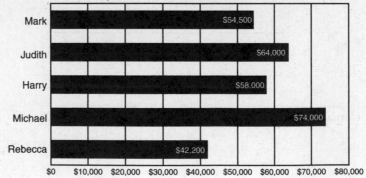

August New Inventory Sales in Dollars
(by Salesperson)

14. Based on the chart, what is the total amount, in dollars, made by the five salespersons during the month of August?

(A) $270,000

(B) $285,000

(C) $292,700

(D) $306,700

15. What is the difference, in dollars, between Michael's sales and Rebecca's sales?

    (A) $10,000
    (B) $16,000
    (C) $19,500
    (D) $31,800

---

16. Simplify the expression.

    $$3a^2 - 3ab + b^2 + 4a^2 + 2ab + 2b^2 =$$

    (A) $7a + ab + b^2$
    (B) $7a^4 - ab + b^4$
    (C) $7a + 5ab + 3b$
    (D) $7a^2 - ab + 3b^2$

17. Simplify the expression. Round your answer to the nearest hundredth.

    $$15 \cdot 16 \div 34 =$$

    (A) 0.9
    (B) 1.1
    (C) 7.06
    (D) 12.6

Question 18 is based on the following passage.

The chess club is baking cookies for the school bazaar. They need the following items from the grocery store. The owner of the store is a school supporter and will give the club a 30% discount on its purchase.

Eggs   15 dozen @$1.50/dozen

Flour   28 lb @ $5.65/5-lb bag

Vanilla   4 bottles @ $1.34/bottle

Sugar   20 lb @ $3.00/10-lb bag

Salt   2 lb @ $1.00/lb

18. How much will the chess club spend at the grocery store?

    (A) $20.93
    (B) $39.76
    (C) $45.23
    (D) $48.83

---

19. What is the length of the hypotenuse, to the nearest inch, when two legs of a right triangle measure 14 inches and 17 inches?

    (A) 21 inches
    (B) 22 inches
    (C) 28 inches
    (D) 45 inches

20. Jason is new to the city and needs to travel from his house to the baseball park. The legend on a city map shows $\frac{1}{2}$ inch = 1 mile. Jason calculates the distance to be 7.5 inches. How many miles will he travel to get to the baseball park from his house?

(A) 5 miles
(B) 15 miles
(C) 20 miles
(D) 22 miles

21. A right angle measures ____ degrees.

(A) 30
(B) 45
(C) 90
(D) 120

22. A man carves wooden birds. He plans to donate 50 birds to a local charity to sell in their annual fundraiser. In his store, the birds sell for $15 each. On average, the man can carve four birds per day. How many days will the man need to carve 50 birds?

(A) 10 days
(B) 13 days
(C) 16 days
(D) 19 days

23. Simplify the expression.

$$(d^3)(d^8) =$$

(A) d^{11}
(B) d^{24}
(C) $2d^{11}$
(D) $2d^{24}$

24. Select the fraction equivalent of 0.06. Reduce to the lowest fraction.

(A) $\frac{3}{50}$

(B) $\frac{4}{50}$

(C) $\frac{5}{50}$

(D) $\frac{6}{50}$

25. Simplify the equation. Solve for x.

$$5x - 14 + 3x - 8 = 10$$

(A) 2
(B) 4
(C) 6
(D) 8

26. Simplify the expression.

$$\frac{3}{4} \cdot \frac{7}{8} =$$

(A) 0.436
(B) 0.656
(C) 0.884
(D) 0.923

27. Simplify the equation.

$$\frac{x}{3} = 7$$

(A) $x = 2.3$
(B) $x = 11.4$
(C) $x = 21$
(D) $x = 42$

28. Samuel and Randi are placemat weavers. Samuel can weave 7 placemats in 8 hours. Randi can weave 5 placemats in 4 hours. How many placemats can they make in 5 days if they worked 8 hours each day?

(A) 24
(B) 60
(C) 79
(D) 85

29. Simplify the following equation. Solve for a.

$$7(5a + 4) - 8 = 29a + 50$$

(A) 5
(B) 9
(C) 13
(D) 15

30. A youth weighs 42 kilograms. What does he weigh in pounds?

(A) 42.0 lb
(B) 76.2 lb
(C) 84.7 lb
(D) 92.4 lb

31. What is the mode in the following set of numbers?

    4　6　12　56　37　6　10　9　13　45　3　19　22

    (A) 4
    (B) 6
    (C) 10
    (D) 56

32. Simplify the expression.

    $\sqrt{144} =$

    (A) 10
    (B) 12
    (C) 18
    (D) 22

33. John is a Registered Nurse who works in surgery. His base pay is $42.17 per hour. In addition, he earns $5.00 per hour for his bachelor's degree in nursing, $6.00 per hour as night supervisor in surgery, and $4.50 per hour for working the night shift. He earns time and a half of his base pay for overtime. For the current pay period, John has worked 80 regular hours and 24 overtime hours. Select the correct formula for John's total earnings for the current pay period.

    (A) Total earnings = $42.17(80) + $5.00(80) + $6.00(80) + $4.50(80) + $63.26(24)
    (B) Total earnings = $42.17(80) + $5.00(80) + $6.00(80) + $4.50(80) + $86.51(24)
    (C) Total earnings = $63.26(104) + $15.00(24)
    (D) Total earnings = $63.26(104) + $5.00(80) + $6.00(80) + $4.00(80)

34. Which of the following would be the least when written in a decimal format?

    (A) $\dfrac{5}{7}$

    (B) $\dfrac{16}{43}$

    (C) $\dfrac{75}{150}$

    (D) $\dfrac{100}{350}$

Question 35 is based on the following chart.

Color Preference

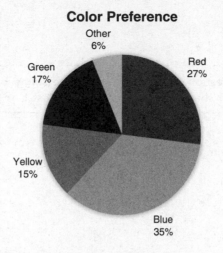

35. What is the mean percentage of the color preferences?

(A) 15%
(B) 20%
(C) 25%
(D) 30%

36. Tom weighs 188.45 pounds. What is his weight in kilograms? Round your answer to the nearest hundredth.

(A) 85.66 kg
(B) 94.23 kg
(C) 106.58 kg
(D) 112.17 kg

SCIENCE

NUMBER OF QUESTIONS: 53

TIME LIMIT: 63 MINUTES

> **Instructions:** Read each question thoroughly. Select the single best answer. Mark your answer (A, B, C, or D) on the answer sheet provided for Practice Test 1.

1. Which of the following is a component of the ear?

   (A) Ciliary process
   (B) Choroid
   (C) Cochlea
   (D) Posterior chamber

2. One function of bile is to

   (A) break down indigestible materials using a fermentation process.
   (B) catalyze biochemical processes.
   (C) emulsify fats.
   (D) facilitate absorption of vitamin B_4 in the large intestine.

3. Select a property of alkali metals such as lithium (Li), sodium (Na), and potassium (K).

   (A) They are commonly used in fireworks.
   (B) They are harder than other metals.
   (C) They are extremely reactive and do not occur in a free form in nature.
   (D) They are poor conductors of electricity.

4. For a substance to be considered a base, it must meet certain criteria. Select the correct criterion.

   (A) A reaction with a metal releases hydrogen.
   (B) It has a pH of 6.5–7.5.
   (C) It is sour to the taste.
   (D) It turns litmus paper blue.

5. Which of the following best describes a dorsal injury?

   (A) A broken tibial plateau
   (B) A contusion of the forebrain
   (C) A gunshot wound to the right upper quadrant of the abdomen
   (D) A torn gastrocnemius

6. Which of the following removes urea from the blood?

   (A) The kidneys
   (B) The liver
   (C) The lungs
   (D) The small intestine

7. The chemical formula for iron disulfide is

(A) $CaCO_3$.
(B) $FeSO_4$.
(C) FeS_2.
(D) PbS.

8. A ball and socket joint is found between which of the following?

(A) Between the anterior iliac spine and iliac crest
(B) Between the femur and pelvis
(C) Between the metatarsals and phalanges
(D) Between the vertebrae

9. An oral temperature of 102.6°F is considered

(A) hypertensive.
(B) hypothermia.
(C) pyrexia.
(D) infectious.

10. Thiamine is also known as vitamin

(A) B_1.
(B) B_2.
(C) B_3.
(D) B_5.

11. Fertilization normally occurs in the

(A) anterior horn of the vagina.
(B) fallopian tube.
(C) urethra.
(D) vagina.

12. What is the relationship between renin and angiotensinogen?

(A) Angiotensinogen is a catalyst that stimulates renin.
(B) Renin is a catalyst that converts angiotensinogen to angiotensin I.
(C) They are catalysts in the liver.
(D) They catalyze proteins.

13. The purpose of the renal system is to support homeostasis

(A) by reabsorbing all inorganic substances, such as glucose and amino acids, back into the systemic circulation.
(B) by regulating urine concentration.
(C) of platelets during hemostatic crisis.
(D) through regulation of water balance and removal of harmful matter from the blood.

14. How many spinal nerves does the human body have?

   (A) 31
   (B) 40
   (C) 62
   (D) 67

15. A cation is a

   (A) negatively charged anion.
   (B) negatively charged atom.
   (C) positively charged anion.
   (D) positively charged atom.

16. According to Archimedes' principle, how much water will a 3,500-ton ship displace?

   (A) 1,700 tons
   (B) 3,500 tons
   (C) 5,300 tons
   (D) 7,000 tons

17. An assemblage of cells of comparable structure working as a unit and executing the same function best describes

   (A) cells.
   (B) organs.
   (C) organ systems.
   (D) tissues.

18. What are the freezing and boiling points of water on a Celsius thermometer, if the freezing and boiling points on a Fahrenheit thermometer are 32°F and 212°F?

   (A) 0°C, 100°C
   (B) 22°C, 72°C
   (C) 65°C, 150°C
   (D) 70°C, 160°C

19. Which of the following glands regulates metabolism?

   (A) Apocrine
   (B) Pancreas
   (C) Pituitary
   (D) Thyroid

20. Epithelial tissue

   (A) is avascular.
   (B) is composed of loosely packed, compressed cells.
   (C) forms between the basement membrane and connective tissue.
   (D) lines external organs.

21. What is the probability that a man with brown eyes (Bb) and a woman with blue eyes (bb) will have a blue-eyed child?

    (A) 25%
    (B) 50%
    (C) 75%
    (D) 100%

22. What type of neuron transmits nerve impulses away from the central nervous system?

    (A) Association
    (B) Memory
    (C) Motor
    (D) Sensory

23. An individual surviving a severe head injury has no sense of proprioception. This means the individual is unable to

    (A) sense touch or pressure.
    (B) recognize visual or photo pigments.
    (C) recognize the position or movement of his/her body.
    (D) understand spoken or written words.

Questions 24–27 are based on the following passage and chart.

Teachers at a private school have been complaining about students falling asleep in their first class after lunch. One teacher postulates that diet is the problem and suggests a study to determine if there is a relationship between diet and sleepiness. The school has a closed campus, and students are not allowed to leave the campus for lunch.

   Twenty students known for falling asleep in the first class after lunch are asked to participate. They are randomly divided into two groups and will eat only food prepared by the cafeteria for lunch. The Light Lunch group will eat salads, raw vegetables, and fruit, and drink noncarbonated sugarless beverages for lunch. The Heavy Lunch group will eat their usual lunch. Data will be collected over a ten-day period. The chart below provides results of their study.

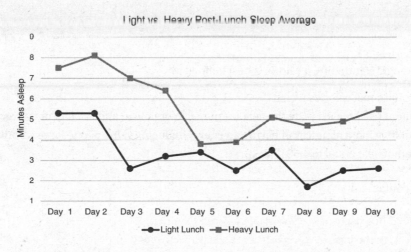

24. What is hypothesized in the passage?

   (A) A correlation exists between diet and sleepiness.
   (B) Students with sleep disorders sleep in class.
   (C) There is a relationship between light and heavy lunches.
   (D) Male students sleep more after consuming a heavy meal than female students after consuming a light meal.

25. As a researcher, would you be comfortable in presenting the results of this study to the faculty at the school?

   (A) Yes, the results are clear. Diet does influence sleepiness.
   (B) Yes, the results are clear. There is no distinct correlation between diet and sleepiness.
   (C) No, there is not enough collected data to draw a conclusion.
   (D) No, there are too many unidentified variables influencing the study to draw any valid conclusion.

26. Which of the following is the dependent variable?

   (A) Light lunches
   (B) Heavy lunches
   (C) Number of days in the study
   (D) Sleep

27. On what day are the sleep minutes lowest for the Light Lunch group?

   (A) Day 1
   (B) Day 6
   (C) Day 7
   (D) Day 8

---

28. What is the most profuse element found in the earth's crust?

   (A) Carbon dioxide
   (B) Oxygen
   (C) Salt
   (D) Water

29. From a physiologic standpoint, a calorie is best defined as

   (A) around 1,500 small calories.
   (B) a component used to designate the heat output of an organism and the fuel or energy value of food.
   (C) the cumulative mass of nutrition having an energy-reducing value of one large calorie.
   (D) an amount of heat equal to 4.52 joules.

30. Erythrocytes contain

   (A) agranulocytes.
   (B) antibodies.
   (C) hemoglobin.
   (D) plasma.

31. Laboratory studies confirm a patient has hypothyroidism. This indicates a deficiency in

    (A) iodine.
    (B) potassium.
    (C) sodium.
    (D) thiamine.

32. There are four basic types of tissue. They are

    (A) cardiac, digestive, pulmonary, and renal.
    (B) glandular, squamous, stratified, and transitional.
    (C) hyaline, lattice, ossified, and spongy.
    (D) muscle, connective, epithelial, and nerve.

33. What type of bone replaces cartilage on the outside of bone?

    (A) Articular
    (B) Compact
    (C) Epiphyseal
    (D) Ossification

34. Antibodies bind to

    (A) antigens.
    (B) macrophages.
    (C) proteins.
    (D) T cells.

35. Functions of the large intestine include all of the following EXCEPT

    (A) absorption.
    (B) bacterial digestion.
    (C) peristalsis.
    (D) storage.

36. Protein synthesis represents enzyme and protein production from DNA. All of the following are steps in this process EXCEPT

    (A) RNA processing.
    (B) sequencing.
    (C) transcription.
    (D) translation.

37. All of the following are commonly accepted functions of the cardiovascular system EXCEPT

    (A) protect.
    (B) regulate.
    (C) storage.
    (D) transport.

38. Bilirubin is a waste product of

    (A) creatine.
    (B) hemoglobin.
    (C) nucleic acids.
    (D) proteins.

39. The purpose of leukocytes is to

    (A) assist the sarcoplasmic reticulum to release calcium during periods of infection.
    (B) bind with specific proteins to combat infection.
    (C) protect the body from toxins and foreign microbes.
    (D) shield erythrocytes from bacterial infection.

40. The diaphragm

    (A) aids in respiration.
    (B) compresses the abdomen during respiration.
    (C) elevates the ribs during respiration.
    (D) stimulates respiration.

41. Which of the following can humans live and function normally without?

    (A) Adrenal glands
    (B) Brain stem
    (C) Right atrium
    (D) Tonsils

42. Proprioceptors are involved with

    (A) blood pressure.
    (B) position of the body.
    (C) tactile stimulation.
    (D) visceral organs.

43. Which of the following carries oxygenated blood?

    (A) Brachial vein
    (B) Carotid vein
    (C) Inferior vena cava
    (D) Pulmonary vein

44. Which of the following anatomical relationships best characterizes the word *ipsilateral*?

    (A) The lumbar spine and the navel
    (B) The nose and the right ear
    (C) The right ankle and left thumb
    (D) The spleen and the descending colon

45. Which of the following is a monosaccharide?

   (A) Fructose
   (B) Glycogen
   (C) Sucrose
   (D) Starch

Question 46 is based on the following cardiac rhythm strip.

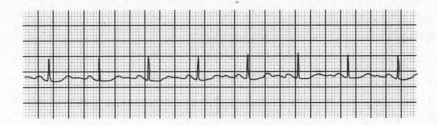

46. The above rhythm strip contains approximately six seconds of cardiac electrical activity. Which of the following would be the best device to aid in determining the heart rate for one minute?

   (A) Calipers
   (B) Chronograph
   (C) Measuring tape
   (D) Ratometer

Question 47 is based on the following chart.

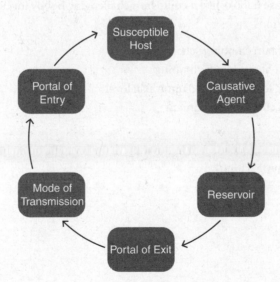

47. The above diagram shows the chain of infection. Which of the following can a nurse use to break this chain?

   (A) Remove the portal of entry from the hospital environment
   (B) Remove the reservoir from the hospital environment
   (C) Instruct patient to wash hands with the appropriate solution upon leaving and reentering the room
   (D) Wash hands with the appropriate solution upon entering and leaving the patients' rooms

Questions 48–49 are based on the Periodic Table of Elements on page 53.

48. Based on information presented in the Periodic Table of Elements, the electrons per shell for boron (B) are

(A) 2, 1.
(B) 2, 3.
(C) 2, 8, 8, 1.
(D) 2, 8, 15, 2.

49. What is the standard atomic weight of manganese (Mn)?

(A) 12.011
(B) 24.305
(C) 40.078
(D) 54.938

50. A person with elevated eosinophilic leukocytosis is commonly suffering from

(A) bacterial/viral infection.
(B) chronic infection.
(C) leukemia.
(D) seasonal allergies.

51. A young woman who has always been interested in mountain activities decides she wants to become a mountain climber because it looks like it could be a challenging hobby for her. Which of the following is her first, most logical action?

(A) Attend a local mountain climbing school
(B) Investigate the sport of mountain climbing
(C) Investigate climbing locations based upon skill level
(D) Purchase mountain climbing equipment

52. Which of the following receptors, located in the walls of the bronchi/bronchioles, are activated when the lungs expand to their physical limit?

(A) Apneustic
(B) Inspiratory
(C) Pneumonic
(D) Stretch

53. Large organic molecules in living organisms are called

(A) macromolecules.
(B) manomolecules.
(C) micromolecules.
(D) monomolecules.

Periodic Table of Elements

1 IA	2 IIA											13 IIIA	14 IVA	15 VA	16 VIA	17 VIIA	18 VIIIA
1 **H** Hydrogen 1.008																	2 **He** Helium 4.002602
3 **Li** Lithium 6.94	4 **Be** Beryllium 9.0121831											5 **B** Boron 10.81	6 **C** Carbon 12.011	7 **N** Nitrogen 14.007	8 **O** Oxygen 15.999	9 **F** Fluorine 18.998403163	10 **Ne** Neon 20.1797
11 **Na** Sodium 22.98976928	12 **Mg** Magnesium 24.305	3 IIIB	4 IVB	5 VB	6 VIB	7 VIIB	8 VIIIB	9 VIIIB	10 VIIIB	11 IB	12 IIB	13 **Al** Aluminium 26.9815385	14 **Si** Silicon 28.085	15 **P** Phosphorus 30.973761998	16 **S** Sulfur 32.06	17 **Cl** Chlorine 35.45	18 **Ar** Argon 39.948
19 **K** Potassium 39.0983	20 **Ca** Calcium 40.078	21 **Sc** Scandium 44.955908	22 **Ti** Titanium 47.867	23 **V** Vanadium 50.9415	24 **Cr** Chromium 51.9961	25 **Mn** Manganese 54.938044	26 **Fe** Iron 55.845	27 **Co** Cobalt 58.93194	28 **Ni** Nickel 58.6934	29 **Cu** Copper 63.546	30 **Zn** Zinc 65.38	31 **Ga** Gallium 69.723	32 **Ge** Germanium 72.630	33 **As** Arsenic 74.921595	34 **Se** Selenium 78.971	35 **Br** Bromine 79.904	36 **Kr** Krypton 83.798
37 **Rb** Rubidium 85.4678	38 **Sr** Strontium 87.62	39 **Y** Yttrium 88.90584	40 **Zr** Zirconium 91.224	41 **Nb** Niobium 92.90637	42 **Mo** Molybdenum 95.95	43 **Tc** Technetium (98)	44 **Ru** Ruthenium 101.07	45 **Rh** Rhodium 102.90550	46 **Pd** Palladium 106.42	47 **Ag** Silver 107.8682	48 **Cd** Cadmium 112.414	49 **In** Indium 114.818	50 **Sn** Tin 118.710	51 **Sb** Antimony 121.760	52 **Te** Tellurium 127.60	53 **I** Iodine 126.90447	54 **Xe** Xenon 131.293
55 **Cs** Caesium 132.90545196	56 **Ba** Barium 137.327	57 - 71 Lanthanoids	72 **Hf** Hafnium 178.49	73 **Ta** Tantalum 180.94788	74 **W** Tungsten 183.84	75 **Re** Rhenium 186.207	76 **Os** Osmium 190.23	77 **Ir** Iridium 192.217	78 **Pt** Platinum 195.084	79 **Au** Gold 196.966569	80 **Hg** Mercury 200.592	81 **Tl** Thallium 204.38	82 **Pb** Lead 207.2	83 **Bi** Bismuth 208.98040	84 **Po** Polonium (209)	85 **At** Astatine (210)	86 **Rn** Radon (222)
87 **Fr** Francium (223)	88 **Ra** Radium (226)	89 - 103 Actinoids	104 **Rf** Rutherfordium (267)	105 **Db** Dubnium (268)	106 **Sg** Seaborgium (269)	107 **Bh** Bohrium (270)	108 **Hs** Hassium (269)	109 **Mt** Meitnerium (228)	110 **Ds** Darmstadtium (281)	111 **Rg** Roentgenium (282)	112 **Cn** Copernicium (285)	113 **Nh** Nihonium (286)	114 **Fl** Flerovium (289)	115 **Mc** Moscovium (289)	116 **Lv** Livermorium (293)	117 **Ts** Tennessine (294)	118 **Og** Oganesson (294)

Atomic Number → 1
H
Name → Hydrogen 1.008
Symbol
Atomic Weight

57 **La** Lanthanum 138.90547	58 **Ce** Cerium 140.116	59 **Pr** Praseodymium 140.90766	60 **Nd** Neodymium 144.242	61 **Pm** Promethium (145)	62 **Sm** Samarium 150.36	63 **Eu** Europium 151.964	64 **Gd** Gadolinium 157.25	65 **Tb** Terbium 158.92535	66 **Dy** Dysprosium 162.500	67 **Ho** Holmium 164.93033	68 **Er** Erbium 167.259	69 **Tm** Thulium 168.93422	70 **Yb** Ytterbium 173.045	71 **Lu** Lutetium 174.9668
89 **Ac** Actinium (227)	90 **Th** Thorium 232.0377	91 **Pa** Protactinium 231.03588	92 **U** Uranium 238.02891	93 **Np** Neptunium (237)	94 **Pu** Plutonium (244)	95 **Am** Americium (243)	96 **Cm** Curium (247)	97 **Bk** Berkelium (247)	98 **Cf** Californium (251)	99 **Es** Einsteinium (252)	100 **Fm** Fermium (257)	101 **Md** Mendelevium (258)	102 **No** Nobelium (259)	103 **Lr** Lawrencium (266)

NUMBER OF QUESTIONS: 28

TIME LIMIT: 28 MINUTES

> **Instructions:** Read each question thoroughly. Select the single best answer. Mark your answer (A, B, C, or D) on the answer sheet provided for Practice Test 1.

1. Select the best meaning of the italicized slang term.

   The police raided the local *cat house* and arrested twelve patrons including the mayor, two city councilmen, and ten prostitutes.

   (A) A bordello
   (B) An illegal gambling house
   (C) A home for felines
   (D) A luxury yacht

2. Which of the following sentences is written in the third-person plural?

   (A) Marcy became lost in the woods and was found by a hiker the next morning.
   (B) The politician, bombarded by the constant questions from the audience, became frustrated and left the stage.
   (C) The teachers told the parents that Martin was a bright student who received low marks because he refused to pay attention and follow directions.
   (D) We took our rain gear with us because the clouds looked dark and threatening.

3. Which of the following is a compound sentence?

   (A) Harry loved spending time in the woods behind his house, yet he feared the woods after sunset.
   (B) Mary and her brother, John, took the 2:30 bus home and arrived before their uncle was scheduled to leave.
   (C) The graduation ceremony lasted longer than expected so the dance started later.
   (D) The man admitted he had taken the car without permission but, said he couldn't remember where he left it.

4. Which of the following sentences is correctly punctuated?

   (A) River stood and said, "Wait a minute before you slam Watson's *Impression of Sunset on a Cold Winter Day*"—read it before you make a judgment!
   (B) The impatient crowd chanted, 'Now, now, now,' when the performer was late in beginning the concert.
   (C) "Wait for me," yelled Samuel, "I'm running as fast as I can."
   (D) "You know said Sarah, I have always wanted to visit the zoo."

5. Which of the following words is correctly spelled?

   (A) Anonamous
   (B) Emberassment
   (C) Phychoanalyses
   (D) Sergeant

6. Select an appropriate synonym for the italicized word in the following sentence.

   The *agile* dog jumped for the ball and landed in the frigid water.

   (A) Apt
   (B) Dexterous
   (C) Felicitous
   (D) Inopportune

7. Select the most appropriate meaning of the root word italicized in the following sentence.

   The nursery worker said to use an insecti*cide* on the trees with wilted leaves.

   (A) Among
   (B) Bind
   (C) Kill
   (D) Spasmodic

8. Select the incorrectly punctuated sentence.

   (A) The armed forces, so the recruiter told them, made boys into men of character and honor.
   (B) Jeff and Tommy went to the bait shop hunting for worms they'd been told the fish on Thomson Creek were biting on worms.
   (C) Were the children excited to visit their grandparent's farm?
   (D) While playing for the Beacon High School baseball team, Josh set many school and state records.

9. Select the incorrectly spelled word.

   (A) Jelous
   (B) Poultry
   (C) Strenuous
   (D) Terse

10. Select the sentence using an incorrect word.

    (A) The affect of the drug altered his perceptions of reality.
    (B) The boy was up, dressed, packed, and ready to go an hour before the bus arrived.
    (C) The city council passed an ordinance requiring microchipping of all dogs and cats prior to administration of yearly rabies shots.
    (D) The rancher said, "I've already sold too many cattle, but I had no choice—the drought's about ruined me."

11. Select the following word equation that correctly adds a suffix to a word ending in *y*.

   (A) Angry + ly = angrily
   (B) Annoy + ance = annoiance
   (C) Bury + ed = buryed
   (D) They + are = there

12. Select the word that has the same spelling but different meanings.

   (A) Date: a point in time, or nonedible fruit
   (B) Desert: a dry place, or to leave without returning
   (C) Entrance: a place to enter, or to repel
   (D) Lead: to go before, or fall behind

13. Select the sentence using an incorrect word.

   (A) After talking with the student's parents, the teacher was sure pomposity ran in the family.
   (B) As an exchange student from Mexico, Pedro was delighted when the teacher asked him to represent the class in the annual spelling bee.
   (C) Her actions during the recent crisis were truly crucible.
   (D) The group had trouble believing what their classmates told them about the vandalized equipment.

14. Select the sentence using an incorrect word.

   (A) Amy's parents were concerned when they discovered she had left home without her driver's license and cell phone.
   (B) While Noah understood the connotations of his name, his friends did not and often teased him.
   (C) Why do you suppose Henry wanted to know where his girlfriend went?
   (D) Where is the campus bookstore at?

15. Which of the following is a simple sentence?

   (A) Although the football team sustained numerous injuries, they still had a winning season.
   (B) Marcus had always wanted to own a fancy sports car, but he had trouble saving his money.
   (C) Politicians say they are interested in the welfare of their constituents even though their actions do not always show it.
   (D) The rescue team and his family looked for the lost hiker.

16. Which of the following is a correctly worded sentence?

   (A) James was offended—he knew his heifer was neither fat nor stupid.
   (B) I love to mountain bike and hiking.
   (C) Tammy's happier and more sociable than me.
   (D) The committee had to approve the change nor they would not be reelected in the fall.

17. Select the incorrectly spelled word.

   (A) Affirmative
   (B) Bounteous
   (C) Kindergarden
   (D) Summarize

18. Select the incorrectly punctuated sentence.

(A) Hawkeye the best skeet shooter in the county finished last in the competition.

(B) Picnicking in the woods, the children spent most of the morning looking for the perfect stick for cooking wieners and marshmallows over a campfire.

(C) The old fisherman and his dog bought a fish for the cat's birthday.

(D) The game was canceled when a severe thunderstorm warning was issued.

19. Select the most appropriate meaning of the root word italicized in the following sentence.

A slim majority of *legis*lators wanted to secede from the country.

(A) Many

(B) Law

(C) Officials

(D) Oppose

20. Select an appropriate synonym for the italicized word in the following sentence.

Harriet Tubman, born Araminta Ross, was an *abolitionist* during the Civil War.

(A) Activist

(B) Conformationist

(C) Restorationist

(D) Validationist

21. Select an appropriate synonym for the italicized word in the following sentence.

Students were instructed to *thoroughly* read the instructions before proceeding to the testing materials.

(A) Carelessly

(B) Conscientiously

(C) Partially

(D) Unpleasantly

22. Select the correctly punctuated sentence.

(A) At the beginning of the long hot summer, not ready for the hot weather.

(B) Alex was seven and he wanted a red wagon and an official NFL football and five different computer games for his eighth birthday.

(C) Sarah, had always wanted to visit Alaska, and she, got her chance, last spring when she won the lottery.

(D) They built their retirement cabin on the lake; it had a dock and boat shed.

23. Select the sentence that uses transition words to enhance clarity.

(A) John went to bed hungry as a result of him being too busy playing at the park to come home for dinner.

(B) The woman took her mother to the supermarket, store, and park.

(C) The child said he didn't have enough money for the purchase and figured the clerk would give him a discount.

(D) "Woe is me," said the student, "I am finished."

24. Select the subject in the following sentence.

    The sponsors of the fishing tournament canceled the event when tornado warnings were issued.

    (A) Canceled
    (B) Fishing
    (C) Sponsors
    (D) Warnings

25. When using the active voice, the subject of the sentence

    (A) indicates what the subject is doing over a period of time.
    (B) is acted upon.
    (C) is indicative of mood.
    (D) performs the action.

26. Select the sentence demonstrating future tense, second person.

    (A) "You will be seeing this information again," the teacher said to the class.
    (B) Everyone knew she had been seeing him for several months.
    (C) "It's not a secret anymore," he said, "we were seen at the lake last evening."
    (D) You have five possible options.

27. The following passage indicates a _____ format.

    I ~~hoped~~ [*find better word*] my vacation to Montana [*should the name of the ranch be included?*] ~~as soon as school~~ three weeks after school was out for the summer. We flew from Chicago to Denver, and then flew on to Billings where we ~~started~~ took a bus to a small town called Roundup [*would it be better to include the names of the states?*]. [*add From there?*] We were taken in four-wheel-drive vehicles to the ranch where our belongings were packed onto mules, and we rode the last six miles on horseback after having our first ranch meal cooked over a fire. [*start a new sentence and discuss the meal?*]

    (A) Brainstorming
    (B) Collaboration
    (C) Draft
    (D) Mind mapping

28. Select the sentence with incorrect subject-verb agreement.

    (A) Sam and Marsha were not surprised when Amy missed the school bus.
    (B) Some of the birds in the forest was noisier than others.
    (C) The Torrance Swim Club offered free swimming lessons each summer.
    (D) City planners thought a larger, updated mall with a better variety of businesses would increase tax revenue for the city.

ANSWER KEY
Practice Test 1

Reading

1.	B	15.	D	29.	B	43.	D
2.	C	16.	B	30.	D	44.	C
3.	C	17.	C	31.	B	45.	C
4.	A	18.	A	32.	C	46.	A
5.	B	19.	B	33.	D	47.	C
6.	A	20.	C	34.	B	48.	D
7.	D	21.	A	35.	A	49.	C
8.	D	22.	A	36.	C	50.	C
9.	B	23.	C	37.	C	51.	B
10.	A	24.	A	38.	D	52.	B
11.	D	25.	B	39.	D	53.	B
12.	B	26.	D	40.	A		
13.	A	27.	B	41.	A		
14.	D	28.	B	42.	C		

Mathematics

1.	D	10.	A	19.	B	28.	D
2.	C	11.	C	20.	B	29.	A
3.	B	12.	D	21.	C	30.	D
4.	B	13.	C	22.	B	31.	B
5.	C	14.	C	23.	A	32.	B
6.	C	15.	D	24.	A	33.	A
7.	D	16.	D	25.	B	34.	D
8.	D	17.	C	26.	D	35.	D
9.	A	18.	D	27.	C	36.	A

ANSWER KEY
Practice Test 1

Science

1.	C	15.	D	29.	B	43.	D
2.	C	16.	B	30.	C	44.	D
3.	C	17.	D	31.	A	45.	A
4.	D	18.	A	32.	D	46.	A
5.	D	19.	D	33.	B	47.	D
6.	A	20.	A	34.	A	48.	B
7.	C	21.	B	35.	D	49.	D
8.	B	22.	C	36.	B	50.	D
9.	C	23.	C	37.	C	51.	B
10.	A	24.	A	38.	B	52.	D
11.	B	25.	D	39.	C	53.	A
12.	B	26.	D	40.	A		
13.	D	27.	D	41.	D		
14.	C	28.	B	42.	B		

English and Language Usage

1.	A	8.	B	15.	D	22.	D
2.	C	9.	A	16.	A	23.	A
3.	A	10.	A	17.	C	24.	C
4.	C	11.	A	18.	A	25.	D
5.	D	12.	B	19.	B	26.	A
6.	B	13.	C	20.	A	27.	C
7.	C	14.	D	21.	B	28.	B

ANSWER EXPLANATIONS
Reading

1. **(B)** *Surmise* is an assumption or deduction. There were no witnesses to the accident, and the driver of the car was not present. Investigators, using evidence found at the scene, *surmised* or *hypothesized* the cause of the accident. *Hypothesize* can be defined as a conjecture or a conclusion. The remaining options are antonyms of *surmise*.

2. **(C)** *Foot* also means the lowest part of something, such as a hill, page, or ladder—the car was found at the deepest part of the ravine. In this case, *foot* and *bottom* are synonyms. The remaining options do not support the information given in the stem.

3. **(C)** The passage, as might be found in a newspaper, is intended to tell readers about an event or accident that happened during a snowstorm. Option (A) asks the reader to make an incorrect assumption that the investigators and search and rescue team are county employees; they may or may not be. Option (B) is unrealistic. Individuals living in areas having treacherous winters understand the increased risk of accidents during bad weather. Option (D) is inaccurate. There is nothing to suggest that the accident could have been prevented if the road were salted or sanded. There may be numerous other causes of the accident, and these will not be known until the driver of the car is found and questioned.

4. **(A)** Bar charts display values in a horizontal format. Column charts display values in vertical or column format. Pie charts resemble a pie and are circular in shape with values shown as pieces of the pie. Line charts join common values together using lines.

5. **(B)** The rose color theme has the shortest time stay of the available color themes and meets a goal of getting truckers in and out as quickly as possible. The remaining color themes indicate longer times spent in the shower facility, with the tan color theme having the longest average time in minutes.

6. **(A)** Of the options, (A) is the most logical. Jenet's grades are borderline at best. How will she manage attending class, studying, and a private life with the addition of the demands of the softball team? She needs a realistic plan she can follow. It may seem like option (B) is the best option, but it is not. A tutor cannot replace sound studying. A tutor is meant to assist a student in the understanding of material, it is not meant as a replacement for studying for the course. Hiring a tutor is a good idea, but only if a realistic plan of study first exists. Option (C) is illogical. Option (D) is vague because there is no way to determine what "work harder on her grades" means since no information is given on why she makes the grades she does.

7. **(D)** *Proposition* is defined as an act of offering or suggesting something. It can also mean something to be considered. *Premise* is defined as a proposition supporting something. The remaining options are antonyms.

8. **(D)** President Lincoln's Gettysburg Address was intended to recognize and honor the Union dead at Gettysburg. No Confederate soldiers are buried in Gettysburg Cemetery. Survivors of the battle were not directly acknowledged. Lincoln spoke of the work ahead of the nation, but not specifically postwar reconstruction. Lee's defeat at Gettysburg was the beginning of the end for the Confederacy.

9. **(B)** Narrative writing provides an account of events and experiences over time or for an isolated event. A narrative can be fiction or nonfiction.

10. **(A)** While you may not be familiar with Wilson's work, the passage gives the answer to the questions when it states, "In the novel, Wilson writes of . . . ." Biographical novels tell an individual's story, but are written by another person based on what he or she has been told or what has been found through research. The remaining options are fictitious.

11. **(D)** True-life or nonfiction writing draws upon fact-based reality and includes autobiography, history, and essay, as opposed to fictional writings, which are made-up, imagined, or invented. The serial section of a library contains items published in installments, such as *National Geographic, Better Homes and Gardens,* or *Rolling Stone.* Reference sections contain items such as dictionaries, encyclopedias, thesauri, manuals, and handbooks.

12. **(B)** The passage is a narrative and tells the story of a young girl frightened by a quarry blast. The passage is meant to entertain. Information in the passage is presented as a series of related events. The passage is not expository because it does not explain or inform the reader. There is nothing argumentative in the passage, and it does not attempt to persuade the reader. No problem is presented in the passage, and no solution is called for.

13. **(A)** The passage heavily suggests that Brenda is a child who does not always listen to what she is told. The passage states that Brenda felt like a fool, but feeling like a fool is not the same as being a fool. The passage does not give enough information to determine if Brenda's parents are good or bad. The last option is an assumption that cannot be accurately determined. The word *vaguely* in the last sentence of the stem means not clear in thought or understanding.

14. **(D)** The persuasive mode is used in the e-mail message. Its purpose is to convince readers that they need the offered home and motor home warranty repair service. The e-mail refers to the readers as valued customers, suggesting as credit account holders they are somehow more special than other customers. The remaining options do not support the mode used in the passage.

15. **(D)** *Valuable* is the only antonym in the options. The remaining options are synonyms of *paltry. Paltry* is defined as something ridiculous or cheap.

16. **(B)** *Locally owned* is a term meaning a business or enterprise owned by a member or members in a community, as opposed to large-scale business chains, such as Home Depot or Albertson's, that are found across specific areas of the country or nationwide. The remaining options do not define *locally owned.*

17. **(C)** The passage is instructional and provides technical information—it gives directions to a celebration to be held at a summer sheep camp and is detailed and precise in nature. The passage is not entertaining or expressive. A distinction must be made between the passage being technical or informative. Informative gives general information, such as one might read in a brochure.

18. **(A)** Based on the map, the shortest, most direct trail is Deer Haven to Devil's Playground to the grocery. The trails presented in the remaining options are not the shortest or most direct.

19. **(B)** The problem can be solved by more than one method. The key to correctly answering the question is noticing the question asks for an *estimation* of the *perimeter* hiking trails on the map. Primitive hiking trails are not shown on the map. The perimeter trails start and end at the Rest Area and include Devil's Playground, Echo's Leap, Laughing Falls, Harmony, Heart Attack Hill, and Bear's Hollar. A rough estimate is 8 to 13 miles. Deer Haven and King's Corner are not perimeter hiking trails.

20. **(C)** Based on information in the brochure, ideal guests are thrill-seeking nature enthusiasts looking for a challenge. The word *audacious* refers to someone bold, daring, adventurous, or reckless—these individuals are more prone to accidental injury because of their attitudes and behaviors. The remaining options are not supportive of information given in the brochure.

21. **(A)** While state parks have strict rules and regulations, they exist for the enjoyment of the public. As such, they are intended for everyday individuals seeking enjoyment. All of the options except (C) could be seen as correct. However, option (A) is the most correct because of the brochure statement, *ultimate camping and trail experiences for thrill-seeking nature*

enthusiasts. The use of the word *average* is also appropriate in the options because the vast majority of individuals are just everyday or run-of-the-mill people. Option (C) cannot be correct because state parks are not structured environments. Do not read information from the previous question (#20) into this question. Each question stands alone and does not influence the answer of any other question.

22. **(A)** The information in the passage is written at a level at which the majority of nonhealth professionals can understand. Even though a number of health-related terms are included in the passage, the information is general and nontechnical in nature. A health-care journal provides technical, in-depth information. Editorials in newspapers generally praise or condemn. New age publications would not address or be supportive of standardized disease management.

23. **(C)** At its simplest level, the heart is a pump. When the heart is unable to pump sufficient blood to meet the demands of the body, pump failure has occurred. Cardiovascular failure involves the heart and vascular systems. Heart disease is seen across the life span, and cardiopulmonary congestion suggests more than heart failure as discussed in the passage.

24. **(A)** Heart failure is a chronic disease and worsens over time with or without treatment. There is no cure. With appropriate medical management, heart failure is not a death sentence, and it is no more or less expensive to treat than any other chronic disorder. All chronic diseases have the potential to put unreasonable demands on an individual's life because a change in lifestyle is usually indicated. Some individuals are unable or unwilling to make lifestyle changes.

25. **(B)** Individuals with anemia have low hemoglobin (red blood cells) in their blood, and their skin color is pale or pallid. The remaining options do not support a definition of anemia.

26. **(D)** Tomatoes are fruits usually eaten as vegetables. The remaining options cannot be addressed since the table of contents is a partial one, and the reader has no way of knowing the subject/content of remaining chapters.

27. **(B)** The mood of the passage is fear, or fear of the unknown. The remaining options are not expressed in the passage.

28. **(B)** An unnerved individual has lost his or her courage, determination, or confidence. Panic often follows being unnerved. The remaining options do not support the activity or behavior occurring in the passage.

29. **(B)** Depending upon the circumstances, the passage could be found in any of the type of novels given. However, when looking for the most likely novel to contain the passage, the mystery novel is most specific and logical. All of the options in this question are potentially correct. To select the correct option, you must employ reasoning skills or critical thinking to determine which option is *most* correct.

30. **(D)** The first step when baking is to always preheat the oven unless the recipe specifically says not to do so. In reading the recipe, the listing of needed ingredients is given first. In the instructions that follow the listing, the first instruction is to preheat the oven. Softening the butter is not an instruction. Baking time and greasing the cookie sheet are instructions, but not the first instruction.

31. **(B)** Imitation or artificial vanilla flavorings may contain numerous natural flavorings. One of these, extracts of cocoa, is found in imitation or artificial vanilla. The remaining cookie ingredients do not contain cocoa extracts.

32. **(C)** According to the order of operations, anything in parentheses is addressed first—multiplying 12 times 3. Options (A) and (D) are not the first action. Option (B) is incorrect because 5 is divided into 30, not 30 divided into 5. It is imperative for you to understand and be able to implement the order of operations—they provide basic instructions on how to approach mathematical problems using more than just addition, subtraction, multiplication, and/or division.

33. **(D)** The graph is a line graph which presents information in a linear format. A bar chart presents information in vertical bars. A cosmo graph maps the features of the universe. A flowchart represents a workflow or problem-solving process.

34. **(B)** Based on information presented in the graph, 13 of the 29 students passed the midterm exam with a grade of 75 or above. Counting the data points is necessary to determine the number of students who passed the exam.

35. **(A)** The steps are as follows:

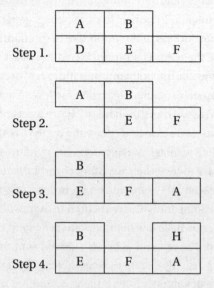

36. **(C)** The purpose of expository writing is to explain and/or inform. Only the facts are presented; opinions are not. There is nothing in the passage to suggest cause and effect. While the passage discusses both girls and boys, the purpose is not to compare or contrast, but again, to explain or inform the reader of childrearing practices in another culture. The passage is not narrative. It was not written to entertain the reader, but to explain or paint a picture of one aspect of life in another culture.

37. **(C)** Understanding the sentence is necessary to correctly answer this question. The phrase *essential avoidance* in the sentence is the key. The word *avoidance* means to stay away from, circumvent, or evade. The word *essential* means important, fundamental, or elementary. Think about what is important for children to avoid. Children should avoid danger—places or events that have the potential to harm them. By the age of six or seven years of age, children should have a sense of what is dangerous. Young girls (and boys) in Samoan society are responsible for younger children and this includes keeping them from harm.

38. **(D)** *Social norms* are unwritten rules of what is considered acceptable behavior in a society. Social norms are shared expectations of behavior, and individuals are expected to conform to these norms. There are negative consequences when nonconformist behavior is shown. The remaining options do not answer the query posed by the stem.

39. **(D)** *Familiarity* is the best answer to the question posed by the stem. The author writes of her observations in Samoa in the 1920s. There is nothing in the passage to suggest there is *cynicism* or *intolerance*. There is no such thing as *communal enjoinment*.

40. **(A)** Primary sources are the original documents, evidence, and objects created at the time under study. *Coming of Age in Samoa* is Mead's written account of her observations in Samoa around 100 years ago. Her writings are considered seminal works in cultural anthropology.

Primary sources are unlike secondary sources, which are accounts or interpretations of events created by someone after the fact. Quaternary sources do not exist.

41. **(A)** Information in the chart is presented in a *column* format, as opposed to a *horizontal* one. The options *horizontal* or *vertical* are incorrect because one means parallel to the ground and the other indicates a direction perpendicular to the horizon—they do not indicate the type of chart. *Stacked* charts have information of the same kind stacked upon each other.

42. **(C)** An estimate of the total number of items sold pre- and post-fair can be obtained by looking at the minor gridlines on the chart. A fairly accurate estimate can be determined because the gridlines are in twos and can be rounded—44 would be rounded down to 40 and 46 would be rounded up to 50. Around 400 items were sold in the week before and week after the fair.

43. **(D)** The chart shows scones as being the poorest seller of items on the chart. The bakers need to determine why scones do not sell as well. Is it their recipe? Do people in the village typically prefer to bake their own scones? Is the price too high? There could be a single reason or numerous reasons why scones are poor sellers.

44. **(C)** The post-fair week had the highest number of items sold. Post-fair items sold are the highest in four of the five categories. Option (B) is incorrect because (1) the number of items sold can be estimated, (2) the exact number of items is not necessary since each bar begins at zero and ends with the highest number of items sold for a given week. The highest number of items sold can also be determined by "eyeballing" the chart.

45. **(C)** It is obvious from the first two paragraphs that Evie is not the writer, and the diary entry is included as an example of Evie's early writings. The excerpt suggests/states Evie was born in the 1940s or 1950s, became a well-known writer, and died in 2014. Since the writer of the excerpt was not present when these things occurred, the piece is a secondary source. Quaternary sources do not exist.

46. **(A)** The diary entry is specific to date and is Evie's chronicle of that day from the viewpoint of a ten-year-old. There is nothing in the entry that suggests secrets, a need for expression, or it being a creative endeavor.

47. **(C)** The relationship type between Evie and her father is implied in the diary entry, and the question must be answered based on this information. Their relationship in the passage is positive. Option (A) asks for comparing and contrasting Evie and her father's relationship to the relationship she has with her mother. The question is not asking for this comparison. A correlation might be found if information regarding father-daughter relationships in the 1950s was provided, but no information is given. The diary entry provides no information supporting the father's preference for one child over the other.

48. **(D)** Evie's writing suggests she is looking forward to walking to work with her father and being able to walk back home by herself. She makes a point to tell her diary that she will be walking home *all by myself,* suggesting or implying this is somehow special. She also restates her father's statement about the sidewalks being cleared. The diary entry provides no information regarding the remaining options.

49. **(C)** The correct option is the most specific and complete summary of the diary entry and provides who, what, when, and where in two brief, meaningful sentences. The remaining options are not specific. One option states the entry is grammatically poor—this is an illogical statement because most ten-year-olds are not stellar writers. The last option is biased and concludes the entry is both preposterous and fabricated. This option is not a summary, but an opinion.

50. **(C)** The graphic represents the state of California. To those living in the United States, the shape is a common one. The remaining options do not have the shape of the state of California.

51. **(B)** The San Andreas fault is well known and is mentioned in the media with each earth-quake in California. The fault is well known because of the destruction caused by the 1906 earthquake. The remaining options are fault lines in the state of Washington that a majority of individuals have never heard of.

52. **(B)** The correct answer to this question is found in the sixth column of the table entitled "National Growth % 2006–2016." Middle school teachers have the lowest growth percentage in the nation at a −11%."

53. **(B)** The fourth column provides information on the average or mean salary for a job. Column one is rank ordering of jobs, column six is national growth rate percentages, and column three is number of local jobs.

Mathematics

1. **(D)** The orders or rules of operation must be followed to correctly solve the problem. They are as follows:

(STEP 1) Parentheses

(STEP 2) Exponents and square roots

(STEP 3) Multiplication and division, whichever comes first working from left to right

(STEP 4) Addition and subtraction, whichever comes first working from left to right

$$4 \cdot 3(7 \div 2) + 75 =$$

(STEP 1) $4 \cdot 3(3.5) + 75 =$

(STEP 2) No exponents or square roots

(STEP 3) $12(3.5) + 75 =$

(STEP 4) $42 + 75 = 117$

2. **(C)** When exponents have the same bases and are divided, the exponents are subtracted. In this equation, the bases (a) are the same. Keep the bases, and subtract 6 from 8 to equal 2.

$$a^8 \div a^6 = a^2$$

3. **(B)** Change the stem to an equation.

Cindy's age $= x$ Marcus's age $= x + 20$ Combined ages $= 66$

$$x + x + 20 = 66$$
$$2x + 20 = 66$$
$$2x = 46$$
$$x = 23$$

4. **(B)** Decimals must be aligned prior to addition.

8,576.00
+ 80.67
8,656.67

5. **(C)** To correctly solve the problem, the units of measurement must agree. The bag of mulch is in meters and the plot is in yards. The answer must be stated in whole bags since a partial bag cannot be purchased. The formula to determine area is used. Once conversions are made the number of bags of mulch can be determined.

- Plot area = 10 yd by 8 yd
  $A = (l)(w) = (10)(8) = 80$ sq yd

- Conversion to meters: 80 sq yd = 73.152 sq m
- 1 bag of mulch = 25 sq m

$$\frac{73.152}{25} = 2.926 = 3 \text{ bags of mulch}$$

6. **(C)** Orders of operation must be followed to correctly solve the equation.

$$14 \div 5\left(\sqrt{36}\right) = 14 \div 5(6) = \frac{14}{5}(6) = \frac{84}{5} = 16.8$$

7. **(D)** Change the sentence to an equation. The problem can be set up a number of ways.

Younger sister $= x - 15$ Older sister $= 1988$

$$x - 15 = 1988$$
$$x = 2003 = \text{birth year of younger sister}$$

8. **(D)** Follow the rules of operation.

$$15x - 30 \cdot 0 + 40 = 89$$
$$15x - 0 + 40 = 89$$
$$15x + 40 = 89$$
$$15x = 49$$
$$x = 3.2666 = 3.3$$

9. **(A)** The contractor will be fencing three sides of the yard since the fence joins to each end of the house. The formula for perimeter $(P) = 2(\text{length}) + 2(\text{width})$. For this problem, there are two lengths but only one width since the fence joins the house on each end.

length $= 50$ ft   width $= 40$ ft
$$P = 2(l) + w$$
$$P = 2(50) + 40$$
$$P = 100 + 40$$
$$P = 140 \text{ ft}$$

10. **(A)** A triangle has three angles equaling 180°. The answer is obtained by adding the two known angles together and subtracting them from 180.

11. **(C)** Multiply the numerators together $(2 \cdot 5 = 10)$ and the denominators together $(9 \cdot 6 = 54)$, which gives $\frac{10}{54} = \frac{5}{27}$ when reduced.

12. **(D)** When multiplying different bases with exponents, first simplify by multiplying the base times their exponent on both sides of the equation, then multiply.

$$2^4 \cdot 3^2 =$$
$$(2 \cdot 2 \cdot 2 \cdot 2)(3 \cdot 3) =$$
$$16 \cdot 9 = 144$$

13. **(C)**

$$69 \div 16 = \frac{69}{16} = 4.3125 = 4.31$$

14. **(C)** The chart allows for easy identification of the August sales for each salesperson. Their amounts are shown in two different ways. The first is the bar itself which extends into the ten thousandths line for each amount. The second is the amount which is indicated numerically at the end of each bar.

Mark	$54,500
Judith	$64,000
Harry	$58,000
Michael	$74,000
Rebecca	+ $42,200
	$292,700

15. **(D)** The difference in dollars between Michael's sales and Rebecca's sales is $31,800. The remaining options are the differences between Michael's sales and the other salespersons.

16. **(D)** Addition of polynomials is the same as regular adding using signed numbers. Exponents are not added.

$$3a^2 - 3ab + b^2$$
$$+ 4a^2 + 2ab + 2b^2$$
$$\overline{7a^2 - ab + 3b^2}$$

17. **(C)** The order of operations must be followed working from left to right. Multiply 15×16, then divide by 34.

$$15 \times 16 \div 34 = \frac{240}{34} = 7.059 = 7.06$$

18. **(D)** The total amount must be determined before the discount can be determined. The discount is subtracted from the total amount.

15 doz eggs @ $1.50	$22.50
6 lb flour @ $5.65	$33.90
4 bottles vanilla @ $1.34	$5.36
2 bags sugar @ $3.00	$6.00
2 lb salt @ $1.00	$2.00
	$69.76

($69.76)(30%) = 20.928 = $20.93

$69.76 − $20.93 = $48.83 total cost of items

19. **(B)** Using a graphic will help visualize the problem. The Pythagorean theorem is used to solve the problem $(a^2 + b^2 = c^2)$.

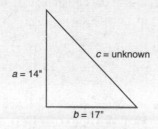

$$a^2 + b^2 = c^2$$
$$14^2 + 17^2 = c^2$$
$$196 + 289 = c^2$$
$$485 = c^2$$
$$\sqrt{485} = c^2$$
$$22.02 = 22" = c$$

20. **(B)** Use ratio and proportion to solve the problem.

$$\text{If } 0.5 \text{ in.} = 1 \text{ mile then } 7.5 \text{ in.} = x \text{ miles}$$
$$0.5 \text{ in.} = 1 \text{ mile} :: 7.5 \text{ in.} = x \text{ miles}$$
$$0.5x = 7.5$$
$$x = 15 \text{ miles}$$

21. **(C)** The hallmark of a right triangle is one of the three angles measures 90°.

22. **(B)** Ratio and proportion can be used to solve the problem.

$$4 \text{ birds} = 1 \text{ day} :: 50 \text{ birds} = x \text{ days}$$
$$4x = 50$$
$$x = 12.5 = 13 \text{ days}$$

23. **(A)** When multiplying base numbers with exponents, the bases remain the same and the exponents are added.

24. **(A)** $0.06 = \dfrac{6}{100} = \dfrac{3}{50}$

25. **(B)**

$$
\begin{array}{l|l}
5x - 14 + 3x - 8 = 10 & 5x - 14 + 3x - 8 = 10 \\
\quad\quad\quad 8x - 22 = 10 & 5(4) - 14 + 3(4) - 8 = 10 \\
\quad\quad\quad\quad\quad 8x = 32 & 20 - 14 + 12 - 8 = 10 \\
\quad\quad\quad\quad\quad\quad x = 4 & 32 - 22 = 10 \\
& 10 = 10
\end{array}
$$

26. **(B)** The problem can be solved by two methods.

$$
\dfrac{3}{4} = 0.75 \quad\quad \dfrac{7}{8} = 0.875
$$
$$
0.75 \times 0.875 = 0.656 \quad\quad\Big|\quad\quad \dfrac{3}{4} \times \dfrac{7}{8} = \dfrac{21}{32} = 0.656
$$

27. **(C)**

$$\dfrac{x}{3} = 7$$
$$\dfrac{x}{3} \bowtie \dfrac{7}{1}$$
$$x = 21$$

20. **(D)** The key to determining the correct answer is making sure the time frames are identical. One weaver's output is given in 4 hours (a half day) and the other is given in 8 hours (1 day). The question asks how many total placemats they can weave in five 8-hour days.

$$\text{Samuel: } 7 \text{ mats in } 8 \text{ hr} \quad\quad \text{Randi: } 10 \text{ mats in } 8 \text{ hr}$$
$$17 \text{ mats} = 8 \text{ hr} :: x \text{ mats in } 40 \text{ hr}$$
$$8x = 680$$
$$x = 85 \text{ placemats}$$

29. **(A)** Since the equation contains more than just addition, subtraction, multiplication, or division, the order of operations must be followed to correctly solve the problem.

$$
\begin{array}{l|l}
7(5a + 4) - 8 = 29a + 50 & 7(5a + 4) - 8 = 29a + 50 \\
35a + 28 - 8 = 29a + 50 & 7(5 \cdot 5 + 4) - 8 = 29(5) + 50 \\
35a + 20 = 29a + 50 & 7(29) - 8 = 29(5) + 50 \\
6a = 30 & 203 - 8 = 145 + 50 \\
a = 5 & 195 = 195
\end{array}
$$

30. **(D)** A conversion must be made to correctly solve the problem.

$$1 \text{ kg} = 2.2 \text{ lb}$$
$$42 \text{ kg} \times 2.2 = 92.4 \text{ lb}$$

31. **(B)** The mode is the number occurring the most times in a series of numbers.

32. **(B)** $\sqrt{144} = 12 \ (12 \times 12 = 144)$

33. **(A)** John receives a base pay plus additional money for his degree, for his position as night supervisor in surgery, and for working the night shift. Since each category has a total number of 80 hours for the pay period, they could be added together and taken times 80 or written as below. He also receives time and a half of his base pay for working over 40 hours per week ($63.26/hour).

$$\text{Total earnings} = \$42.17(80) + \$5.00(80) + \$6.00(80) + \$4.50(80) + \$63.26(24)$$

34. **(D)** Divide the numerator by the denominator. If there is more than one number to the right of the decimal, look at the number in terms of hundredths, such as 0.71, 0.37, 0.50, and 0.28, to determine the smallest.

$$\frac{5}{7} = 0.714 \qquad \frac{16}{43} = 0.372 \qquad \frac{75}{150} = 0.500 \qquad \frac{100}{350} = 0.286$$

35. **(B)** This pie chart presents information in percentages, meaning the total of added components of the chart should equal 100 percent. To determine the mean or average percent, add the percentages together and divide by the number of components, five.

$$6 + 27 + 35 + 15 + 17 = \frac{100}{5} = 20\%$$

36. **(A)** Ratio and proportion can be used to solve the determination.

$$\text{If } 1 \text{ kg} = 2.2 \text{ lb, then } x \text{ kg} = 188.45 \text{ lb}$$
$$1 = 2.2 :: x = 188.45$$
$$2.2x = 188.45$$
$$x = 85.659 = 85.66 \text{ kg}$$

Science

1. **(C)** The cochlea is the auditory portion of the inner ear that translates sound into nerve impulses to be sent to the brain. The cochlea is in the mastoid bone of the skull behind each ear. The remaining options are components of the eye.

2. **(C)** Bile has a number of functions: (1) emulsify fats; (2) assist with the absorption of fat in the intestines; and (3) release bilirubin and excess cholesterol into the intestinal tract for elimination with other waste products. Bile is not a catalyst. Vitamin B_4 does not exist.

3. **(C)** Alkali metals have the following common properties: (1) low melting and boiling points; (2) low densities; (3) extremely reactive with water; (4) malleable and easily cut; (5) do not occur in a free form in nature; and (6) excellent conductors of electricity. Alkali metals are not used in fireworks.

4. **(D)** The criteria for a base are as follows: (1) phenolphthalein turns pink and litmus paper turns blue when exposed to a base; (2) has a slippery feel; (3) conducts electricity in aqueous solutions; (4) reacts with fats to create soap compounds; and (5) bases and acids neutralize each other and form water and salt; (6) have a pH of 8–14; and (7) are bitter to taste.

5. **(D)** The back of an individual is considered the dorsal aspect. The gastrocnemius is a calf muscle and is located on the back or dorsal aspect of the lower leg. All of the other options are located on the front or ventral aspect of the body. One way to remember dorsal is to think of

the shark which has a dorsal fin. It is often the dorsal fin of a shark that announces its presence because it can be seen out of the water.

6. **(A)** Urea is a waste product. Nephrons in the kidney filter the blood and remove urea. The remaining options cannot perform this function.

7. **(C)** All of the options are compounds. FeS_2 is iron disulfide or pyrite (fool's gold). $CaCO_3$ is calcium carbonate. $FeSO_4$ is iron sulphate, and PbS is lead sulfide.

8. **(B)** The hip joint, located between the femur and pelvis, is a ball and socket joint. A condyloidal joint is between the metatarsals and phalanges. The remaining options do not contain joints.

9. **(C)** *Pyrexia* is a synonym for an elevation in temperature. *Hypertensive* refers to elevated blood pressure. *Hypothermia* refers to a sub or below body temperature. While something infectious can cause hyperthermia, it has nothing to do with the question. *Infectious* is usually an adjective. The question calls for a noun.

10. **(A)** Vitamins may be referred to by their name or vitamin designation. Thiamine is vitamin B_1, riboflavin is vitamin B_2, niacin is vitamin B_3, and pantothenic acid is vitamin B_5. There is no vitamin B_4.

11. **(B)** Fertilization normally occurs in the fallopian tubes. The remaining options are not involved in fertilization.

12. **(B)** The enzyme renin converts angiotensinogen to angiotensin I. Renin stimulates angiotensinogen. Neither are catalysts in the liver, and they do not catalyze proteins. Angiotensin is a hormone, not a catalyst.

13. **(D)** The renal system is a major supporter of homeostasis because it regulates water balance and removes harmful matter from the blood. The renal system does not support hemostasis of platelets, or reabsorb inorganic substances. While the renal system does regulate urine concentration, it is one mechanism in the system. Note: Hemostasis and homeostasis are not synonyms.

14. **(C)** The body has 62 individual spinal nerves, or 31 pairs of spinal nerves. The question asks for the number of spinal nerves, not the number of pairs of spinal nerves.

15. **(D)** A cation is a positively charged atom and has more protons than electrons (definition). Iron, lead, and sodium are cations. Anions are the opposite of cations. Bromide, chloride, and fluoride are anions.

16. **(B)** Archimedes' principle has to do with buoyancy. "If the weight of the water displaced is less than the weight of the object, the object will sink. Otherwise the object will float, with the weight of the water displaced equal to the weight of the object." *http://physics.weber.edu/carroll/archimedes/principle.htm*

17. **(D)** The stem of the question is a definition of tissue. The human body is composed of hierarchical levels: atoms $\Rightarrow$ molecules $\Rightarrow$ cells $\Rightarrow$ tissue $\Rightarrow$ organs $\Rightarrow$ organ systems $\Rightarrow$ human body.

18. **(A)** Using the Celsius scale, the freezing point for water is 0 °C, and the boiling point is 100 °C. Both can be calculated. Formulas for Fahrenheit to Celsius are $T_{(°C)} = (T_{(°F)} - 32)\left(\dfrac{5}{9}\right)$ or $T_{(°C)} = (T_{(°F)} - 32) \div 1.8$. Formulas for Celsius to Fahrenheit are $T_{(°F)} = T_{(°C)} \times \dfrac{9}{5} + 32$ or $T_{(°F)} = T_{(°C)} \times 1.8 + 32$.

19. **(D)** Thyroxine (T_4) and triiodothyronine (T_3) are polypeptide hormones that regulate metabolism. The remaining options do not regulate the body's metabolism.

20. **(A)** Epithelial tissue has no blood vessels. Exchange of nutrients and water occurs through diffusion. Epithelial tissue is composed of tightly packed, compressed cells. Epithelial tissue

lines internal organs. The basement membrane forms between epithelial tissue and connective tissue.

21. **(B)** Use a Punnett square to make the determination.

Bb = brown eyes   bb = blue eyes

Father (Bb)

	B	b
b	Bb	bb
b	Bb	bb

Mother (bb)

22. **(C)** Motor neurons send nerve impulses away from the central nervous system to target cells and effectors to produce a response. Sensory neurons do the opposite and send impulses from the sensory organs toward the central nervous system. Located in the central nervous system, association neurons send impulses from sensory neurons to motor neurons. Nearly 100 percent of the neurons in the human body are association neurons. Memory neurons do not exist.

23. **(C)** One method of classifying sensory receptors is by location. Proprioceptors respond to stimulation occurring in the musculoskeletal system and have to do with position and movement. Exteroceptors are on or near the surface of the skin and have to do with sensations of touch and pressure. Visual pigment has to do with vision. Understanding written and spoken words has to do with Wernicke's area in the brain.

24. **(A)** Correlation suggests a relationship exists between variables, but it is not a cause and effect relationship. Synonyms are words such as *similarly*, *matching*, *parallelism*, *interdependence*, and *interconnection*. There is no suggestion that sleep disorders might be part of the problem. The study is interested in sleepiness after a light or heavy meal, not what the meal is composed of. Gender was not included in the study, so such a determination cannot be made.

25. **(D)** As a researcher, you should not be comfortable in presenting this study to anyone. It has numerous flaws and is a weak study. A ten-day period is too short a time to discern any patterns in days or students who suffered from sleepiness after a meal. Overall, this study has too many unidentified variables that could influence a student's sleepiness in the first class after lunch—the time of year, the number of hours slept each night by each student, gender, medications, health issues, lack of interest in the subject or education in general, what each group normally eats for lunch, and many others.

26. **(D)** The dependent variable is sleep or sleepiness. It is the variable the researcher is interested in as a possible effect of some action or thing.

27. **(D)** The sleep minutes for the Light Lunch group on Day 8 is less than two minutes. The remainder of sleep minutes for this group are above two minutes.

28. **(B)** The key to correctly answering this question is the word *element* in the stem. Oxygen is the only element in the options; the remainder are compounds.

29. **(B)** The question is specific in the type of calorie, and asks to define a calorie from a physiologic viewpoint (option (B)). Options (A), (C), and (D) do not define a calorie from a physiologic standpoint.

30. **(C)** Erythrocytes are often called red blood cells. They are responsible for transport of carbon dioxide and oxygen in the blood. Erythrocytes contain hemoglobin that carries oxygen. Erythrocytes (mature) do not contain a nucleus or many organelles. This increases their oxygen carrying capacity. The remaining options are not found in erythrocytes.

31. **(A)** Iodine is an element that is essential to the production of the thyroid hormones thyroxin and triiodothyronine. The body does not produce iodine, and it is supplied by the food we eat. An insufficient intake of iodine results in hypothyroidism. An insufficient amount of dietary intake of iodine during pregnancy can cause mental retardation in infants. Nondietary causes of hypothyroidism include autoimmune disease, thyroidectomy, and radiation treatment. The remaining options are not key in hypothyroidism.

32. **(D)** The human body has four types of tissue that perform specialized physiologic roles. The skin, as an organ, is composed of epithelial tissue. It also forms the linings of most body cavities. The body has three types of muscle tissue: cardiac, skeletal, and smooth. Each type has a unique composition. Connective tissue is the most abundant in the body and supports and protects as part of its many functions. Nerve tissue conducts impulses. The remaining options are not one of the four identified types of body tissues.

33. **(B)** Fibrous membranes and hyaline cartilage form the beginning of the human skeleton during early embryonic development. Two different bone-building processes replace these tissues: intramembranous ossification and endochondral ossification. During the endochondral process, compact bone replaces the hyaline cartilage on the outsides of the bone. This process forms all bones below the skull, except for the clavicles. Compact bone, also called cortical bone, covers most bones and most of the composition of long bones. Articular has to do with joints, epiphyseal has to do with epiphyses or ends of long bones, and ossification is the process of conversion to bone.

34. **(A)** The immune response is the third and final line of defense of the immune system and involves an antibody-antigen complex. Antibodies, produced by B lymphocytes, bind to specific antigens (proteins attached to the surface of pathogens). Think of this as a mobile antibody army protecting the body against invading antigens. Macrophages are phagocytes found in various tissues of the body, proteins are a class of molecules that have various functions, and T cells are a type of lymphocyte.

35. **(D)** The large intestine has four functions: absorption, bacterial digestion, defecation, and peristalsis.

36. **(B)** Protein synthesis occurs during the S phase of interphase during mitosis. The steps in this ordered process are (1) transcription; (2) RNA processing; and (3) translation. Sequencing of nucleotides is the termination point of transcription.

37. **(C)** While blood is in the cardiovascular system at all times, it does not store blood. The remaining options are functions of the cardiovascular system.

38. **(B)** Hemoglobin is contained in erythrocytes which have no cellular organelles or physiologic ability to maintain themselves. As a result, their life span is approximately 120 days or around 4 months. Old, deteriorating erythrocytes are broken down in the liver and spleen. After iron is removed from the hemi group of the erythrocyte, it is broken down into bilirubin. The liver changes bilirubin into bile. Creatine, nucleic acids, and proteins are not waste products.

39. **(C)** Leukocytes, also called white blood cells, are cells of the immune system that work to protect the body from toxins and foreign microbes. They are classified as agranulocytes or granulocytes. Lymphocytes and monocytes are agranulocytes. Basophils, eosinophils, and neutrophils are granulocytes. The remaining options are not purposes of leukocytes.

40. **(A)** The diaphragm separates the thoracic cavity from the abdominal cavity. It moves down on inspiration increasing the volume of the thoracic cavity. This allows for expansion of the lungs. On expiration, it moves up and decreases the thoracic cavity volume. The diaphragm is enervated by the phrenic nerve and is attached to the six lower ribs on the left and right sides, the sternum on the anterior of the body, and the spine on the posterior.

41. **(D)** The tonsils, or palatine tonsils, are soft tissue masses located at the rear of the pharynx. The tissue in tonsils is similar to lymph node tissue. The tonsils are part of the lymphatic system, which supports the immune system. Tonsillectomy, a common childhood surgical procedure, does not seem to increase vulnerability to infection or affect well-being. The remaining options are necessary for life.

42. **(B)** Proprioception is an awareness of the position of parts of the body. For example, an individual turns his head. The individual knows both the direction the head was turned as well as the position of the head. The brain merges data from proprioceptors (sense organs) and from the vestibular system (in the ear) into its overall sense of body position, movement, and acceleration. The cerebellum is largely responsible for coordinating the unconscious aspects of proprioception.

43. **(D)** The pulmonary vein, located in the heart, is the only vein in the body that carries oxygenated blood. Likewise, the pulmonary artery is the only artery in the body that carries deoxygenated blood. The remaining options carry deoxygenated blood.

44. **(D)** *Ipsilateral* means on the same side, as opposed to contralateral which means on the opposite side. The spleen and descending colon are on the same side of the body. The remaining options are contralateral.

45. **(A)** Monosaccharides, such as fructose, are classified as carbohydrates and have a single sugar molecule. Other carbohydrates are disaccharides which contain two linked sugar molecules, and polysaccharides are chains of monosaccharides. Sucrose is a disaccharide composed of one glucose and one fructose molecule. Starch and glycogen are polysaccharides.

46. **(A)** Calipers are the most logical instrument to use with a rhythm strip. Calipers are frequently used to measure small distances where precision, not given by other instruments such as rulers and tape measures, is needed. Chronographs measure time, and a ratometer is fictitious.

47. **(D)** Good handwashing breaks the chain of infection and is one key to infection control in the health care setting. The portal of entry and reservoir cannot be removed from the hospital environment because medicine treats illness and disease. Option (C), which addresses patient handwashing is logical, but it does not answer the question of what a nurse can do to break the chain.

48. **(B)** All atoms of an element have the same atomic number, and the *atomic number is equal to the number of electrons*. Each shell or energy level has a maximum number of electrons. Filling of levels begins with the lowest level. The first level has a maximum number of 2 electrons, the second 8 electrons, the third 18 electrons, the fourth 32 electrons, the fifth 50 electrons, and the sixth 72 electrons. In most instances, it is not necessary to memorize each element's electrons per shell. The atomic number is included on most Periodic Tables. The correct answer, boron, has an atomic weight of 5 and electrons per shell of 2, 3. Lithium has an atomic number of 3 and electrons per shell of 2, 1. Potassium has an atomic number of 19 and electrons per shell of 2, 8, 8, 1, and cobalt has an atomic weight of 27 and electrons per shell of 2, 8, 15, 2.

49. **(D)** Manganese (Mn) has a standard atomic weight of 54.938. Carbon (C) has a standard atomic weight of 12.011, magnesium has a standard atomic weight of 24.305, and calcium has a standard atomic weight of 40.078.

50. **(D)** Seasonal allergies are a common cause of elevated eosinophils. Neutrophils are elevated when you have an acute bacterial infection, monocytes are elevated when you have a chronic

infection, and in certain types of leukemia different leukocytes are elevated. Bacterial and viral infections are not the same thing.

51. **(B)** From one viewpoint, all of the options for this question are correct. However, the question asks for the first, most logical action and that is learning more about mountain climbing. Having increased her knowledge base will either increase or squelch her desire to be a mountain climber.

52. **(D)** When the physical limits of the lungs are reached, stretch receptors communicate with the respiratory center to deactivate respiratory muscles. The remaining options do not have this capability.

53. **(A)** Organic systems have large molecules called macromolecules. There are four classes of organic molecules: carbohydrates, lipids, proteins, and nucleic acids. A key to selecting the correct answer to this question is recognizing that the word *macro* is a prefix that means large or long. The remaining options are not organic molecules, or do not exist.

English and Language Usage

1. **(A)** *Cat house* is a slang term from the 1930s meaning a bordello, also known as a house of prostitution or a brothel. The sentence gives clues to the meaning of the word. The most notable clue is prostitutes. A police raid suggests something illegal, a synonym for patron is client, and prominent individuals in the community were arrested. A home for felines and a luxury yacht can be excluded as possible answers since they do not seem related to the context of the sentence. Both bordello and illegal gambling house fit the sentence context, but one is more logical than the other. Individuals frequenting a bordello or cat house may be referred to as patrons or clients.

2. **(C)** Third person is used when referring to any person, place, or thing other than the speaker and the person who is being addressed. The teachers or "they" denotes third-person plural. Marcy or "she" denotes first-person singular, the politician or "he/she" denotes first-person singular, and "we" denotes first-person plural.

3. **(A)** Compound sentences contain separate pairs of subjects and verbs. A coordinating conjunction preceded by a comma is used to join the two phrases or sentences together to form a compound sentence. Option (A) meets this criterion. A comma connects the two sentences after the word *house* and before the word *yet* (the coordinating conjunction). Other coordinating conjunctions include the words *for, or, not, and,* and *but.* Option (B) uses an incorrect punctuation, option (C) is a simple sentence (no comma), and option (D) has misplaced punctuation—the comma should come after the word *permission*, not after *but*.

4. **(C)** Direct quotes are enclosed in double quotation marks (". . ."), one set at the beginning of the statement and the other set at the end of the statement. Option (A) has improper use of double quotation marks. Single quotations ('. . .') are used inside of double quotations. Option (B) uses single quotations instead of double quotations to enclose the quote. Option (D) includes the speaker as well as the direct quote in double quotations. The speaker (Sarah) is never included in the quotations.

5. **(D)** Sergeant is spelled correctly. Option (A) should be *anonymous*, option (B) *embarrassment*, and option (C) *psychoanalysis.*

6. **(B)** *Agile* means being quick and well-coordinated. *Dexterous* means *skill* or *adroitness.* The words are synonyms. The remaining options are not synonyms. *Apt* means likely or inclined, *felicitous* means well-suited or appropriate, and *inopportune* means inconvenient or inappropriate.

7. **(C)** The root word *-cide* comes from Latin and means killer or an act of killing. The remaining options do not support the context of the sentence.

8. **(B)** Option (B) is a run-on sentence. The problem can be corrected by making two separate sentences: *Jeff and Tommy went to the bait shop hunting for worms. They'd been told the fish on Thompson Creek were biting on worms.* The remaining options are punctuated correctly. If you missed this question, did you miss it because you misread *incorrectly* as *correctly*? If so, you need to slow down and make sure you understand the stem before proceeding.

9. **(A)** The word is correctly spelled *jealous*. The remaining options are spelled correctly.

10. **(A)** The word *affect* is incorrectly used and should be *effect*. The two words are frequently misused. *Affect*, usually a verb, means to influence or produce a change. *Effect* is the result or a consequence of something. The remaining sentences are correct.

11. **(A)** *Angrily* is correct, adding *ly* to *angry*. The remaining options are incorrect and should read *annoyance, buried,* and *they're.*

12. **(B)** Homographs are words that have the same spelling but different meaning. Only option (B) meets this criterion. A *date* is an edible fruit, not a nonedible one. The words *entrance* and *to repel* are antonyms, as are *lead* and *fall behind.*

13. **(C)** *Crucible* is the incorrect word, meaning a container that can withstand high temperatures. The correct word is *credible*, meaning believable, aboveboard, or honest.

14. **(D)** *At* is the incorrect word in the sentence. *At* and *where* are redundant (unnecessary repetition). Sentences rarely end with the word *at*. The remaining sentences are correct.

15. **(D)** A simple sentence is the simplest or most basic sentence form and generally contains one subject and one verb. Subjects and verbs can also be multiple or compound. The simple sentence is a complete thought. The correct option has two subjects (*team* and *family*) and a single verb (*looked*).

16. **(A)** The correct option demonstrates the correct use of *neither* and *nor*. The verbs *bike* and *hiking* do not agree in option (B). The word *I* instead of *me* is the correct word in option (C), and the word *nor* is incorrect and should be *or* in option (D).

17. **(C)** The correct spelling is *kindergarten*. The remaining options are spelled correctly.

18. **(A)** The phrase, *the best skeet shooter in the county,* is a nonrestrictive appositive and should be set off between commas. Appositives are words or groups of words that mean the same thing. They are found together in sentences. They explain or identify the words they modify. The sentence should read, *Hawkeye, the best skeet shooter in the county, finished last in the competition.* The remaining options are punctuated correctly.

19. **(B)** The root word *legi* means law. Legislators are governmental law makers. The remaining options are not definitions of the root word.

20. **(A)** Synonyms are words that have the same or nearly the same meaning. They are equivalent. In the years before the Civil War, *abolitionists*, like Harriet Tubman, advocated the end of slavery. The remaining options are not synonyms of *abolitionist.*

21. **(B)** Synonyms are words that have the same or nearly the same meaning. Something done *thoroughly* is done comprehensively or consummately. The remaining options do not support the context of the sentence and are not synonyms of *thoroughly.*

22. **(D)** Semicolons are used to separate independent clauses and indicate some sort of relationship between the two clauses. The remaining options are incorrectly punctuated. Option (A) is not a sentence but two dependent clauses, option (B) is a run-on sentence, and option (C) is incorrectly punctuated.

23. **(A)** The phrase *as a result* is transitional and clarifies/enhances the sentence. The remaining options do not contain transitional words or phrases.

24. **(C)** A subject is the part or component of a sentence or clause that indicates what the sentence is about or who or what performs an action—in this case, the sponsors canceled the event. The word *canceled* is a verb, and *fishing* and *tornado* are adjectives.

25. **(D)** The correct option defines "active voice." An example is *the child stumbled*. The remaining options do not correctly define active voice.

26. **(A)** The correct option contains "you" indicating second-person plural, and "will be seeing" indicates future action. Options (B) and (C) are past tense. Option (D) is present tense.

27. **(C)** A writing draft is a work in progress that changes and improves over time. There are numerous instances in the passage where the original writing has been changed or questioned. The passage does not suggest brainstorming, a conference technique used to problem solve or develop new ideas. There is no evidence that the writer of the passage is collaborating or working with others. Mind mapping and brainstorming are synonyms.

28. **(B)** The correct option (B) should use the plural form "were" instead of the singular "was." "Of the birds" and "in the forest" are phrases that identify or explain the subject of the sentence (some). If the phrases were removed, the sentence would correctly read, "Some were noisier than others." The remaining options have correct subject-verb agreement.

Practice Test 2

ANSWER SHEET
Practice Test 2

Reading

1. Ⓐ Ⓑ Ⓒ Ⓓ	15. Ⓐ Ⓑ Ⓒ Ⓓ	29. Ⓐ Ⓑ Ⓒ Ⓓ	43. Ⓐ Ⓑ Ⓒ Ⓓ
2. Ⓐ Ⓑ Ⓒ Ⓓ	16. Ⓐ Ⓑ Ⓒ Ⓓ	30. Ⓐ Ⓑ Ⓒ Ⓓ	44. Ⓐ Ⓑ Ⓒ Ⓓ
3. Ⓐ Ⓑ Ⓒ Ⓓ	17. Ⓐ Ⓑ Ⓒ Ⓓ	31. Ⓐ Ⓑ Ⓒ Ⓓ	45. Ⓐ Ⓑ Ⓒ Ⓓ
4. Ⓐ Ⓑ Ⓒ Ⓓ	18. Ⓐ Ⓑ Ⓒ Ⓓ	32. Ⓐ Ⓑ Ⓒ Ⓓ	46. Ⓐ Ⓑ Ⓒ Ⓓ
5. Ⓐ Ⓑ Ⓒ Ⓓ	19. Ⓐ Ⓑ Ⓒ Ⓓ	33. Ⓐ Ⓑ Ⓒ Ⓓ	47. Ⓐ Ⓑ Ⓒ Ⓓ
6. Ⓐ Ⓑ Ⓒ Ⓓ	20. Ⓐ Ⓑ Ⓒ Ⓓ	34. Ⓐ Ⓑ Ⓒ Ⓓ	48. Ⓐ Ⓑ Ⓒ Ⓓ
7. Ⓐ Ⓑ Ⓒ Ⓓ	21. Ⓐ Ⓑ Ⓒ Ⓓ	35. Ⓐ Ⓑ Ⓒ Ⓓ	49. Ⓐ Ⓑ Ⓒ Ⓓ
8. Ⓐ Ⓑ Ⓒ Ⓓ	22. Ⓐ Ⓑ Ⓒ Ⓓ	36. Ⓐ Ⓑ Ⓒ Ⓓ	50. Ⓐ Ⓑ Ⓒ Ⓓ
9. Ⓐ Ⓑ Ⓒ Ⓓ	23. Ⓐ Ⓑ Ⓒ Ⓓ	37. Ⓐ Ⓑ Ⓒ Ⓓ	51. Ⓐ Ⓑ Ⓒ Ⓓ
10. Ⓐ Ⓑ Ⓒ Ⓓ	24. Ⓐ Ⓑ Ⓒ Ⓓ	38. Ⓐ Ⓑ Ⓒ Ⓓ	52. Ⓐ Ⓑ Ⓒ Ⓓ
11. Ⓐ Ⓑ Ⓒ Ⓓ	25. Ⓐ Ⓑ Ⓒ Ⓓ	39. Ⓐ Ⓑ Ⓒ Ⓓ	53. Ⓐ Ⓑ Ⓒ Ⓓ
12. Ⓐ Ⓑ Ⓒ Ⓓ	26. Ⓐ Ⓑ Ⓒ Ⓓ	40. Ⓐ Ⓑ Ⓒ Ⓓ	
13. Ⓐ Ⓑ Ⓒ Ⓓ	27. Ⓐ Ⓑ Ⓒ Ⓓ	41. Ⓐ Ⓑ Ⓒ Ⓓ	
14. Ⓐ Ⓑ Ⓒ Ⓓ	28. Ⓐ Ⓑ Ⓒ Ⓓ	42. Ⓐ Ⓑ Ⓒ Ⓓ	

Mathematics

1. Ⓐ Ⓑ Ⓒ Ⓓ	10. Ⓐ Ⓑ Ⓒ Ⓓ	19. Ⓐ Ⓑ Ⓒ Ⓓ	28. Ⓐ Ⓑ Ⓒ Ⓓ
2. Ⓐ Ⓑ Ⓒ Ⓓ	11. Ⓐ Ⓑ Ⓒ Ⓓ	20. Ⓐ Ⓑ Ⓒ Ⓓ	29. Ⓐ Ⓑ Ⓒ Ⓓ
3. Ⓐ Ⓑ Ⓒ Ⓓ	12. Ⓐ Ⓑ Ⓒ Ⓓ	21. Ⓐ Ⓑ Ⓒ Ⓓ	30. Ⓐ Ⓑ Ⓒ Ⓓ
4. Ⓐ Ⓑ Ⓒ Ⓓ	13. Ⓐ Ⓑ Ⓒ Ⓓ	22. Ⓐ Ⓑ Ⓒ Ⓓ	31. Ⓐ Ⓑ Ⓒ Ⓓ
5. Ⓐ Ⓑ Ⓒ Ⓓ	14. Ⓐ Ⓑ Ⓒ Ⓓ	23. Ⓐ Ⓑ Ⓒ Ⓓ	32. Ⓐ Ⓑ Ⓒ Ⓓ
6. Ⓐ Ⓑ Ⓒ Ⓓ	15. Ⓐ Ⓑ Ⓒ Ⓓ	24. Ⓐ Ⓑ Ⓒ Ⓓ	33. Ⓐ Ⓑ Ⓒ Ⓓ
7. Ⓐ Ⓑ Ⓒ Ⓓ	16. Ⓐ Ⓑ Ⓒ Ⓓ	25. Ⓐ Ⓑ Ⓒ Ⓓ	34. Ⓐ Ⓑ Ⓒ Ⓓ
8. Ⓐ Ⓑ Ⓒ Ⓓ	17. Ⓐ Ⓑ Ⓒ Ⓓ	26. Ⓐ Ⓑ Ⓒ Ⓓ	35. Ⓐ Ⓑ Ⓒ Ⓓ
9. Ⓐ Ⓑ Ⓒ Ⓓ	18. Ⓐ Ⓑ Ⓒ Ⓓ	27. Ⓐ Ⓑ Ⓒ Ⓓ	36. Ⓐ Ⓑ Ⓒ Ⓓ

ANSWER SHEET
Practice Test 2

Science

1. Ⓐ Ⓑ Ⓒ Ⓓ	15. Ⓐ Ⓑ Ⓒ Ⓓ	29. Ⓐ Ⓑ Ⓒ Ⓓ	43. Ⓐ Ⓑ Ⓒ Ⓓ
2. Ⓐ Ⓑ Ⓒ Ⓓ	16. Ⓐ Ⓑ Ⓒ Ⓓ	30. Ⓐ Ⓑ Ⓒ Ⓓ	44. Ⓐ Ⓑ Ⓒ Ⓓ
3. Ⓐ Ⓑ Ⓒ Ⓓ	17. Ⓐ Ⓑ Ⓒ Ⓓ	31. Ⓐ Ⓑ Ⓒ Ⓓ	45. Ⓐ Ⓑ Ⓒ Ⓓ
4. Ⓐ Ⓑ Ⓒ Ⓓ	18. Ⓐ Ⓑ Ⓒ Ⓓ	32. Ⓐ Ⓑ Ⓒ Ⓓ	46. Ⓐ Ⓑ Ⓒ Ⓓ
5. Ⓐ Ⓑ Ⓒ Ⓓ	19. Ⓐ Ⓑ Ⓒ Ⓓ	33. Ⓐ Ⓑ Ⓒ Ⓓ	47. Ⓐ Ⓑ Ⓒ Ⓓ
6. Ⓐ Ⓑ Ⓒ Ⓓ	20. Ⓐ Ⓑ Ⓒ Ⓓ	34. Ⓐ Ⓑ Ⓒ Ⓓ	48. Ⓐ Ⓑ Ⓒ Ⓓ
7. Ⓐ Ⓑ Ⓒ Ⓓ	21. Ⓐ Ⓑ Ⓒ Ⓓ	35. Ⓐ Ⓑ Ⓒ Ⓓ	49. Ⓐ Ⓑ Ⓒ Ⓓ
8. Ⓐ Ⓑ Ⓒ Ⓓ	22. Ⓐ Ⓑ Ⓒ Ⓓ	36. Ⓐ Ⓑ Ⓒ Ⓓ	50. Ⓐ Ⓑ Ⓒ Ⓓ
9. Ⓐ Ⓑ Ⓒ Ⓓ	23. Ⓐ Ⓑ Ⓒ Ⓓ	37. Ⓐ Ⓑ Ⓒ Ⓓ	51. Ⓐ Ⓑ Ⓒ Ⓓ
10. Ⓐ Ⓑ Ⓒ Ⓓ	24. Ⓐ Ⓑ Ⓒ Ⓓ	38. Ⓐ Ⓑ Ⓒ Ⓓ	52. Ⓐ Ⓑ Ⓒ Ⓓ
11. Ⓐ Ⓑ Ⓒ Ⓓ	25. Ⓐ Ⓑ Ⓒ Ⓓ	39. Ⓐ Ⓑ Ⓒ Ⓓ	53. Ⓐ Ⓑ Ⓒ Ⓓ
12. Ⓐ Ⓑ Ⓒ Ⓓ	26. Ⓐ Ⓑ Ⓒ Ⓓ	40. Ⓐ Ⓑ Ⓒ Ⓓ	
13. Ⓐ Ⓑ Ⓒ Ⓓ	27. Ⓐ Ⓑ Ⓒ Ⓓ	41. Ⓐ Ⓑ Ⓒ Ⓓ	
14. Ⓐ Ⓑ Ⓒ Ⓓ	28. Ⓐ Ⓑ Ⓒ Ⓓ	42. Ⓐ Ⓑ Ⓒ Ⓓ	

English and Language Usage

1. Ⓐ Ⓑ Ⓒ Ⓓ	8. Ⓐ Ⓑ Ⓒ Ⓓ	15. Ⓐ Ⓑ Ⓒ Ⓓ	22. Ⓐ Ⓑ Ⓒ Ⓓ
2. Ⓐ Ⓑ Ⓒ Ⓓ	9. Ⓐ Ⓑ Ⓒ Ⓓ	16. Ⓐ Ⓑ Ⓒ Ⓓ	23. Ⓐ Ⓑ Ⓒ Ⓓ
3. Ⓐ Ⓑ Ⓒ Ⓓ	10. Ⓐ Ⓑ Ⓒ Ⓓ	17. Ⓐ Ⓑ Ⓒ Ⓓ	24. Ⓐ Ⓑ Ⓒ Ⓓ
4. Ⓐ Ⓑ Ⓒ Ⓓ	11. Ⓐ Ⓑ Ⓒ Ⓓ	18. Ⓐ Ⓑ Ⓒ Ⓓ	25. Ⓐ Ⓑ Ⓒ Ⓓ
5. Ⓐ Ⓑ Ⓒ Ⓓ	12. Ⓐ Ⓑ Ⓒ Ⓓ	19. Ⓐ Ⓑ Ⓒ Ⓓ	26. Ⓐ Ⓑ Ⓒ Ⓓ
6. Ⓐ Ⓑ Ⓒ Ⓓ	13. Ⓐ Ⓑ Ⓒ Ⓓ	20. Ⓐ Ⓑ Ⓒ Ⓓ	27. Ⓐ Ⓑ Ⓒ Ⓓ
7. Ⓐ Ⓑ Ⓒ Ⓓ	14. Ⓐ Ⓑ Ⓒ Ⓓ	21. Ⓐ Ⓑ Ⓒ Ⓓ	28. Ⓐ Ⓑ Ⓒ Ⓓ

READING

NUMBER OF QUESTIONS: 53

TIME LIMIT: 64 MINUTES

> **Instructions:** Read each question thoroughly. Select the single best answer. Mark your answer (A, B, C, or D) on the answer sheet provided for Practice Test 2.

1. The information guides at the top of a page in a dictionary are *gender discrimination* and *genocide*. Which of the following will be found on this page?

   (A) Gender
   (B) Generic social processes
   (C) Globalization
   (D) Goffman

2. Which of the following best describes historicism? [-*ism* means doctrine]

   (A) An approach in biophysical anatomy that assumes historical references played heavily in the moral and social development of the human species
   (B) An approach to the social sciences that views historical prediction as a fundamental objective. It assumes this objective can be achieved by discerning the patterns, sequences, laws, or bearings that underlie the evolution of history.
   (C) An upcoming biological perspective that supports studying the size and configuration of a population and its relationship to other heterogeneous populations
   (D) A worldview supporting the concept that the psychological perspective of a generation calculates what future generations will do. The doctrine was popular prior to World War II, but fell out of favor with the defeat of the Third Reich.

Questions 3–6 are based on the following passage.

Prohibition (1920–1933) was brought about as a solution to (a) improve the well-being of citizens, (b) lessen crime and exploitation in the public and private sectors, (c) resolve social problems, and (d) decrease the tax encumbrance created by prisons and government-administered facilities sustaining and furnishing housing for the dependent and/or needy. It was influenced by the widespread temperance movement present in the United States at the beginning of the twentieth century. The *ratification* of the Eighteenth Amendment to the U.S. Constitution in 1919 and implementation in 1920 heralded an era that outlawed producing, shipping, and/or selling of alcoholic spirits in the United States. While promising in the beginning, Prohibition fell out of favor by the end of the 1920s. Among the factors leading to a declining support for Prohibition were (a) the illegal manufacturing, distributing, and selling of alcohol leading to an increase in consumption, (b) the explosion of illegal drinking locations, (c) the escalation of gang violence and other crimes, (d) the spiraling costs for enforcement, jails, and penitentiaries to maintain Prohibition, and (e) the loss of millions of dollars in liquor taxes paid to the government. The ratification of the Twenty-first Amendment in 1933 ended Prohibition. The *noble experiment,* as it has been called, was a profound failure that did more damage than good.

3. Based upon the passage, which of the following best describes *ratification*?

(A) Conceding or concession
(B) Denial or negation
(C) Enactment or authorization
(D) Reject or repudiate

4. Of the following identified problems, which would be most supportive of the temperance movement?

(A) Improving the well-being of citizens
(B) Lessening crime and exploitation
(C) Resolving social problems
(D) Slashing the tax burden

5. Which of the following had the greatest negative effect on the general public during Prohibition?

(A) Escalation of gang violence and other crimes
(B) Explosion of illegal drinking locations
(C) Illegal manufacturing, distributing, and selling of alcohol
(D) Loss of millions of dollars in liquor taxes paid to the government

6. Select the statement that best summarizes the passage.

(A) Citizens did not understand the need for Prohibition, causing it to fail.
(B) Experiments often miscarry.
(C) Governments make mistakes.
(D) In theory, Prohibition was feasible; in practice, it was a fiasco.

Questions 7–10 are based on the following passage.

Taken from *The Submariner and Life on the Boats in World War II.*

On board an informal, but professional, attitude prevailed. Although we had an evaporator to make fresh water, battery watering was primary. In the design and scheme of things, personal hygiene or washing of clothes did not seem to be considered. One Engineering Petty Officer, called the Water King, ran the evaporator. Personal hygiene or washing of clothing was an afterthought. The use of after-shave lotions, deodorants (called Foo-Foo juice), and especially talcum powders prevailed. Large cans of Lilac were the norm, purchased inexpensively in local 5&10 stores and sprinkled liberally.

7. Is the passage based on fact or opinion?

(A) Fact. Information can be verified.
(B) Fact. No stereotypical presentation is in the passage.
(C) Opinion. Information cannot be verified.
(D) Opinion. Information is biased.

8. What is the author's likely purpose of writing the passage?

(A) To entertain the reader
(B) To illustrate one aspect of life on a submarine during the World War II
(C) To persuade the reader of the hardships of Navy life
(D) To provide information on the value of the submarine during World War II

9. What type of magazine publication is most appropriate for this type of writing?

   (A) Autobiographical
   (B) Biographical
   (C) Historical
   (D) Science fiction

10. What logical conclusion can be drawn from the passage?

    (A) Hygiene was not a priority for everyone.
    (B) Life aboard a submarine during World War II required sacrifice.
    (C) Living conditions in the armed forces have improved since World War II.
    (D) Members of the U.S. Navy endured sacrifice during World War II.

Questions 11–13 are based on the following table.

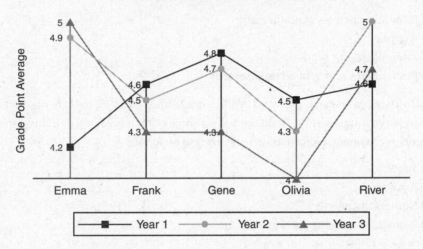

11. Which of the following students had the highest grade point average for the three academic years?

    (A) Emma
    (B) Gene
    (C) Olivia
    (D) River

12. Of the following students, which had the lowest potential for receiving the GPA Science/Math award?

    (A) Emma
    (B) Frank
    (C) Gene
    (D) Olivia

13. Which of the five students had the greatest variance in GPAs over the three-year period?

    (A) Emma
    (B) Frank
    (C) Gene
    (D) Olivia

Questions 14–15 are based on the following from the Dewey decimal classification.

510 Mathematics

- 511 General principles of mathematics
- 512 Algebra
- 513 Arithmetic
- 514 Topology
- 515 Analysis
- 516 Geometry
- 517 *Not assigned or no longer used*
- 518 Numerical analysis
- 519 Probabilities and applied mathematics

14. Mick, an engineering major, is having problems understanding statistics. A classmate told him the school library has excellent books on statistics that might help him. He finds the above when looking at the Mathematics section of the Dewey decimal classification. What subdivision of the section would offer him the most logical assistance?

    (A) 511 General principles of mathematics
    (B) 512 Algebra
    (C) 515 Analysis
    (D) 519 Probabilities and applied mathematics

15. A student's assigned research project is to address attributes of space that are preserved under continuous distortions (stretching, twisting, bending, and warping, but not breaking or pulling apart). In which subcategory is the needed information most likely to be found?

    (A) 514 Topology
    (B) 515 Analysis
    (C) 518 Numerical analysis
    (D) 519 Probabilities and applied mathematics

Questions 16–21 are based on the following passage.

Memorandum #165

To: Employees
From: Legal Services
Date: March 10
Re: E Lot parking

As seems to happen every year, there is unauthorized parking in the E Lot. The problem, however, has skyrocketed this year, and the Board of Directors has requested a new policy to alleviate the problem. This memorandum includes a summary of the new policy (online Employee Handbook, Parking #34.3.a).

At present, 650 employees park in the E Lot. Of these 650 spaces, 400 are reserved for employees who have paid an annual fee of $56 for 24-hour/7-day access for an assigned parking space. The remaining 250 employees parking in the E Lot park in unassigned spaces. The E Lot is gated, and

---

only employees with E Lot identification on their automobiles are admitted to the lot. In the past 15 workdays, security has issued 283 written warnings to employees parking in spaces assigned to other employees. There has also been an average of 17 employee complaints per day during the same time frame.

Effective Monday, April 12, any employee improperly parked in the E Lot will immediately forfeit their ability to park in the E Lot, and their automobile will be impounded until a $400 release fee is paid. The release fee will be deducted from the next paycheck. *Forfeiture* of E Lot parking will require said employee(s) to park in the F Lot which is approximately 2 miles away from the office and take the free company shuttle bus to and from the office—time schedules are available on the company website.

Please contact Legal at extension 4588 for clarification or additional information.

16. The purpose of the memorandum is to

 (A) chastise.
 (B) entertain.
 (C) inform.
 (D) persuade.

17. The memorandum implies a specific group of individuals is responsible for the unauthorized parking. Who are these individuals?

 (A) Employees parking for free in the E Lot
 (B) Visitors
 (C) Employees assigned to other parking lots
 (D) Part-time/temporary employees

18. The word *forfeiture* is used in the memorandum. What is the most logical antonym for this word?

 (A) Deprivation
 (B) Expense
 (C) Loss
 (D) Retribution

19. Which of the following best abridges the memorandum?

 (A) All employees suffer because of the actions of a few.
 (B) The Board of Directors is unsympathetic to employee needs.
 (C) Parking has always been a problem and the new policy was needed.
 (D) Unauthorized parking will have negative consequences.

20. What evidence suggests the need for change?

 (A) A sharp increase in the amount of unauthorized parking
 (B) The Board of Directors' request for policy regarding unauthorized parking
 (C) Long-standing unauthorized parking
 (D) No evidence is given.

21. What is the logical conclusion from reading the memorandum?

(A) Company employees will unite and demand a revocation of the new policy.

(B) Employees who do not see unauthorized parking as an issue will continue to park dishonestly.

(C) Unauthorized companywide parking will decrease sharply.

(D) Unauthorized parking in the E Lot will decrease sharply.

Questions 22–23 are based on the following.

The Annual Mountain Bike-a-Thon is a statewide event for Children's Charity that benefits the four children's hospitals in the state. The event not only draws heavily from the state but from the surrounding six states in the catchment area of the four hospitals. Overhead cost is approximately 7.34% with the remainder of money split equally among the hospitals. Advertising has increased each year and the long-time advertising company has withdrawn its support of the event stating it can no longer afford to give a discount. As a result, event organizers developed and printed the advertising flyer (below) and mailed 2,800 copies to various places and organizations in the five states.

18th Annual Mountain Bike-a-Thon for Children's Charity
Thompson Recreational Area
June 2–3

- Alcohol-free event
- General admission
  - Adults - $25
  - Adults >50 - $15
  - Children - $10
  - Children <10 - Free (accompanied by adult)
- Entries
  - $50 child >10/entry
  - $75 adult/entry
  - $300 adult team/entry (5 members or less)
  - 5, 10, 15, & 30-mile child/adult routes

- Level-appropriate trails
- Aid stations (EMT staffed)
- Handicap accessible
- Prizes
- Food & game booths
- Free entertainment
- Close parking
- Child care available
- Donations accepted

22. What is implied in the passage and advertising flyer?

(A) The event is successful in raising money for the children's hospitals.

(B) The event must make extravagant sums of money since its overhead is so high.

(C) High costs of admission and entry fees are targeted at the upper middle class.

(D) A decrease in admission and entry fees would increase the number of attendees at the event.

23. What major criterion is omitted from the flyer?

(A) Aid station capabilities

(B) Contact information

(C) How close is close parking

(D) Event registration

24. Select the correct *hierarchy* of the biological classification system.

    (A) Domain ⇒ Class ⇒ Phylum ⇒ Kingdom ⇒ Order ⇒ Genus ⇒ Family ⇒ Species ⇒ Subspecies
    (B) Domain ⇒ Kingdom ⇒ Family ⇒ Class ⇒ Phylum ⇒ Order ⇒ Genus ⇒ Species ⇒ Subspecies
    (C) Domain ⇒ Kingdom ⇒ Phylum ⇒ Class ⇒ Order ⇒ Family ⇒ Genus ⇒ Species ⇒ Subspecies
    (D) Domain ⇒ Phylum ⇒ Kingdom ⇒ Class ⇒ Order ⇒ Family ⇒ Genus ⇒ Species ⇒ Subspecies

25. Which of the following is a primary source?

    (A) An earthquake expert's commentaries on the San Francisco earthquake of 1906
    (B) A historical writer's memorable quotes of Benjamin Franklin
    (C) A researcher's results of clinical trials
    (D) A Vietnam veteran's analysis of Vietnam War battles

26. A treatise entitled *Terrorism in America, 1980–2015* is an example of a _____ commentary.

    (A) devotional
    (B) humanistic
    (C) indirective
    (D) social

27. *The Shining,* a 1980 film about supernatural forces that influence a man's sanity, belongs to which of the following genres?

    (A) Eco-thriller
    (B) Mystery thriller
    (C) Psychological thriller
    (D) Techno thriller

Questions 28–35 are based on the following two memos and chart.

Confidential Memo #1

To: Marsha Franks, Lead Junior/Senior Counselor
From: Thad Wilson, Principal
Date: April 7
Subject: William Denny, junior student

It has recently come to my attention that we have a student in *jeopardy*. William Denny transferred from an out-of-state high school at the beginning of this semester. According to his transfer records, William was an *exemplary* student who was involved in extracurricular activities and served as a mentor/tutor to other students. However, since coming to AHS, William has been anything but what his records suggest. I would appreciate your looking into this matter.

Confidential Memo #2

To: Thad Wilson, Principal

From: Marsha Franks, Lead Junior/Senior Counselor

Date: April 25

Subject: Follow-up William Denny, junior student

We do, indeed, have a student in *jeopardy*. No one at his previous school was aware of William having problems—many suggested he saw his move to Anthony Junction and transfer to AHS as an adventure he was looking forward to. I did a home visit and talked with Louise Martini (William's mother) on a day William was in school and discovered the following:

- Louise married Joseph Martini four years ago, and they have a two-year-old daughter and five-month-old son. Her first husband, Robert Denny, was killed by a drunk driver in 2013. They had six children. William is the oldest. Step-son/father relationship was so-so.
- Joseph Martini died suddenly before Christmas (five months ago).
- The Martini family moved to Anthony Junction at the end of the fall semester.
- William works 10- to 12-hour nights Monday through Friday and 12-hour shifts on Saturday and Sunday to support the family.

I have scheduled a conference with William and his mother next week. I believe there are a number of options to be investigated that can be instrumental in getting William back on track. I shall keep you posted. Below is a chart demonstrating William's present trend.

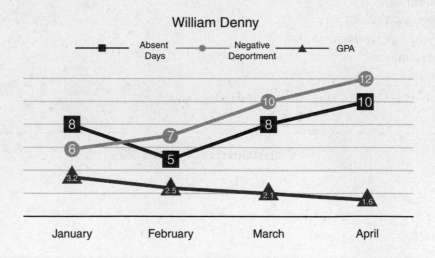

28. What is an antonym for the word *jeopardy* in the first memo?

(A) Precarious

(B) Protection

(C) Trouble

(D) Vulnerable

29. What is a synonym for the word *exemplary* in the first memo?

    (A) Culpable
    (B) Inferior
    (C) Praiseworthy
    (D) Reproachable

30. Which of the following words best describes *deportment* as shown on the chart?

    (A) Avoidance of school-related issues
    (B) Behavior or conduct at school
    (C) Need to leave school
    (D) Include in group work

31. Based on information in the memos and chart, what appears to be the root of William's problems at school?

    (A) Anger, grief, and lack of respect for authority
    (B) Excessive work load and lack of study and personal time
    (C) Expression of pent-up emotions about moving to new state
    (D) Homesick for friends, school involvement, and lack of social support

32. What is the implied end result for William if his downward trend is not halted?

    (A) Everyone will ultimately support him and he will improve.
    (B) His school deportment will end in suspension and time in jail.
    (C) He will not graduate from high school.
    (D) Once out of school, he will find a better job and not have to work so many hours.

33. In which month has William had the lowest number of absent days?

    (A) April
    (B) February
    (C) March
    (D) January

34. In which month has William had the highest number of deportment issues?

    (A) April
    (B) February
    (C) March
    (D) January

35. What is the rationale for the second memo?

    (A) To demonstrate that the job is being completed
    (B) To meet policy requirements
    (C) To provide information
    (D) To validate competency

36. Follow the instructions to change *teacher* into a new word.

   1. Replace *t* with *b*.
   2. Remove *cher*.
   3. Add *ley* after *a*.
   4. Drop *ea*.
   5. Add *ar* before *l*.

   The new word is

   (A) barely.
   (B) barley.
   (C) result is not a legitimate word.
   (D) rarely.

Questions 37–39 are based on the following passage.

Emily's actual age was unknown, but she was old, really old. People in the nursing home said she'd been there as long as anyone could remember. She'd outlived her family by many years. Sometimes her short-term memory failed and she was *short* with her caregivers, but her long-term memory was amazing. She remembered leaving Pennsylvania with her parents, older brother, and four younger sisters in a covered wagon pulled by oxen. Two of her sisters died from the summer *flux* somewhere in what is now Nebraska. After months of traveling west, her family finally settled and started farming in a *lush* valley surrounded by mountains in the Wyoming Territory. When she was 15, a family from Kentucky camped on a creek a few miles from their farm to rest their stock and rebuild their wagon. After a few months, the family left to continue their journey to the Pacific Northwest and Emily left with them—she and the family's middle son, Andrew, had "taken a liking" to each other. They were never officially married but had sworn their commitment to each other in front of their parents. Emily thinks she and Andrew were together for 70 or so years. She doesn't remember seeing her parents or siblings again, but she remembers three of her ten children reaching adulthood.

37. Two of Emily's younger sisters died from what was referred to as the summer *flux*. What possible condition could this be in today's terms?

   (A) Encephalitis
   (B) Heat madness
   (C) Respiratory infection
   (D) Watery diarrhea

38. What does the word *lush* suggest in terms of the valley where Emily and her family settled?

   (A) Numerous heavy drinkers of alcohol lived in the valley.
   (B) The economy of the valley was depressed.
   (C) The valley was bleak and impoverished.
   (D) The valley was green, luxuriant, and fertile.

39. What is a synonym for *short* in terms of Emily's relationship with her caregivers?

   (A) Brusque
   (B) Circuitous
   (C) Long-winded
   (D) Voluble

Question 40–41 are based on the following table.

Hoffman Terrace Multiplex				
Open 10:30 AM		Movies beginning at 11:00 AM		
Movie Name	Puff's Birthday Party	Summer Thunder	Monster from the Ice	Immortal Kingdom
Times	11:00	12:00	11:15	11:00
	1:15	2:30	1:15	14:30
	3:45	5:00	3:15	6:00
		7:30	5:15	21:30
		11:00	7:15	
			9:15	
<13 Ticket	$5.50	$5.50	$5.50	$6.00
Adult Ticket	$8.00	$8.00	$8.00	$8.50
55+ Ticket	$2.00	$2.00	$2.00	$2.00
With Season Pass	$4.50*	$4.50*	$4.50*	$5.00*

*Price per person regardless of age

40. What is the cost for a 12-year-old to see "Immortal Kingdom" at 6:00 P.M.?

(A) $2.00
(B) $5.00
(C) $6.00
(D) $8.50

41. Philip purchased a season pass for his family because they see a new movie every week. His mother, aged 62, usually accompanies them, and Philip always pays for her admission. Is it more economical for him to pay for a 55+ ticket for his mother, or to include her in the season ticket price?

(A) Buy a separate 55+ ticket for his mother
(B) Include her as a part of the season ticket price
(C) Let his mother decide which she would prefer
(D) Split the difference with his mother

Questions 42–46 are based on the following passage.

Families are social systems that function within larger societal systems. Within the family system are numerous smaller systems called subsystems. Families have the following characteristics: They (1) live together, (2) interact and communicate on a regular basis, (3) have common interests and concerns, (4) have strong emotional bonds, and (5) have recognized roles and responsibilities.

Families undergo predictable change over time. Each change requires *adaptation* for family members. A task for newlyweds is learning to negotiate and developing a new family system. As children enter school, parents and their children must adapt to interacting with the educational system outside of the home—there are new rules to apply and potential negative consequences when these rules are broken. The family with teenage children must address dependence and independence issues. Families in the late stages of aging must adapt not only to physiological loss but also the loss of family members, friends, and relationships.

Families can be broadly categorized as functional or dysfunctional. These labels are not static. Developmental and/or situational crises affect the functional health of a family. Over the lifetime of a family, as it is influenced by inside and outside forces, it will move from one category to another. *Adaptation* is necessary for resolution of any crisis.

42. The passage can best be described as

(A) expository.
(B) narrative.
(C) persuasive.
(D) technical.

43. Which of the following is the best logical conclusion of the passage?

(A) Families are either functional or dysfunctional.
(B) Families are static systems.
(C) Families, as subsystems within a larger society, are social systems that change over time.
(D) Family roles and responsibilities are identical for all families.

44. What is the biggest change facing a family when the breadwinner is involved in an accident that results in a permanent disability?

(A) Letting go of the past and building a new future
(B) Living on a reduced income
(C) Modifying roles and responsibilities
(D) Redefining family needs

45. The passage states that physiological loss occurs with aging. Select the best example of this type of loss in older adults.

(A) Depression
(B) Loss of muscle mass
(C) Loss of teeth
(D) Premature aging

46. What is meant by the term *adaptation*?

(A) Confuse
(B) Disarrange
(C) Remodel
(D) Renegotiate

Questions 47–50 are based on the following graphic of the United States.

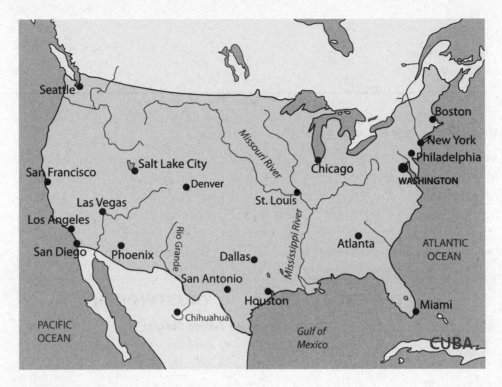

47. What is the northernmost river labeled on the map?

    (A) Columbia River
    (B) Missouri River
    (C) Ohio River
    (D) Rio Grande River

48. Select the city located on the Mississippi River.

    (A) Chihuahua
    (B) San Diego
    (C) St. Louis
    (D) Seattle

49. Which westernmost city is located on a well-known bay?

    (A) Boston
    (B) New York
    (C) San Francisco
    (D) Vancouver

50. Select the city east of the Rio Grande River.

   (A) Dallas
   (B) Denver
   (C) Salt Lake City
   (D) Winnipeg

---

51. Which is an example of a tertiary source?

   (A) Architecture
   (B) Audio recordings
   (C) Biographies
   (D) Chronologies

Question 52 is based on the following flyer.

DEPENDABLE   **TRUSTWORTHY**

Cindy's Graduate Typing Service

(Not a writing service)

555-555-5555

- Thesis & Dissertation Projects (Graduate School Style Guide)
- Professional resumes with cover sheet
- Home-based within walking distance from campus
- 99% accuracy
- Available 6.5 days/week and most holidays
- References available from faculty and students
- Make <u>free</u> appointment to discuss your project and determine your individual needs

---

52. The focus of the typing service

   (A) is broad.
   (B) cannot be determined; not enough information given.
   (C) could be narrow or broad depending on university enrollment.
   (D) is narrow.

---

53. Marie is doing a compare and contrast project for the school chemistry fair. She is planning an oral presentation supported by a slide presentation. Her project has a 30-minute minimum and a 40-minute maximum. Which of the following is most logical for Marie's project?

   (A) Atoms and genes
   (B) Alkali and alkaline earth metals
   (C) Biology and chemistry majors
   (D) Horses and humans

MATHEMATICS

NUMBER OF QUESTIONS: 36

TIME LIMIT: 54 MINUTES

Instructions: Read each question thoroughly. Select the single best answer. Mark your answer (A, B, C, or D) on the answer sheet provided for Practice Test 2.

1. Dawn is baking cookies and cakes for the student nursing association fundraiser. She plans on making six batches of sugar cookies that require two eggs per batch; five batches of coconut-chocolate cookies that require two eggs per batch; four ice cream cakes requiring three eggs per cake; and two pineapple cakes requiring five eggs per cake including eggs needed for icing. How many dozens of eggs does she need to purchase?

    (A) 3 dozen
    (B) 3.5 dozen
    (C) 4 dozen
    (D) 4.5 dozen

Questions 2–3 are based on the following information.

A shop owner packages his own trail mix. He sells 8-ounce and 1-pound bags of mix. Each bag contains 12% peanuts, 20% almonds, 3 ounces of pecans, 30% cashews, 10% sunflower seeds, and the remainder are walnuts.

2. About what percentage of a 1-pound bag is pecans?

    (A) 6%
    (B) 10%
    (C) 15%
    (D) 19%

3. How many ounces of cashews are in the 8-ounce bag of mix?

    (A) 2.0 oz
    (B) 2.4 oz
    (C) 2.8 oz
    (D) 3.2 oz

---

4. What number is its own opposite?

    (A) −2
    (B) −1
    (C) 0
    (D) 1

5. Write the following in an expression format.

    5 subtract a negative 2

    (A) 5 + (−2)
    (B) 5 − (−2)
    (C) 5 − 2
    (D) (5)(−2)

6. Mathematical statements can be written in various ways. Select the option that demonstrates the following:

43 divided by 62

(A) $\frac{62}{43}$ $43\overline{)62}$ $62 \div 43$

(B) $\frac{43}{62}$ $62\overline{)43}$ $43 \div 62$

(C) .6935 $43 + 62$ 1.144

(D) (62)(43) $62 + 43$ $62 - 43$

7. A long-distance runner is 15 miles west of the finish line. He runs an additional 10 miles. How far is he from the finish line and in what direction is he running?

(A) $\frac{10}{15}$, northwest

(B) $\frac{15}{10}$, southeast

(C) 5 miles, east

(D) 5 miles, west

8. What number plus 4 equals −20?

(A) −5

(B) −6

(C) −16

(D) −24

9. Reduce the following to place value.

5,693.419

(A) $(5 \times 1,000) + (6 \times 100) + (9 \times 10) + (3 \times 1) + (4 \times 1) + \left(1 \times \frac{1}{10}\right) + \left(9 \times \frac{1}{100}\right)$

(B) $(5 \times 1,000) + (6 \times 100) + (9 \times 10) + (3 \times 1) + \left(4 \times \frac{1}{10}\right) + \left(1 \times \frac{1}{100}\right) + \left(9 \times \frac{1}{1,000}\right)$

(C) $(5 \times 10,000) + (6 \times 1,000) + (9 \times 10) + (3 \times 1) + \left(4 \times \frac{1}{10}\right) + \left(1 \times \frac{1}{100}\right) + \left(9 \times \frac{1}{1,000}\right)$

(D) $(5 \times 1,000) + (6 \times 100) + (9 \times 10) + (3 \times 1) + \left(4 \times \frac{1}{1}\right) + \left(1 \times \frac{1}{10}\right) + \left(9 \times \frac{1}{100}\right)$

10. Arrange the following numbers in order from the least to the greatest.

0.76   0.308   0.2435446   0.319   0.4883

(A) 0.2435446, 0.308, 0.319, 0.4883, 0.76

(B) 0.2435446, 0.76, 0.319, 0.308, 0.4883

(C) 0.308, 0.319, 0.76, 0.2435446, 0.4883

(D) 0.4883, 0.2435446, 0.308, 0.319, 0.76

11. What is the approximate percent decrease from $6,500 to $5,000?

(A) 3%

(B) 8%

(C) 15%

(D) 23%

12. Simplify the following.

$$5^5 \div 5^2$$

(A) 5^3
(B) 5^7
(C) 1^7
(D) 1^{10}

13. Compute the following.

$$(2^4)^3$$

(A) 192
(B) 4,096
(C) 13,824
(D) 331,776

14. A health care provider's order reads: Give PediMed 20 mg/kg/day orally. The PediMed dosage label reads 5 ml = 50 mg. How many total milliliters of medication will be administered in a 24-hour period to an infant who weighs 15 pounds? Do NOT round your answer.

(A) 4.5 ml
(B) 6.7 ml
(C) 13.6 ml
(D) 14.0 ml

15. A teacher has 42 students in a work-study program. How many students attend the school if these 42 students are equal to 5.85% of the student population?

(A) 717.94
(B) 718
(C) 720
(D) 720.34

16. The numerator in a fraction is 15 and the value of the fraction is 65. What is the denominator?

(A) 0.23
(B) 4.32
(C) 5.0
(D) 9.78

17. A sack of marbles contains 150 marbles. Thirteen marbles are blue. What percentage of the marbles is blue?

(A) 4.6%
(B) 8.7%
(C) 10.2%
(D) 12.3%

18. Marshall has been saving his money to purchase a new suit for his parents' anniversary party. He has saved $143.49. Each of his four older siblings gave him $15.00 for his birthday, his uncle gave him $25.00, and he can earn an additional $40.00 by mowing lawns this weekend. The cost of the suit, including alterations, is $247.95 plus tax of 14.875%. Does Marshall have enough money to purchase the suit?

   (A) No, he still needs almost $17.00 to make the purchase.
   (B) No, he is short by several dollars and decides to wait until the suit is on sale.
   (C) Yes, he has almost $21.00 more than he needs.
   (D) Yes, he can ask his uncle for the needed amount.

19. What is the numerator in a fraction where 250 is the denominator and simplification of the fraction equals 50?

   (A) 50
   (B) 750
   (C) 10,050
   (D) 12,500

20. Convert 0.024 to a fraction.

   (A) $\dfrac{12}{50}$

   (B) $\dfrac{24}{1,000}$

   (C) $\dfrac{125}{3}$

   (D) $\dfrac{250}{6}$

21. A contractor is preparing to seed a lawn. One sack of grass seed covers 2,000 square feet. How many sacks are needed for an area 200 feet by 250 feet?

   (A) 15 bags
   (B) 20 bags
   (C) 25 bags
   (D) 30 bags

22. 4,578 is divisible by

   (A) 2, 3, 6, 7
   (B) 3, 5, 7
   (C) 3, 8, 9
   (D) 3, 6, 8, 9

23. For a company to remain competitive in a robust economy, it decides to increase its number of manufacturing plants from 115 to 120. What is the percent increase? Round your answer to the nearest hundredth.

   (A) 1.96%
   (B) 2.04%
   (C) 3.38%
   (D) 4.35%

24. Arrange the following from greatest to the least.

$$0.3 \quad -\frac{3}{4} \quad 0.427 \quad \frac{5}{8} \quad 0.734 \quad 0.0$$

(A) $0.734, \frac{5}{8}, 0.427, 0.3, 0.0, -\frac{3}{4}$

(B) $0.0, 0.3, 0.427, \frac{5}{8}, 0.734, -\frac{3}{4}$

(C) $-\frac{3}{4}, 0.734, \frac{5}{8}, 0.427, 0.3, 0.0$

(D) $0.3, 0.0, -\frac{3}{4}, 0.734, \frac{5}{8}, 0.427$

Questions 25–29 are based on the following passage and table.

It is tradition at Weissach College to have its annual Welcome Back picnic and "Student Assistance Bank" fundraiser together at the beginning of each fall semester. Ninety percent of the money raised funds the Student Assistance Bank. Weissach students attending the picnic and fundraiser receive a 100% discount, while faculty, staff, and the public pay full price for the dinners. The cost of admission is included in the dinner price. There is minimal cost (10%) to the college since everything needed for the picnic is donated by community businesses and organizations.

	Number Attending	Beef Dinners*	Chicken Dinners**	Vegetarian Dinners***
Students	348	170	136	42
Faculty/Staff	150	82	42	26
Public	496	292	133	71
Totals	994	544	311	139

*Beef Dinner—$15.00

**Chicken Dinner —$12.50

***Vegetarian Dinner—$10.00

25. How many total individuals will be attending the annual Welcome Back picnic?

(A) 150
(B) 348
(C) 646
(D) 994

26. What is the total amount, in dollars, of beef dinners sold?

(A) $1,890.00
(B) $3,780.00
(C) $5,610.00
(D) $8,160.00

27. What percentage of attendees ordered chicken dinners? Round your answer to the nearest whole number.

   (A) 17%
   (B) 19%
   (C) 26%
   (D) 31%

28. What percentage of attendees did not pay for their dinners?

   (A) 34%
   (B) 35%
   (C) 37%
   (D) 39%

29. What is the total amount of dollars that will go to the Student Assistance Bank?

   (A) $7,890.75
   (B) $9,550.00
   (C) $11,047.50
   (D) $12,093.44

30. Change $\frac{5}{2}$ to a mixed number.

   (A) $2\frac{1}{2}$

   (B) $2\frac{3}{2}$

   (C) $3\frac{1}{2}$

   (D) $4\frac{1}{2}$

31. Change $15\frac{5}{7}$ to an improper fraction.

   (A) $\frac{22}{7}$

   (B) $\frac{27}{7}$

   (C) $\frac{105}{7}$

   (D) $\frac{110}{7}$

32. The star player on the football team scored $\frac{2}{3}$ of the 76 total points in the homecoming game. How many points did the remainder of the team score? Round your answer to the nearest whole number.

   (A) 21
   (B) 25
   (C) 64
   (D) 76

33. Solve for x in the following equation. Round your answer to the nearest hundredth.

$$15x + (14 - 3) - 2[(2)(7)] = 80$$

(A) 0.87
(B) 2.38
(C) 6.47
(D) 8.38

34. Fifteen multiplied by the sum of y plus 8 is equal to 145. Solve for y. Round your answer to the nearest hundredth.

(A) 1.67
(B) 2.60
(C) 3.75
(D) 7.50

35. What is the remaining number if the sum of two numbers is 108 and one of the numbers is 84?

(A) 24
(B) 65
(C) 109
(D) 133

Question 36 is based on the following passage and chart.

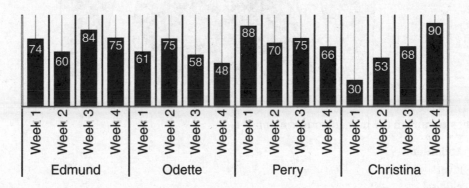

Student Body President
(votes/week)

A civics class is monitoring the race for student body president at a high school. Four qualified students are running. The class has been conducting weekly polls in an effort to predict the winner of the race. Students participating in the poll were asked one question, "Who would you vote for if the election were held today?" The chart shows the number of votes each student received each week of the poll.

36. Which student had the highest average of votes for the four-week period?

(A) Christina
(B) Edmund
(C) Odette
(D) Perry

SCIENCE

NUMBER OF QUESTIONS: 53

TIME LIMIT: 63 MINUTES

Instructions: Read each question thoroughly. Select the single best answer. Mark your answer (A, B, C, or D) on the answer sheet provided for Practice Test 2.

Questions 1–4 are based on the following diagram.

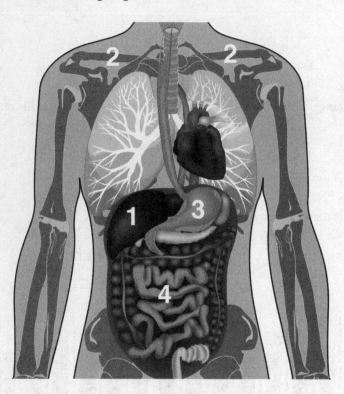

1. What structure in the human body is number **1**?

   (A) Abdomen
   (B) Liver
   (C) Pancreas
   (D) Spleen

2. The number **2** identifies two bones in the upper part of the torso. Select the name of these bones.

   (A) Auricular surface
   (B) Clavicles
   (C) Lateral malleolus
   (D) Scapula

3. What structure of the human body is number **3**?

   (A) Duodenum
   (B) Pancreas
   (C) Stomach
   (D) Transverse colon

4. What structure of the human body is number **4**?

   (A) Ascending colon
   (B) Large intestine
   (C) Pancreas
   (D) Small intestine

___

5. What are the reactants in the following equation?

   $$NH_4NO_3 \rightarrow N_2O + H_2O$$

   (A) NH, NO, and HO
   (B) NH_4NO_3
   (C) $N_2O + H_2O$
   (D) $NH_4NO_3 \rightarrow N_2O + H_2O$

6. Select the best, most logical definition of physiology.

   (A) A subsystem of biology having to do with normal functioning groups of isolated organs within living creatures. Within living bodies are additional subsystems with unique nonspecialized functions beginning with atoms and molecules $\Rightarrow$ cells $\Rightarrow$ tissues $\Rightarrow$ organ systems $\Rightarrow$ organism. Physiology is a normal process that goes on inside of the body to keep living creatures alive.
   (B) Often referred to as the biology of life, physiology consists of groups of independent organ systems within living creatures. Within the living body are additional subsystems with unique and specialized functions beginning with atoms and molecules $\Rightarrow$ tissues $\Rightarrow$ cells $\Rightarrow$ organs $\Rightarrow$ organ systems $\Rightarrow$ organism. Depending upon circumstances, physiology is the study of normal or abnormal processes with the body.
   (C) Once considered a subsystem of biology, physiology is now seen as a stand-alone science such as chemistry, physics, and geology. Physiology studies abnormal functioning groups of organs within both living and extinct creatures. Physiology is a normal process that not only goes on inside of the body, but also provides valuable information about the evolution of a species.
   (D) Physiology, a subsystem of biology, is the study of normal functioning groups of organs and their various parts within living creatures. Within living bodies are additional subsystems with unique and specialized functions beginning with atoms and molecules $\Rightarrow$ cells $\Rightarrow$ tissues $\Rightarrow$ organs $\Rightarrow$ organ systems $\Rightarrow$ organism. Physiology is a normal process that goes on inside of the body to keep living creatures alive.

7. Dry ice is an example of solid

   (A) anhydride.
   (B) amalgam.
   (C) carbon dioxide.
   (D) water.

8. Which of the following is NOT an example of a chemical reaction occurring?

   (A) A new element is formed.
   (B) A new material is generated.
   (C) Gas is produced.
   (D) Heat is taken in or given off.

9. Milk turning sour is an example of a chemical

   (A) change.
   (B) expansion.
   (C) reactant.
   (D) substitution.

10. The thoracic cage consists of all of the following EXCEPT the

   (A) costal cartilage.
   (B) ribs.
   (C) sternum.
   (D) vertebral column.

11. The running clubs in the area petitioned the city to provide safe running areas for runners of all ages, skill levels, and distances. They have specifically asked for a running trail/route from the city park to the lake recreational area (around 14 or 15 miles). What is the most appropriate unit to determine the distance from the park to the recreational area?

   (A) Centimeter
   (B) Decimeter
   (C) Kilometer
   (D) Meter

Questions 12–13 are based on the following passage.

A researcher, employed by the local sugar manufacturer, is interested in the long-term effects of a new sugar substitute produced by a competitor. He wants to recruit 500 individuals from attendees at the Foxworth County Fourth of July Beach Shindig since over 10,000 men, women, and children usually attend the three-day activity each year. He plans to walk the beach and hand out participant forms to individuals and families. The form specifically asks for parents to complete the forms for their children under 15 years of age. Participants in the study will be the first 500 individuals returning forms.

12. Is there a bias inherent in the design of this study?

   (A) No bias exists.
   (B) No bias exists providing the researcher carefully screens the returned forms for duplicates and gross inaccuracies.
   (C) A bias exists because the researcher is employed by a manufacturer of sugar products, and he will be studying the effects of a competitor's product.
   (D) A bias exists because children cannot participate in a research study without their parents' permission.

13. Select a design flaw in this study.

    (A) Adults and children should never participate in the same study.
    (B) No logical reason exists for a sugar producer to study a sugar substitute product.
    (C) The population from which participants will be selected
    (D) The researcher's qualifications to conduct the study

---

14. Mass is the amount of matter in an object. Four liters of water has a mass of

    (A) 1.0 kg.
    (B) 2.2 kg.
    (C) 3.7 kg.
    (D) 4.0 kg.

15. Based on information presented in the Periodic Table of Elements (page 53), the electrons per shell for calcium (Ca) are

    (A) 2, 8, 7.
    (B) 2, 8, 8, 2.
    (C) 2, 8, 15, 2.
    (D) 2, 8, 18, 1.

16. The antidiuretic hormone (ADH) elevates blood pressure by stimulating the kidneys to

    (A) hold water, consequently elevating blood pressure, by expanding blood volume.
    (B) release water and stabilize blood pressure by hemostasis.
    (C) vasoconstrict the arterial and venous systems.
    (D) vasodilate the arterial and venous systems.

17. Diffusion of oxygen occurs across the

    (A) adventitia.
    (B) alveoli.
    (C) costal surface of the inside of the lungs.
    (D) oxygen receptors.

18. All of the following are types of teeth EXCEPT

    (A) cuspids.
    (B) gingivae.
    (C) incisors.
    (D) premolars/molars.

19. Spermatogenesis begins

    (A) at puberty.
    (B) during the eighth month of pregnancy.
    (C) shortly after the onset of sexual activity.
    (D) within two to three months after birth.

20. Select the enzyme that catalyzes fats.

    (A) Amylase
    (B) Lactase
    (C) Lipase
    (D) Pepsin

21. Which of the following is an inorganic compound?

    (A) $C_6H_8O_6$ (ascorbic acid)
    (B) Lipids
    (C) Fe_2O_3 (iron oxide)
    (D) Saccharides

22. All of the following are examples of biological negative feedback EXCEPT

    (A) blood sugar regulation.
    (B) body temperature.
    (C) childbirth.
    (D) control of endocrine hormones.

23. What is the difference between strong and weak acids?

    (A) Strong acids release many ions and are strong conductors of electricity. Weak acids are the opposite and release few ions and are weak conductors of electricity.
    (B) Strong acids release few ions and are strong conductors of electricity.
    (C) Weak acids are the opposite and release many ions and are weak conductors of electricity.
    (D) Strong acids release many ions and are weak conductors of electricity. Weak acids are the opposite and release few ions and are weak conductors of electricity.

24. Margaret Mead, a cultural anthropologist in the 1920s, lived in Samoa for an extended period of time conducting field study research in Samoan society. Her research method is considered

    (A) empirical.
    (B) experimental.
    (C) participatory.
    (D) retrospective.

25. Which of the following habitual lifestyles can contribute to liver failure?

    (A) A diet high in fat, salt, sugar, and cholesterol
    (B) Excessive consumption of alcohol
    (C) Physical inactivity
    (D) Smoking tobacco products

Recommendations for Total Weight Gain During Pregnancy by Prepregnancy BMI*

Prepregnancy BMI (kg/m²)	Category	Total Weight Gain Range	Total Weight Gain Range for Pregnancy with Twins
<18.5	Underweight	28–40 lbs.	
18.5–24.9	Normal Weight	25–35 lbs.	37–54 lbs.
25.0–29.9	Overweight	15–25 lbs.	31–50 lbs.
≥30.0	Obese	11–20 lbs.	25–42 lbs.

Weight Gain During Pregnancy: Reexamining the Guidelines. The Institute of Medicine of the National Academies, May 26, 2009

26. A woman of childbearing age has a BMI of less than 18.5 prior to pregnancy. To stay within recommended guidelines, her weight gain during pregnancy should not exceed

(A) 11–20 lbs.
(B) 15–25 lbs.
(C) 25–35 lbs.
(D) 28–40 lbs.

27. What criterion determines a woman's category?

(A) BMI
(B) Genetic predisposition for twins
(C) The information is not on the table.
(D) Weight during pregnancy

---

28. Which of the following antibodies induces basophils and mast cells to secrete histamine?

(A) IgA
(B) IgD
(C) IgE
(D) IgM

29. Select the major component of the cardiovascular system that carries blood to the body.

(A) Arterial system
(B) Capillary system
(C) Cardiac system
(D) Venous system

30. What is the ratio of hydrogen to oxygen in water?

(A) 1:1
(B) 1:2
(C) 2:1
(D) 2:2

31. The nervous system is composed of two systems. They are the

(A) afferent and efferent systems.
(B) autonomic and somatic systems.
(C) central and peripheral systems.
(D) sympathetic and parasympathetic systems.

32. The following is a list of serial events that occur with the patellar reflex. List the events in the correct order of occurrence.

1. Impulse goes across the synapse
2. Impulse travels via the efferent nerve tract
3. Lower leg extends
4. Muscle contracts
5. Muscle stretches
6. Nerve signal goes to spinal cord
7. Tendon tapped

(A) 7, 2, 4, 6, 1, 5, 3
(B) 7, 2, 5, 6, 4, 1, 3
(C) 7, 4, 1, 5, 2, 6, 3
(D) 7, 5, 6, 1, 2, 4, 3

33. Which of the following is the correct sequence of cardiac conduction?

(A) Atrioventricular node ⇒ Sinoatrial node ⇒ Purkinje fibers ⇒ Bundle of His
(B) Bundle of His ⇒ Sinoatrial node ⇒ Atrioventricular node ⇒ Purkinje fibers
(C) Sinoatrial node ⇒ Atrioventricular node ⇒ Bundle of His ⇒ Purkinje fibers
(D) Sinoatrial node ⇒ Atrioventricular node ⇒ Purkinje fibers ⇒ Bundle of His

Questions 34–35 are based on the following diagram.

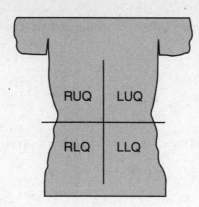

34. All of the following are found in the left upper quadrant EXCEPT

(A) gallbladder.
(B) pancreatic duct.
(C) pancreas.
(D) stomach.

35. Which of the following is technically found in all four abdominal quadrants?

    (A) Anus
    (B) Colon
    (C) Ileum
    (D) Liver

---

36. What is the product in the following chemical equation?

    $$Ca(H_2PO_4)_2 + CaSO_4 + HF \rightarrow Ca_{10}F_2(PO_4)_6 + H_2SO_4$$

    (A) $Ca(HPO) + CaSO + HF$
    (B) $Ca(H_2PO_4)_2 + CaSO_4 + HF$
    (C) $CaF(PO) + HSO$
    (D) $Ca_{10}F_2(PO_4)_6 + H_2SO_4$

37. The fight-or-flight response is triggered by which of the following hormones?

    (A) Epinephrine
    (B) Oxytocin
    (C) Somatotropin
    (D) Testosterone

38. Broadly speaking, homeostasis depends upon all of the following EXCEPT

    (A) acids/bases.
    (B) electrolytes.
    (C) fluids.
    (D) ions.

39. Select the *true* statement.

    (A) An increase in plasma protein level is a frequent etiology of edema in the lower extremities.
    (B) A pH of 7.2 indicates metabolic alkalosis.
    (C) The body's acid-base condition is evaluated in systemic venous blood.
    (D) The trachea is supported by rings called the hyaline cartilage.

40. _____ is a compensatory mechanism for metabolic acidosis.

    (A) Capillary impermeability
    (B) Excessive water in the kidneys
    (C) Hyperventilation
    (D) Osmotic pressure

41. The tube extending from the urinary bladder to the tip of the penis is the

    (A) accessory duct.
    (B) ejaculatory duct.
    (C) ureter.
    (D) urethra.

42. What is one function of the ovaries?

   (A) Delivers egg cell to the uterus
   (B) Production of female sex hormones
   (C) Protection of internal reproductive organs
   (D) Site of fertilization

43. A newly discovered species of butterfly is found to have both long wing and short wing varieties as opposed to other species having either long or short wings. A three-year quantitative field study, performed in the only area where the butterflies are found, demonstrated a preponderance of long winged butterflies. This suggests that butterflies with short wings carry a _____ for wing length.

   (A) dominant trait
   (B) hereditary trait
   (C) Punnett trait
   (D) recessive trait

44. Which of the following is a true statement regarding atomic structure?

   (A) Atoms have an overall positive charge because there is one in each orbital shell.
   (B) Electrons are arranged in orbital shells.
   (C) The nucleus is composed of negative protons and positive neutrons.
   (D) The valence is the inside orbital shell.

45. Crude oil can be deadly hazards to water birds because it coats the bird's feathers. Why does crude oil stick to bird feathers?

   (A) Hydrocarbons found in crude oil overwhelm the base elements covering the oil on bird feathers.
   (B) The aggregate weight of the oil on the bird feathers is less than that of crude oil.
   (C) The aggregate weight of the oil on the bird feathers is greater than that of crude oil and attracts it.
   (D) The feathers of birds are coated with a natural oil which mixes with the crude oil.

46. Digestion of food begins

   (A) in the esophagus.
   (B) in the stomach.
   (C) in the mouth.
   (D) in the posterior pharynx.

47. Expressive language and social functioning are considered functions of the _____

   (A) cerebellum.
   (B) frontal lobe.
   (C) parietal lobe.
   (D) temporal lobe.

48. _____ may be defined as meiotic cell division that leads to the production of ova in females.

   (A) Cell succession
   (B) Graafian phase
   (C) Oogenesis
   (D) Ovarian cycle

49. Which of the following smooth muscles produces "goose bumps" in the skin when the muscle contracts and the hair becomes upright?

(A) Arrector pili
(B) Hyperdermis
(C) Matrix
(D) Stratum lucidum

50. What gives hair its strength?

(A) Irregular shaped osteons
(B) Keratin
(C) Sesamoid fibers
(D) Thin, irregular shaped cartilage

51. Mitochondria carry out _____ respiration.

(A) aerobic
(B) anaerobic
(C) both aerobic and anaerobic
(D) Mitochondria do not have a respiratory component.

52. Taking aspirin to reduce pain _____ the production of _____.

(A) increases, glucose
(B) modulates, pain sensation at nerve roots
(C) regulates, cortisol
(D) suppresses, prostaglandins

53. What is the name of the appendage found at the beginning of the large intestine?

(A) Appendix
(B) Cecum
(C) Ileum
(D) Jejunum

ENGLISH AND LANGUAGE USAGE

NUMBER OF QUESTIONS: 28

TIME LIMIT: 28 MINUTES

Instructions: Read each question thoroughly. Select the single best answer. Mark your answer (A, B, C, or D) on the answer sheet provided for Practice Test 2.

1. Select the correctly punctuated sentence.

   (A) Although, Karen was worried by the news of the impending storm she still went to the concert.
   (B) Around 95 percent of the money goes to school funding; the remaining five percent seems to vanish like the wind.
   (C) Biology, is the study of, life and living things.
   (D) The candy mixture contained jaw breakers bubble gum lemon balls and sour twists.

2. Select the simple sentence.

   (A) Alex and Sierra are training for long distance running.
   (B) He told his friends he would probably be late, but no one anticipated he'd be four hours late.
   (C) I returned to the grocery even though I left without buying anything.
   (D) The children forfeited their weekly allowance when they failed to complete their chores.

3. Select the sentence with the correct correlative conjunctions.

   (A) John told his father he didn't finish mowing the lawn for the reason that he twisted his ankle.
   (B) She was demoted when production fell because she refused to follow company policy.
   (C) When the truth was known, neither boy wanted to go alone or be seen as afraid.
   (D) Whether you run in the marathon or decide to work in the support team is your choice.

4. Select an appropriate synonym for the italicized word in the following sentence.

   The campers had seen sunset after *boring* sunset on their journey.

   (A) Amusing
   (B) Animated
   (C) Burrowing
   (D) Platitudinous

5. Select the sentence that uses an incorrect word.

   (A) John was in a quandary and he knew it.
   (B) She suffered from spasmodic episodes in her muscles since the accident.
   (C) The lost watch was found among the rocks alongside the trail.
   (D) The scent of his colon lingered long after he'd left the room.

6. Select the incorrectly spelled word.

   (A) Aerospace
   (B) Bulleten
   (C) Rescue
   (D) Yacht

7. Select the sentence that uses an incorrect word.

(A) Apples picked before the first freeze are not as sweet as those picked after the freeze.
(B) Fifteen of the students attending the festival developed gastrointestinal disturbances after eating at the chili booth.
(C) Gauging the affect of the death of a classmate is best done by professional counselors.
(D) Professional athletes are made, not born.

8. Select the sentence that uses an incorrect word.

(A) New students were required to have the following to register for the fall semester: (1) state-issued birth certificate; (2) up-to-date immunization record; (3) official transcript(s) from schools previously attended; and (4) proof of residence in the school district (current utility bill).
(B) The mother was displeased when she read the teacher's note stating her daughter had been sent to the principle's office because she repeatedly misbehaved in class.
(C) Mark's plan was to repaint the outside of the house over the weekend if weather permitted.
(D) Tommy had saved his allowance to buy marbles to add to his collection, but he ended up paying for a new bathroom window because he was told not to hit the ball toward the house.

9. A compound sentence is best described as

(A) two independent clauses joined by a coordinating conjunction, conjunctive adverb, or semicolon.
(B) one dependent clause joined to an independent clause.
(C) a stand-alone independent clause with appropriate punctuation.
(D) two independent clauses joined to one or more dependent clauses.

10. Select the best meaning of the italicized phrase in the following sentence.

Leo bragged he had *dodged a bullet* when he was caught breaking curfew because his father was a big financial supporter of the football team.

(A) Calm and relaxed
(B) Lucky and eschewed misfortune
(C) Strong and tough
(D) Truthful and dependable

11. Select the mnemonic for the correct order of the Great Lakes from west to east.

(A) Large Animals Jump Slowly
(B) Smart Boys do Fine Always
(C) Royal Houses of Stuart and Lancaster
(D) Super Man Helps Every One

12. Select an appropriate synonym for the italicized word in the following sentence.

The newest version of the computer game was *rad*.

(A) Detestable
(B) Ordinary
(C) Second-rate
(D) Stupendous

13. Select the most appropriate meaning of the root word italicized in the following sentence.

   The most popular major at the small college this semester was *agri*business.

   (A) Agent
   (B) Condition
   (C) Farm
   (D) Knowledge

14. Select the most appropriate meaning of the root word italicized in the following sentence.

   The *inscript*ion on the tombstone read, "Beloved daughter of H.L. and R.E. Adamson."

   (A) Addition
   (B) Before
   (C) Caricature
   (D) Write

15. Select the sentence that uses an incorrect word.

   (A) Emma was saving her money to buy the bicycle the coach of the mountain biking team suggested.
   (B) Friend's Market had a sale on fruits and vegetables every year before Memorial Day.
   (C) The parents of the young man were relieved when he passed his competency exams for advanced prep courses at the local high school.
   (D) The young man had dreams of becoming an allusionist.

16. Select an appropriate antonym for the italicized word in the following sentence.

   The politician's speech was awash with *benign* statements.

   (A) Auspicious
   (B) Despicable
   (C) Passive
   (D) Promising

17. Adding the suffix *-ful* to the word *loathe,* it becomes

   (A) loathful.
   (B) loatheful.
   (C) loathfull.
   (D) loathe-ful.

18. The root word *capit* means

   (A) around.
   (B) before.
   (C) head.
   (D) state of being.

19. Select the dependent clause in the following sentence.

Although I have been nodding off all day, I still feel like I could work another ten hours.

(A) Although I have been nodding off all day
(B) I still feel like I could work another ten hours
(C) Nodding off all day
(D) Work another ten hours

20. Which of the following is a compound-complex sentence?

(A) Albert Leo, Madison Abel, Joseph Eugene, Francis Henry, and George Thomas Sullivan were brothers who joined the Navy after Pearl Harbor, served together on the light cruiser *USS Juneau*, and died when their ship was sunk during the Naval Battle of Guadalcanal.
(B) If I were young, I think I would want to be a doctor or I would want to be a poet.
(C) Melville's published works include *Moby Dick* and *Billy Budd*.
(D) To earn extra money, Marge worked mornings in the school cafeteria, Sarah worked afternoons in the self-serve laundry, and Amy worked nights in a nursing home.

21. Select the sentence with correct capitalization.

(A) Rome is often referred to as the holy city.
(B) Many believe the Valley of the Mississippi is the most beautiful area in the state.
(C) The eighty-sixth congress adjourned for summer break.
(D) Zach could never remember which was the Tropic of Cancer and which was the Tropic of Capricorn.

22. Select the writing process that best completes the following sentence.

Henry, the production team manager, called a _____ session because the team failed to meet the deadline by working individually.

(A) brainstorming
(B) freewriting
(C) mind mapping
(D) stream of consciousness

23. Select the most appropriate meaning of the root word italicized in the following sentence.

The instructions said to include a *bibli*ography at the end of the paper.

(A) Book
(B) Connect
(C) Reference
(D) Write

24. Select the most appropriate meaning of the root word italicized in the following sentence.

There were so many re*strict*ions that Henry questioned his decision to live on the island.

(A) Bind
(B) Boundary
(C) Contingent
(D) Theology

25. Select the incorrectly punctuated sentence.

    (A) Multicolored leggings had become the rage in the elementary school.
    (B) The community hospital having been supported by community donations for so long had to revamp many of its practices when it became the county hospital.
    (C) The family-owned market advertised the freshest melons and vegetables in town.
    (D) "I just can't believe it—the curling team lost the championship."

26. Select the sentence that uses an incorrect word.

    (A) Deb's grades in nursing soared after she started working with a tutor.
    (B) Of the eighteen students in the program, six were admitted to Harvard.
    (C) The old woman's routine was to walk her dog every morning around 8:00 A.M.
    (D) The politician's illusions to health care for the infirmed angered many of his supporters.

27. Babby has an assignment to write a paper on a historic event happening in the county during the nineteenth century. The first step in her writing process is to

    (A) check out books at the local library.
    (B) develop an idea.
    (C) search the Internet.
    (D) write a broad topical outline.

28. Select the well-developed paragraph from the following.

    (A) After several weeks of writing, Katrine has numerous pages of what she hopes will be her first children's book. A friend of many years she frequently communicates with suggested she try writing since her long letters read more like entertaining stories instead of a list of happenings. Katrine is 56 years old. She had dreamed of writing a children's book since she was a teenager, but she didn't think she had the knowledge and skill to be a writer. Katrine took her friend's advice and decided to give writing a try.
    (B) Katrine is 56 years old. She took her friend's advice and decided to give writing a try. After several weeks of writing, she has numerous pages of what she hopes will be her first children's book. She had dreamed of writing a children's book since she was a teenager, but she didn't think she had the knowledge and skill to be a writer. A friend of many years she frequently communicates with suggested she try writing since her long letters read more like entertaining stories instead of a list of happenings.
    (C) Katrine is 56 years old. She had dreamed of writing a children's book since she was a teenager, but she didn't think she had the knowledge and skill to be a writer. A friend of many years she frequently communicates with suggested she try writing since her long letters read more like entertaining stories instead of a list of happenings. Katrine took her friend's advice and decided to give writing a try. After several weeks of writing, she has numerous pages of what she hopes will be her first children's book.
    (D) She had dreamed of writing a children's book since she was a teenager, but she didn't think she had the knowledge and skill to be a writer. Katrine took her friend's advice and decided to give writing a try. After several weeks of writing, she has numerous pages of what she hopes will be her first children's book. A friend of many years she frequently communicates with suggested she try writing since her long letters read more like entertaining stories instead of a list of happenings. Katrine is 56 years old.

ANSWER KEY
Practice Test 2

Reading

1.	B	15.	A	29.	C	43.	C
2.	B	16.	C	30.	B	44.	C
3.	C	17.	A	31.	B	45.	B
4.	C	18.	D	32.	C	46.	C
5.	A	19.	D	33.	B	47.	B
6.	D	20.	A	34.	A	48.	C
7.	A	21.	D	35.	C	49.	C
8.	B	22.	A	36.	B	50.	A
9.	C	23.	B	37.	D	51.	D
10.	B	24.	C	38.	D	52.	D
11.	D	25.	C	39.	A	53.	B
12.	D	26.	D	40.	C		
13.	A	27.	C	41.	A		
14.	D	28.	B	42.	A		

Mathematics

1.	C	10.	A	19.	D	28.	B
2.	D	11.	D	20.	B	29.	A
3.	B	12.	A	21.	C	30.	A
4.	C	13.	B	22.	A	31.	D
5.	B	14.	C	23.	D	32.	B
6.	B	15.	B	24.	A	33.	C
7.	C	16.	A	25.	D	34.	A
8.	D	17.	B	26.	C	35.	A
9.	B	18.	A	27.	D	36.	D

Science

1.	B	15.	B	29.	A	43.	D
2.	B	16.	A	30.	C	44.	B
3.	C	17.	B	31.	C	45.	D
4.	D	18.	B	32.	D	46.	C
5.	B	19.	A	33.	C	47.	B
6.	D	20.	C	34.	A	48.	C
7.	C	21.	C	35.	B	49.	A
8.	A	22.	C	36.	D	50.	B
9.	A	23.	A	37.	A	51.	A
10.	D	24.	A	38.	D	52.	D
11.	C	25.	B	39.	D	53.	A
12.	C	26.	D	40.	C		
13.	C	27.	A	41.	D		
14.	D	28.	C	42.	B		

English and Language Usage

1.	B	8.	B	15.	D	22.	A
2.	A	9.	A	16.	B	23.	A
3.	D	10.	B	17.	A	24.	A
4.	D	11.	D	18.	C	25.	B
5.	D	12.	D	19.	A	26.	D
6.	B	13.	C	20.	B	27.	B
7.	C	14.	D	21.	D	28.	C

ANSWER EXPLANATIONS
Reading

1. **(B)** *Generic social processes* fall within the guidelines; the remaining options do not. *Gender* is listed before *gender discrimination,* and *globalization* and *Goffman* are listed after *genocide.*

2. **(B)** Without knowing the definition of *historicism,* each option must be critically read and considered. Each incorrect option gives specific misinformation that must be identified to select the correct option (which is a definition of *historicism*). Option (A) references the relationship between biophysical anatomy and the moral and social development of the human species. There is no relationship between anatomy and moral/social development. What is biophysical anatomy? Option (C) mentions a biological perspective studying the size and configuration of a population as it relates to dissimilar or unrelated populations. Biology is the science or study of life or living matter and has nothing to do with the size and configuration or structure of a population—biology considers the structure of the organism, not a population. Option (D) references the psychological perspective of one generation determining what a future generation will do. Psychology is the study of behavior or the science of the mind. A generation is a group of people born and living during the same time. Each generation is influenced by occurrences within that generation with things falling into and out of vogue. Examples are Generations X, Y, Z, and the Baby Boomers.

3. **(C)** *Enactment* or *authorization* are synonyms of *ratification.* The remaining options are antonyms.

4. **(C)** Temperance movements were organized efforts to bring about partial or complete abstinence of alcohol consumption. They viewed alcohol use as detrimental to the family and marriage. As such, they supported resolution of societal problems. The health of citizens is included under the umbrella of social issues or problems. The remaining options were not the focus of temperance movements.

5. **(A)** In terms of options, which is the worst or costliest in relation to the general public? The escalation of gang violence and other crimes, including senseless killing of innocent children and adult citizens, increases in alcohol-related offenses, and gang wars. When present on a national level, these activities affect the general public on a personal level. An increase in the number of places to drink and the availability of alcohol was a response to public demand. Taxes lost by the government did not have a direct negative effect on the public.

6. **(D)** Prohibition sounded good in theory, but it was a failure in practice.

7. **(A)** The passage deals with factual material and happenings. These can be verified in records, diaries, and official communication of individuals serving on submarines during World War II. No stereotypes are presented in the passage. The Allies (the nations that fought against the Axis) and the Axis (Germany, Italy, and Japan) are examples of World War II stereotypes. Allied soldiers were envisioned as honest, upstanding, and everything a good person wanted to be. Axis soldiers were envisioned as devious, dishonest, and dishonorable—everything seen in individuals with questionable morals. No biases are evident in the passage.

8. **(B)** The passage presents a glimpse of life on board a wartime submarine more than 70 years ago. The passage presents a slice of life in a long past era—something that people of today can read about, but never truly understand or experience. The remaining options do not address why the passage was written.

9. **(C)** The historical publication is the most logical since the passage is factual in nature and deals with a specific event in the past. The remaining options are not supportive of the passage.

10. **(B)** Based on the passage, life on a World War II submarine was hard, demanding, and required sacrifice. It can be assumed that living conditions in the armed forces have improved over time, but is illogical because there is nothing accurate to compare it to since the country is not involved in a world war. The phrase *members of the U.S. Navy* implies or suggests *all of the Navy* endured sacrifice and this is not true. Wars are managed and numerous members of the armed forces served from behind desks and never left the United States, fired a rifle, or spent a night separated from their loved ones. Regarding hygiene, the passage is clear that hygiene was an issue they had little control over.

11. **(D)** The key to correctly answer this question is visually comparing GPAs—no calculations are needed. An estimate of his GPA is at least a 4.5. This can be visualized on the chart. All of River's GPAs are above 4.6. None of the other students fall into this range for the three-year period. The remaining GPAs are below 4.60.

12. **(D)** The overall GPA trend is downward. Olivia has the lowest potential with a highest GPA of 4.5 or less.

13. **(A)** Emma had the greatest variance in GPAs over the three-year period. Her variance is 0.8 $(5.0 - 4.2 = 0.8)$. The remaining variances range from 0.4 to 0.5. Calculations are not needed to determine the answer. *Change* is a synonym for *variance*. The change in GPAs can be visualized on the chart.

14. **(D)** Books on statistics would be found in 519 Probabilities and applied mathematics. Statistics is considered applied mathematics because it is a combination of mathematical knowledge. Statistics is also used in numerous fields such as engineering, industry, science, and business.

15. **(A)** The definition of topology is presented in the stem. The answer can be determined by three methods: first, by breaking the word into its parts; second, by having previous knowledge of topology; and third, by a process of eliminating what you know is incorrect. The definition of topology does not fit into any of the other mathematical categories. Topology remains as the only feasible option.

16. **(C)** The memorandum is informative and provides employees with information about and measures to alleviate a specific problem. The word *chastise* means to castigate, punish, or penalize. The passage speaks of negative consequences for those employees who choose to disregard policy, but it does not chastise. The memorandum is not meant to entertain or persuade the reader.

17. **(A)** The memorandum provides specific information regarding the E Lot. The lot is gated, and employees seeking entry must have the appropriate identification on their automobiles. Since two groups of employees (paying and nonpaying) use the lot, employees who park in the lot for free are the most likely to park illegally.

18. **(D)** *Retribution* is an antonym for *forfeit* and *forfeiture*. The remaining options are synonyms for *forfeit* and *forfeiture*.

19. **(D)** The word *abridge* means to condense, abbreviate, or put in a nutshell. The correct response (D) is the most specific. The memo briefly identifies the problem and provides a condensed version of the new policy. If an E Lot employee parks in an unauthorized area, there will be negative consequences. There is nothing in the memorandum suggestive of the Board of Directors being unsympathetic to employee needs; if anything, they are sympathetic. The new policy affects only those employees who presently park in the E Lot, and does not have any bearing on employees parking in other lots. All employees are notified because

the policy is companywide. Referring simply to parking as a problem in option (C) is vague. The same is true for a new policy in option (C). It also is vague.

20. **(A)** The sharp increase in unauthorized parking in the E Lot has brought about a need for change. The Board of Directors is responding to an escalating problem. The statement *long-standing unauthorized parking* suggests it has not been seen as a problem until the present.

21. **(D)** The most logical conclusion is that there will be a sharp decrease in unauthorized parking in the E Lot. There is a harsh penalty for E Lot employees who disregard the new policy. Only a fool would risk a $400 fine for one day of unauthorized parking when a reserved space is available 24/7 for $56 a year. It is doubtful employees will unite and demand a revocation of the policy since the policy only affects employees parking in a specific lot. Employees who disregard the new policy will be penalized. The memorandum does not provide information on unauthorized parking in other lots.

22. **(A)** It is doubtful that the event would be in its eighteenth year if it were not successful in raising money for the Children's Charity. The Mountain Bike-a-Thon draws attendees and entrants from the home state as well as the surrounding states. The overhead is low and reasonable considering it is a charity event. The cost of admission and event entry will discourage potentially problematic individuals from attending. There is nothing in the cost of attending or participating in event activities that targets any class. There is nothing to suggest that decreasing admission and entry fees would increase the number of attendees.

23. **(B)** While the flyer provides pertinent information, there is no contact information for individuals with questions. The remaining options (such as event registration) address information individuals may need to know, but this information cannot be obtained without first having contact information.

24. **(C)** Option (C) is the correct order for the hierarchy of the biological classification system.

25. **(C)** A researcher's results of clinical trials are a primary source; the remaining options are secondary sources of information.

26. **(D)** A *social* commentary provides analysis, interpretation, or observation on social issues within a society. *Devotional*, *indirective*, and *humanistic* are not topics likely to be associated with terrorism.

27. **(C)** The movie genre *thriller* has numerous subheadings. *The Shining* is an example of a *psychological thriller* in which an individual faces situations that threaten his or her sanity. *Eco-thrillers* concern man-made or natural threats to society. *Mystery thrillers* involve murder or other puzzling events that have to be unraveled. *Techno-thrillers* involve technology of some sort.

28. **(B)** An antonym is a word that has the opposite meaning of another word. *Jeopardy* can be used to indicate trouble or danger. *Protection* is an antonym of *jeopardy*. The remaining options are not antonyms of *jeopardy*.

29. **(C)** A synonym is a word that has the same or similar meaning as another word. An *exemplary* individual is honorable, good, commendable, or worthy. *Exemplary* and *praiseworthy* are synonyms.

30. **(B)** *Deportment* has to do with behavior or conduct. The word is often used to describe the conduct or behavior of students in school. The remaining options do not describe *deportment*.

31. **(B)** Information presented in the passage and on the chart make it easy to read into this question. To correctly answer the question, answers must be based on what is present, not what is assumed. Information in the memo indicates William has an excessive workload, little time

for studying, and little time for himself. The chart presents information heavily suggestive of a student with problems. His absence days and deportment have steadily worsened since the beginning of the semester, and his grade point average has steadily fallen from a passing to a failing average. The remaining options are assumptions trying to explain William's behavior.

32. **(C)** Using information presented in the memos and looking at the trends on the chart both suggest William will not graduate from high school. The use of the word *everyone* in the first option disqualifies the option. Words like *everyone*, *always*, and *never* are usually clues that a testing statement is incorrect. There is nothing to suggest that his deportment is to the point of suspension, or that his behavior is breaking the law. In most instances, there is a positive relationship between education and earning power. At this point in time, William has neither.

33. **(B)** William's absence days are lowest in February; the remaining months have a higher number of absence days.

34. **(A)** William's deportment issues are trending upward, with April being the highest month.

35. **(C)** The second memo from the Lead Junior/Senior Counselor to the school principal is a follow-up memo providing information regarding the principal's concerns presented in the first memo. It states what new information has been discovered and provides a possible explanation for the increased absence days, deportment issues, and decreasing grade-point average. It also states what the counselor plans to do and her belief that William's situation can be modified. The remaining options have to do with the counselor's performance.

36. **(B)** The new word is *barley*, the grain of a cereal plant.

37. **(D)** This question is more difficult because it requires you to take the basic meaning of a word and generalize it as a new concept. This is similar to taking the word *cup* and extending it to mean a measuring cup, tea cup, athletic cup, or brassiere cup. In each example, the cup holds something. In regard to the question, the word *flux* has numerous meanings. Simply put, *flux* has to do with flowing, passage, or movement. Another definition has to do with usually fatal bloody and/or watery diarrhea frequently seen in children in the summer months before the advent of modern medicine. The remaining options do not incorporate *flux* into their meanings.

38. **(D)** The word *lush* is described as something that is succulent, has luxuriant vegetation, or is fertile or opulent. There is nothing in the passage to suggest intoxicated individuals lived in the valley. The passage is also not supportive of the valley being bleak, impoverished, or depressed.

39. **(A)** *Brusque* is a synonym for *short*. The remaining options are antonyms for *short*.

40. **(C)** The cost of tickets for "Immortal Kingdom" is $6.00 for all people under 13 years of age. The remaining options are incorrect.

41. **(A)** It is more economical for Phillip to buy his mother a senior ticket for $2.00. Her ticket, when included in the season ticket price, is $4.50.

42. **(A)** Expository passages explain or elucidate. In the case of this passage, the author is providing information or explaining to the reader how families are social systems. Narratives tell stories, entertain, or inform. Persuasive articles seek to change viewpoints or opinions. Technical material is scientific, specialized, high-tech, or scholarly.

43. **(C)** The passage has three main points: (1) families are subsystems in larger societal systems; (2) families are social systems; and (3) families change over time. Functional or dysfunctional families are subsystems of the family system. Families are dynamic, not static. Use of the word *all* in the last option disqualifies it as a correct answer.

44. **(C)** Family roles and responsibilities are one of the characteristics of a family system. Roles and responsibilities are solidified early in the life of a family and change as the family

changes. The passage provides examples of normal, expected changes in families over time. This question requires thinking outside of the box—if these changes normally occur, then what happens when something unexpected occurs? Modification of roles and responsibilities must occur for the family to continue. The remaining options are possibilities, but cannot be adequately addressed until roles and responsibilities are modified.

45. **(B)** Physiological loss has to do with loss or reduction of function. Loss of muscle mass begins in the 30s and progresses throughout the life span. This phenomenon is most obvious in older adults in terms of loss of strength. Depression, tooth loss, and premature aging are not expectations of aging.

46. **(C)** Simply put, *adaptation* means a change in structure or remodeling. It can also mean a conscious or unconscious modification. The remaining options do not support *adaptation.*

47. **(B)** Making assumptions could influence selecting an incorrect answer. The Columbia River in the Pacific Northwest runs more northward than the Missouri River in the central United States. However, the Missouri River is *labeled* on the map, and the Columbia River is not. The remaining options run south of the Missouri River.

48. **(C)** St. Louis is the only city on the map located on the Mississippi River. The remaining options are incorrect.

49. **(C)** San Francisco is located on the San Francisco Bay and is the only city that meets the criterion of a westernmost city located on a well-known bay. Boston and New York are on the east coast of the United States. Vancouver is in British Columbia, Canada.

50. **(A)** Dallas is the only city located east of the Rio Grande River. Denver is north, Salt Lake City is northwest, and Winnipeg is in Manitoba, Canada.

51. **(D)** Chronologies are tertiary sources. They are summaries or condensed versions of past events and are usually based on primary and secondary sources. Architecture and audio recordings are primary sources. Biographies are secondary sources.

52. **(D)** The focus of the typing service is narrow. It is intended for graduate students and focuses on theses, dissertations, and résumés. A broadly focused typing service would be intended for all college/university students and, perhaps, the general public. There is little, if any, relationship between university enrollment and the typing service. The typing service is not owned or controlled by the institution.

53. **(B)** Comparing and contrasting the alkali and alkaline earth metals from the Periodic Table is the only project that satisfies the criteria—the project must be a chemistry project. It cannot be a chemistry project if it addresses anything outside of chemistry. The remaining options are not appropriate for comparing and contrasting, or they only partially meet the criteria.

Mathematics

1. **(C)** The recipes require a total of 44 eggs, which equals 3.7 dozen. Eggs are typically sold in dozens, so Dawn must purchase 4 dozen eggs.

2. **(D)** Each item in the mix is given in percentages except for pecans (3 ounces) and an unknown percentage of walnuts. Use ratio and proportion to determine the percentage of pecans in a one-pound mixture.

$$\text{If } 16 \text{ oz} = 100\%, \text{ then } 3 \text{ oz} = x\%$$
$$16 = 100 :: 3 = x$$
$$16x = 300$$
$$x = 19\%$$

3. **(B)** The correct answer can be determined using ratio and proportion since the percentage of cashews in the mix is known. Note the question asks for an 8-ounce package, not a 16-ounce package.

$$100\% = 8 \text{ oz} :: 30\% = x \text{ oz}$$
$$1 = 8 :: 0.3 = x$$
$$x = 2.4 \text{ oz}$$

4. **(C)** Every number has an opposite. The addition of a positive number and its opposite always equals zero. For example, +5 plus −5 equals 0 or −7 + 7 = 0. The numbers cancel each other out. The exception is zero, which is neither positive nor negative, and is its own opposite.

5. **(B)** It is important to note that −2 is being subtracted from 5. There are two negatives in the equation. To change the statement into a logical equation, it is important to make distinctions between subtraction and a negative number. Parentheses are added to clarify.

$$5 - (-2)$$

Subtracting a negative number changes it to a positive number.

$$-(-a) = a$$

6. **(B)** In this question, three different expressions can be made with each indicating the same action. The fraction bar, $\overline{)}$, and the division sign, ÷, all indicate the same action. Number placement is important because it indicates what is being divided into what. Options (C) and (D) are obviously incorrect because they do not contain an expression indicating division. Option (A) is incorrect because all three divide 43 into 62.

7. **(C)** The runner is 15 miles from the finish line and runs 10 additional miles making him 5 miles from the finish line. He is west of the finish line and must run east to reach it.

8. **(D)**

$$x + 4 = -20 \qquad\qquad x + 4 = -20$$
$$x = -24 \qquad\qquad -24 + 4 = -20$$
$$-20 = -20$$

9. **(B)**

1,000	100	10	1	Decimal point	$\dfrac{1}{10}$	$\dfrac{1}{100}$	$\dfrac{1}{1,000}$
5	6	9	3	.	4	1	9

10. **(A)** When determining rank order of numbers, it is important to remember that numbers get larger to the left of the decimal point, and smaller to the right of the decimal point. Fifty is greater than 5, and 0.05 is smaller than 0.5. One method of determining a rank order of decimals is to look at the tenths position of each number in the series. This makes the order 0.2, 0.3, 0.3, 0.4, and 0.7, and it would be correct for ordering least to greatest if it weren't for two 0.3s. In this case, the hundredths place needs to be considered. They are 0.30 and 0.31, with 0.30 being the smaller of the two. The thousandths place can be considered if the order is still equivalent, such as 0.520 and 0.521.

11. **(D)** The formula for percent change must be used.

$$\text{Percent change (PC)} = \frac{\text{change}}{\text{starting point}}$$

$$\text{PC} = \frac{\$6,500 - \$5,000}{\$6,500}$$

$$PC = \frac{1,500}{6,500}$$

$$PC = 0.2308 = 23\%$$

It doesn't matter if addition or subtraction is used to determine the amount of change.

$$6,500 - 5,000 = x \qquad \text{or} \qquad 5,000 + x = 6,500$$

$$1,500 = x \qquad\qquad\qquad x = 1,500$$

12. **(A)** When dividing identical bases with exponents, subtract the exponents.

$$5^5 \div 5^2 = \frac{(5 \times 5 \times 5 \times 5 \times 5)}{(5 \times 5)} = 5^3$$

$$5^5 \div 5^2 = 5^{5-2} = 5^3$$

13. **(B)** When a base number with an exponent is taken to another power, multiply the exponents and perform the function.

$$(2^4)^3 = 2^{12} = 4,096$$

The problem can also be solved using the following method.

$$(2^4)^3 = (2 \times 2 \times 2 \times 2)^3 = 16^3 = (16 \times 16 \times 16) = 4,096$$

14. **(C)** Medication doses for infants and children are rarely rounded to a whole number unless there is no other option. This problem can be solved using a number of methods. Dimensional analysis and ratio and proportion are shown. The following is taken from the question:

Order: 20 mg/kg/day	On hand: 5 ml = 50 mg
Weight: 15 lb	Wanted: ml/day

<u>Dimensional analysis:</u>

$$\frac{\text{ml}}{\text{day}} = \frac{5\,\text{ml}}{50\,\text{mg}} \times \frac{20\,\text{mg}}{\text{kg/day}} \times \frac{1\,\text{kg}}{2.2\,\text{lb}} \times \frac{15\,\text{lb}}{1} = 13.6\,\text{ml/day}$$

Note that the mg cancels mg, kg cancels kg, and lb cancels lb leaving ml/day.

<u>Ratio and proportion:</u>

Step 1. Change pounds to kilograms.
$$1\,\text{kg} = 2.2\,\text{lb} :: x\,\text{kg} = 15\,\text{lb}$$
$$2.2x = 15$$
$$x = 6.8\,\text{kg}$$

Step 2. Determine milligrams/kilogram/day.
$$20\,\text{mg} = 1\,\text{kg} :: x\,\text{mg} = 6.8\,\text{kg}$$
$$x = 136.4\,\text{mg}$$

Step 3. Determine milliliters per day.
$$5\,\text{ml} = 50\,\text{mg} :: x\,\text{ml} = 136.4\,\text{mg}$$
$$50x = 682$$
$$x = 13.6\,\text{ml/day}$$

15. (B) Ratio and proportion can be used to solve the problem.

$$\text{If } 42 \text{ students} = 5.85\%, \text{ then } x \text{ students} = 100\%$$
$$42 = 5.85 :: x = 100$$
$$5.85x = 4{,}200$$
$$x = 717.94 = 718 \text{ students}$$

The answer to the problem must be rounded up to the next whole number since it is impossible to have a partial student.

16. (A) The number above the fraction line is the numerator, and the number below the line is the denominator. Ask what number (d) divided into 15 is equal to 65.

$$\frac{n}{d} = \frac{15}{d} = 65$$
$$15 = 65d$$
$$0.23 = d$$

17. (B)

$$100\% = 150 \text{ marbles} :: x\% = 13 \text{ marbles}$$
$$150x = 1{,}300$$
$$x = 8.666 = 8.7\%$$

18. (A) You are being asked to answer a specific question—based on the given information, does Marshall have enough money to buy the suit? He has $268.49, and needs $284.83. He is around $17.00 short of his goal. Option (C) subtracts the amount Marshall has saved from the cost of the suit. The tax on the purchase is not included. The remaining options make assumptions and do not address the posed question. Option (B) assumes the suit will be on sale. The passage does not stipulate that the suit is selling for its regular price or a sale price. Option (D) assumes the money can be borrowed.

Saved	$143.49
Siblings	$60.00
Uncle	$25.00
Yards	+$40.00
Total	$268.49

Cost of suit × tax = $247.95 × 14.875% = $36.88

Cost of suit + tax = $247.95 + $36.88 = $284.83

Cost of suit − amount available = $284.83 − $268.49 = $16.34 still needed

19. (D) The number above the fraction line is the numerator and the number below the line is the denominator.

$$\frac{n}{d} = \frac{n}{250} = 50$$
$$n = 12{,}500$$

20. (B) Numbers to the left of the decimal point are whole numbers. Numbers to the right of the decimal points are fractions.

$$0.024 = \text{twenty-four thousandths} = \frac{24}{1{,}000}$$

21. (C) The formula for area is used to determine square feet.

$$\text{Area } (A) = \text{length } (l) \times \text{width } (w) = 200 \times 250 = 50{,}000 \text{ sq ft}$$
$$1 \text{ bag} = 2{,}000 \text{ sq ft} :: x \text{ bags} = 50{,}000 \text{ sq ft}$$
$$2{,}000 \, x = 50{,}000$$
$$x = 25 \text{ bags}$$

22. **(A)** The quotients of the division must be a whole number. 4,578 is divisible by

$$4,578 \div 2 = 2,289$$
$$4,578 \div 3 = 1,526 \text{ The sum of the digits is divisible by 3 } (24 \div 8 = 3).$$
$$4,578 \div 6 = 763$$
$$4,578 \div 7 = 654$$

23. **(D)** The formula for percent change is used.

Percent change = change/starting point

$$\text{Percent change} = \frac{120-115}{115} = \frac{5}{115} = 0.04348 = 4.35\%$$

24. **(A)** When determining rank order of numbers, it is important to remember that numbers get larger to the left of the decimal point and smaller to the right. Fifty is greater than 5, and 0.05 is smaller than 0.5. Also, remember negative numbers are less than zero. One method of determining a rank order of decimals is to look at the tenths position of each number in the series. If there are identical tenths, move to the hundredths, and so on. The fraction $\frac{5}{8}$ needs to be changed to a decimal (0.625). The fraction $-\frac{3}{4}$ is automatically the smallest number since a positive number divided into a negative number gives a negative answer (−0.75). The order from greatest to least based on tenths is now 0.7, 0.6, 0.4, 0.3, 0.0, and −0.7 or 0.734, $\frac{5}{8}$, 0.427, 0.3, 0.0, and $-\frac{3}{4}$.

25. **(D)** The answer is located at the bottom of the second column of the table.

26. **(C)** A key to this question is making sure you understand what the question is asking. The question asks how many dinners were sold (not the number prepared, which would include the college students).

$$\text{Beef dinners: } 82 \text{ faculty} \times \$15 = \$1,230$$
$$292 \text{ public} \times \$15 = \underline{+ 4,380}$$
$$\$5,610$$

27. **(D)** Understanding what the question asks is key to obtaining the correct answer. The question asks for the percentage of individuals ordering chicken dinners, not the percentage paying for chicken dinners. Three hundred and eleven chicken dinners were ordered.

$$\frac{311}{994} = 31.3 = 31\%$$

28. **(B)** The answer is determined by dividing 348 students by 994, the total number of attendees at the picnic.

$$\frac{348}{994} = 35.01 = 35\%$$

29. **(A)** Total Amount Made − 10% = Amount to Student Assistance Fund (SAF)

$$(\$ \text{ Beef dinners}) + (\$ \text{ Chick dinners}) + (\$ \text{ Veg Dinners}) = \$ \text{ Total}$$
$$(374 \times \$15.00) + (175 \times \$12.50) + (97 \times \$10.00) = \$ \text{ Total}$$
$$\$5,610.00 + 2,187.50 + 970 = \$8,767.50$$
$$\text{Dollar Total} \times 10\% = \$8767.50 \times 10\% = \$876.75$$
$$\$8,767.50 - \$876.75 = \$7,890.75 \text{ to SAF}$$

30. **(A)** Two can be divided into 5 two times with 1 remaining, or $2\frac{1}{2}$.

$$\frac{5}{2} = 2\frac{1}{2}$$

31. **(D)** An improper fraction is greater than one, and the numerator is larger than the denominator. A proper fraction is less than one, and the numerator is less than the denominator.

$$15\frac{5}{7} = 15 \times 7 + 5 = 105 + 5 = \frac{110}{7}$$

32. **(B)** There is more than one way to solve the problem.
$$(76)(0.3333) = 25.33 = 25 \text{ pts}$$
$$\text{or}$$
$$76 \text{ pts} = 100\% \therefore x \text{ pts} = 33\%$$
$$1.0x = (76 \times 0.3333)$$
$$x = 25.33 = 25 \text{ pts}$$

33. **(C)** The rules of operation must be used to correctly determine x.

$$
\begin{array}{l|l}
15x + (14 - 3) - 2[(2)(7)] = 80 & 15x + (14 - 3) - 2[(2)(7)] = 80 \\
15x + (11) - 2(14) = 80 & 15(6.47) + 11 - 28 = 80 \\
15x + 11 - 28 = 80 & 97.05 - 17 = 80 \\
15x - 17 = 80 & 80.05 = 80 \\
15x = 97 & 80 = 80 \\
x = 6.46667 = 6.47 &
\end{array}
$$

34. **(A)** The sentence must first be changed into an equation. The rules of operation must be followed to determine y.

$$(15)(y + 8) = 145$$
$$15y + 120 = 145$$
$$15y = 25$$
$$y = 1.66666 = 1.67$$

35. **(A)** The sentence must be changed into an equation format.

$$x + 84 = 108$$
$$x = 24$$

36. **(D)** Perry had the highest average for the four-week period with 74.75 votes.

$$\frac{88 + 70 + 75 + 66}{4} = 74.75$$

Science

1. **(B)** The liver, the largest gland in the body, is located in the right upper quadrant (RUQ) of the abdomen under the diaphragm. It is of primary importance as an accessory organ to the gastrointestinal tract. The liver is divided into the caudate, left, quadrate, and right lobes. As an accessory organ, it has numerous vital functions in the process of digestion: (a) carbohydrate metabolism, (b) fat metabolism, (c) protein metabolism, (d) production of bile, (e) removal of toxic and hormone substances from the circulation, and (f) vitamin storage (A, B_{12}, D, E, and K). The pancreas and spleen are located in the left upper quadrant (LUQ), and they, with the liver, are all located in the abdominal cavity. Drug metabolism also occurs in the liver.

2. **(B)** The clavicles are two of the 126 bones in the appendicular skeleton. The clavicles (located on the ventral side of the body) and scapula (located to the left and right of the spinal column and on the dorsal aspect of the body) form the pectoral girdle that connects the bones of the arm to the rib cage. The remaining options are not associated with the clavicles. The auricular surface of the ilium, the L- or J-shaped surface found on the medial aspect of the ilium, articulates with the sacrum. The lateral malleolus, located at the end of the fibula, forms the lateral part of the ankle.

3. **(C)** The stomach, a large sac-like organ, is located in the left upper quadrant of the abdomen. It is located between the esophagus and the small intestine and lies inferior to the diaphragm. Functions of the stomach include chemical and physical breakdown of food, mixing, and storage. The pancreas, duodenum, and transverse colon are part of the gastrointestinal system.

4. **(D)** The small intestine, located in the right and left lower abdominal quadrants, is composed of the duodenum, jejunum, and ileum. Approximately 20 feet in length, its functions include absorption of nutrients and mechanical and chemical digestion. The pancreas is located in the left upper quadrant. The ascending colon is part of the large intestine, which is the only organ found in all four abdominal quadrants.

5. **(B)** In chemical equations, the reactants are located to the left of the arrow, and the products are located to the right of the arrow. The arrow indicates a chemical reaction has occurred. Chemical reactions create new substances; they do not create new elements. This occurs with nuclear reactions. The remaining options do not meet the criteria for a reactant.

6. **(D)** To satisfy the definition of physiology, it must contain the following: (a) subsystem of biology, (b) study of normal functioning, (c) focus on living creatures or individuals, (d) composed of systems and subsystems, and (e) a normal process. Physiology does not provide information about the evolution of a species. Pathophysiology is the study of abnormality in organisms or their parts.

7. **(C)** Dry ice is the solid form of carbon dioxide, which sublimes at −109.26°F. Its chief purpose is refrigeration. Sublimation is the process of changing from a solid to a gas without passing through a liquid state. Snow sublimes on cold, sunny days. Deposition is the opposite of sublimation and is the process through which dry ice is made. Anhydrides are organic compounds formed when water is removed from more complex compounds. Amalgams are combinations of mercury and other metals usually used in filling cavities in teeth. Dry ice is not frozen water.

8. **(A)** All of the options are correct except (A). New elements are formed through nuclear reactions.

9. **(A)** The souring of milk is a chemical change because the end product is lactic acid, a sour-tasting substance. The souring of milk is literally the rotting of milk. It is also impossible to reverse this change. The remaining options are illogical.

10. **(D)** While the thoracic vertebrae are a part of the thoracic cage, the vertebral column also includes the cervical and lumbar vertebrae which are not a part of the thoracic cage. Ribs attach posteriorly to their corresponding thoracic vertebrae.

11. **(C)** Understanding metric unit terms is essential to correctly answering this question. Meters are used to measure length. Kilometers are the most appropriate units of measure. The distance given in the question is 14 to 15 miles. Using 14.5 miles as the midpoint,

$$14.5 \text{ miles} = 2{,}333{,}548.8 \text{ cm}$$
$$14.5 \text{ miles} = 23{,}335.488 \text{ m}$$
$$14.5 \text{ miles} = 23.335 \text{ km}$$

The following are important to know:

$$10 \text{ millimeters (mm)} = 1 \text{ centimeter (cm)}$$
$$10 \text{ centimeters} = 1 \text{ decimeter (dm)}$$
$$100 \text{ centimeters} = 1 \text{ meter (m)}$$
$$1,000 \text{ meters} = 1 \text{ kilometer (km)}$$

12. **(C)** A researcher, employed by a sugar manufacturer, plans on performing a study of the sugar substitute produced by a competitor. As an employee of a sugar manufacturer, the researcher brings either known or unknown bias to the study—his role includes championing the sugar manufacturer that employs him. Children participating in a study is not a bias; it is a legal issue.

13. **(C)** The designated population from which participants will be selected is a design flaw and has the potential to color the results. The researcher should be looking at a specific group (perhaps individuals who have no option except to use a sugar substitute, or individuals allergic to sugar) or a cross section of the population (a group larger than individuals who attend the event) who use this particular substitute. There are also other design flaws present. Adults and children participating in the same study is not a design flaw—it depends upon the specific study. Reason does exist for a sugar manufacturer to study a sugar substitute product. The researcher's qualifications are not provided in the passage.

14. **(D)** If the weight of one liter of water is known, the weight of four liters is easily determined. The key is recognizing that the question asks for the weight of four liters, not one liter. One liter of water is equal to one kilogram.

15. **(B)** The atomic number of an element is equal to the total number of electrons in the element. The atomic number of calcium (Ca) is 20. The electrons per shell for calcium are 2, 8, 8, 2. The electrons per shell of chlorine (Cl) are 2, 8, 7; cobalt (Co) 2, 8, 15, 2; and copper (Cu) 2, 8, 18, 1.

16. **(A)** Antidiuretic hormone (ADH), produced by the hypothalamus and released by the posterior pituitary, has to do with water regulation in the body. As such, it influences blood pressure. ADH stimulates the kidneys to retain water thus increasing blood volume, which raises blood pressure. ADH does not vasoconstrict or vasodilate. Hemostasis has to do with the clotting of blood after vessel injury.

17. **(B)** The alveoli are small sac-like structures where the exchange of oxygen and carbon dioxide takes place in the lungs. The remaining options have nothing to do with diffusion. The adventitia is the outer section of the trachea. The costal surface is on the outside of the lungs. The body has numerous receptors, but oxygen receptors are not one of them.

18. **(B)** The gingiva are gums, not teeth.

19. **(A)** Spermatogenesis, the process of sperm production via meiosis, begins with the onset of puberty and continues throughout the life span.

Pituitary gland $\Rightarrow$ FSH $\Rightarrow$ Testes $\Rightarrow$ Sertoli cells $\Rightarrow$ Sperm cells $\Rightarrow$ Spermatogenesis

20. **(C)** Lipase, a digestive enzyme produced in the pancreas and small intestine, is used to catalyze fats. The remaining options are also digestive enzymes. (a) amylase (produced in the pancreas, salivary glands, and small intestine) catalyzes starch, (b) lactase (produced in the small intestine) catalyzes lactose, and (c) pepsin (produced in the pancreas, small intestine, and stomach) catalyzes protein.

21. **(C)** Inorganic compounds typically do not contain carbon. Salt (NaCl) and water (H_2O) are two other examples of inorganic compounds. The remaining options are organic compounds.

22. **(C)** The body has feedback systems to regulate and protect the body. Positive feedback systems work to meet a specific end as in the clotting of blood (vessel injury begins the clotting process which stops when the clot has been formed), and childbirth (oxytocin is released to intensify and speed up contractions which causes more oxytocin to be released; the cycle ends with the birth of the child). The remaining options are examples of negative feedback systems that work to maintain homeostasis.

23. **(A)** The correct answer is the difference between strong and weak acids. The remaining options are incorrect.

24. **(A)** Empirical research is based upon observation. Mead's research is not experimental because she did not manipulate the actions or behaviors of the Samoans she observed. Her research is not participatory because Mead did not interject herself into the Samoan society; again, she merely observed. Retrospective research is done after the fact; Mead's research was based in the present.

25. **(B)** All of the options can contribute negatively to an individual's well-being. Alcohol consumption is the only option with a known relationship to liver failure.

26. **(D)** According to the table, a weight gain of 28–40 pounds is acceptable for a woman with a prepregnancy BMI of less than 18.5. The information is found in the first row under the heading in columns one and three. The remainder of the table addresses prepregnancy BMI of 18.5 and greater.

27. **(A)** The title provides this information as does the first column of the table. The BMI for each weight class provides specific information under the headings of Category, Total Weight Gain Range, and Total Weight Gain Range for Pregnancy with Twins.

28. **(C)** IgE is one of five types of antibodies in the body. Antibodies are proteins. IgE is found in the blood and lymph tissues. It does not cross the placenta and functions in allergic reactions by inducing basophils and mast cells to secrete histamine. The antibodies in the remaining options have different functions. Of the five antibodies, only IgG has the ability to cross the placenta.

29. **(A)** The word *major* is key to correctly answering this question. Two separate but interdependent systems circulate blood through the body—the arterial system and the venous system. The arterial system carries oxygenated blood from the heart to the body, and the venous system carries deoxygenated blood back to the heart. The remaining options do not carry blood to the body or the heart.

30. **(C)** H_2O is the chemical formula for dihydrogen monoxide, commonly known as water. Each molecule of water is composed of two hydrogen atoms and one oxygen atom, providing a 2:1 ratio. The remaining options are incorrect ratios.

31. **(C)** The physiologic role of the nervous system is receiving information (stimuli), integrating it, and coordinating functions of the body. Major components of the nervous system are the sense organs, nerves, spinal cord, and brain. The system is divided into hierarchal systems beginning topmost with the central nervous system (CNS) and the peripheral nervous system (PNS). The CNS is the "command Center" for the body and is composed of the brain and spinal cord. The PNS serves as the "go-between" between the body and the CNS. It is composed of nerves (including cranial nerves) outside of the CNS. The remaining options are components of either the CNS or PNS.

32. **(D)** The patellar reflex occurs as follows: Tendon tapped $\Rightarrow$ Muscle stretches $\Rightarrow$ Nerve signal goes to spinal cord $\Rightarrow$ Impulse goes across the synapse $\Rightarrow$ Impulse travels via the different nerve tract $\Rightarrow$ Muscle contracts $\Rightarrow$ Lower leg extends.

33. **(C)** The sinoatrial (SA) node, the primary pacemaker of the heart, located in the right atrium, generates an action potential to the atrioventricular (AV) node located within the triangle of

Koch, a region at the base of the right atrium. The action potential is then generated to the Bundle of His located in the intraventricular septum that separates the right and left ventricles. Last, the action potential is generated to the Purkinje fibers located in the interventricular walls of the ventricles.

34. **(A)** Of the options, the gallbladder is the only organ found in the right upper quadrant; the remaining options are found in the left upper quadrant.

35. **(B)** Of the options, the colon is the only organ found in all four quadrants. The anus is in the midline and is not found in any of the four quadrants. The ileum or small intestine is found in the lower left and right quadrants. The liver is in the right upper quadrant.

36. **(D)** The product is located to the right of the arrow in a chemical equation. The arrow indicates a reaction has taken place. The remaining options are incorrect.

37. **(A)** The fight-or-flight response is a natural response when the body is threatened or stressed in some fashion (pain, fear, drop or increase in blood pressure or blood sugar, potential or actual physical injury). The response includes physical, nervous system, and endocrine changes. Activation of the autonomic nervous system leads to a chain of events that includes release of epinephrine by the adrenal medulla. The remaining option hormones are not involved with the fight-or-flight response. Oxytocin stimulates contractions during labor and promotes milk release, somatotropin is a growth hormone, and testosterone is responsible for secondary sex characteristics in males.

38. **(D)** There must be active involvement of body acids, bases, electrolytes, and fluids for homeostasis to be maintained. An ion is an electrically charged atom or group of atoms.

39. **(D)** The hyaline cartilage keeps the trachea from collapsing during inspiration. The remaining options are false. A decrease in plasma protein can cause edema in the extremities. A pH of 7.4 or greater indicates metabolic alkalosis. Acid/base is evaluated using arterial blood (think of arterial blood gases and what they measure).

40. **(C)** Metabolic acidosis and hyperventilation go hand in hand. Metabolic acidosis occurs when there is an excessive absorption/retention of acid or excessive excretion of bicarbonate. Hyperventilation is a compensatory process employed to decrease the acidity of the blood. Vigorous or excessive activity is one example of the etiology of lactic acid buildup in the blood that can produce a metabolic imbalance in the body. The remaining options are not compensatory mechanisms.

41. **(D)** All of the options have to do with the male urinary/reproductive system. The stem of the question is the definition of urethra.

42. **(B)** The ovaries are responsible for female reproductive health and have a role in both the reproductive and endocrine systems. Their reproductive function is to produce ova (egg cells). The function of the ovaries (as an endocrine gland) is secretion of estrogen and progesterone.

43. **(D)** In terms of genetic traits, the presence of a dominant gene masks that of a recessive gene when both are present. Dominant traits are outwardly present even when only one copy of the gene is present. Recessive traits are outwardly obvious when two copies of the recessive gene are present. In the case of butterfly wing length, the greater number of long wings over short wings suggests long wings are dominant and short wings are recessive.

44. **(D)** Of the options, only (D) is correct, the remaining are false statements. Atoms have an overall neutral charge with one electron for each proton. Protons in the nucleus are positive and neutrons are neutral. The valence is the outer shell, not the inner.

45. **(D)** Birds distribute a natural oil on their feathers when they preen. The oil provides for waterproofing and buoyancy. Crude oil coats bird feathers, adds weight, and affects buoyancy.

The mixing of crude oil and the natural oil on bird feathers has to do with polarity—polar substances mix. The remaining options have nothing to do with mixing of oils.

46. **(C)** Digestion begins in the mouth. Included in the components of saliva are digestive enzymes. The remaining options are incorrect.

47. **(B)** Functions of the frontal lobe include voluntary movement, motor integration, expressive language, social functioning, impulse inhibition, emotions, and short-term memory. The cerebellum controls muscle tone and motor coordination, equilibrium, and balance. Parietal lobe functions include cognition, visual perception, touch sensation, reading and writing, and mathematical computation. Temporal lobe functions include auditory perception, memory, speech, facial recognition, and visual perception.

48. **(C)** The stem of the question is the definition of oogenesis.

49. **(A)** The arrector pili is the smooth muscle attached to a hair follicle. Smooth muscles are innervated by nerve cells and fibers, nonvoluntary in nature, and respond to stimulation from hormones and nerve cells.

50. **(B)** Keratin, a fibrous structural protein and an essential component of hair, originates in the hair follicle. Elements in the hair are proteins, amino acids, melanin, and keratin. Keratin in the hair is considered "hard hair" because it is insoluble in water and incredibly strong. Keratin gives hair its strength.

51. **(A)** Mitochondria are the largest organelles in the cell. They are found in most eukaryotic cells and contain (a) enzymes needed for metabolism and (b) genetic material. Mitochondria are responsible for energy production using aerobic respiration. Mitochondria have their own DNA that comes through the maternal line.

52. **(D)** Aspirin reduces fever, inflammation, and pain by suppressing the production of prostaglandins, which cause fever, inflammation, and pain. Aspirin reduces glucose production, does not modulate pain, and reduces cortisol.

53. **(A)** One key to correctly answering this question is defining the word *appendage*—a subordinate part attached to something. What, at the beginning of the large intestine, could be considered an appendage? The appendix is the only logical answer. The appendix is attached to the cecum, the beginning area of the large intestine. None of the remaining options are considered appendages. The ileum and jejunum are part of the small intestine.

English and Language Usage

1. **(B)** The use of a semicolon indicates that the phrase or words that follow contain information related to what was previously stated in the sentence. The remaining options are incorrectly punctuated with each having comma-related errors. Option (A): delete comma after *although* and add comma after *storm*. Option (C): delete commas after *biology* and *of*. No commas are needed. Option (D): add comma after *breakers*, *gum*, and *balls*.

2. **(A)** A simple sentence contains a subject and a verb. The sentence is a completed thought that has one independent clause. There may be more than one subject and verb in a simple sentence. Option (B) is a compound sentence, and options (C) and (D) are complex sentences.

3. **(D)** Correlative conjunctions are always in pairs and are treated as being grammatically equal. Use of *whether . . . or* is correct in option (D). Examples are *neither . . . nor*, *either . . . or*, and *not only . . . but*. Options (A) and (B) do not contain correlative conjunctions, and option (C) should contain *neither . . . nor*.

4. **(D)** The word *platitude* is defined as something dull, common, or overused. *Platitudinous* and *boring* are synonyms. The remaining options are not synonyms of *boring*.

5. **(D)** The incorrect word is *colon,* which is part of the intestines and is located in the abdominal cavity. The word should be *cologne,* which is a fragrance such as a perfume or aftershave. The remaining options are correct.

6. **(B)** *Bulleten* is incorrectly spelled; it should read *bulletin*. The remaining options contain correctly spelled words.

7. **(C)** The word *affect* is incorrectly used in the sentence. *Effect* is the appropriate word. *Affect* denotes influencing, impressing, acting on, or producing a change. *Effect* stands for the result, outcome, accomplishment, or intention. Grief is the outcome of loss. A death has occurred, and the question asks about the outcome or end result. The remaining options use the appropriate verbiage.

8. **(B)** The correct word is *principal,* not *principle*. A *principal* is a school administrator; a *principle* is a law or standard. The remaining options are correct. Try to remember that a *principal* is a *pal* to students.

9. **(A)** The correct option is the definition of a compound sentence. The remaining options do not satisfy the definition of a compound sentence.

10. **(B)** *Dodge a bullet* is a slang term originating in the sixties meaning lucky or fortunate in sidestepping trouble or adversity. The sentence suggests Leo wasn't punished for breaking curfew because of his father's financial influence on the football team.

11. **(D)** Mnemonics are tools used to help remember information. The Great Lakes, going from west to east, are Superior (Super), Michigan (Man), Huron (Helps), Erie (Every), and Ontario (One). Other examples include the mnemonic for the order of operations (Please Excuse My Dear Aunt Sally) and the 12 cranial nerves (On Old Olympus' Towering Top A Fin And German Viewed Some Hops). The remaining options are not mnemonics for the Great Lakes.

12. **(D)** Something referred to as *rad* is first-rate, out-of-the-ordinary, awesome, or incredible. Something *stupendous* is fantastic, astonishing, phenomenal, or spectacular. The remaining options are not synonyms of *rad*.

13. **(C)** The root word *agri-* has to do with farming or ranching. Agribusiness is a college major that has to do with the business of ranching or farming. The remaining options are not realistic when their various meanings are considered.

14. **(D)** Inscriptions are often found on tombstones and provide information about the person buried there. *Inscript* means to write. The remaining options do not apply. A *caricature* is a drawing or a figure.

15. **(D)** *Allusionist* is incorrect; it should be *illusionist*, a person who creates illusions or magic by sleight of hand. The word *allude* means to imply or insinuate; *allusionist* is not a word. The remaining options are worded correctly.

16. **(B)** *Despicable* is the only antonym listed for *benign*. In the sentence, *benign* statements are kind, gracious, or innocent statements.

17. **(A)** The correct spelling is *loathful*. The *e* is dropped and the suffix, *-ful*, is added. The remaining options are spelled incorrectly.

18. **(C)** The root word *capit* stands for head. An example is *capital* meaning assets or headquarters. The remaining options are not definitions of *capit*.

19. **(A)** A dependent clause defines itself. While dependent clauses contain a subject and verb, they are not complete sentences. They are dependent on another sentence to be reasonable and complete. The word *although* is a subordinating conjunction that comes at the beginning of a dependent clause. It communicates that a relationship exists between the dependent clause and the attached independent clause or sentence. *I still feel like I could work another ten hours* is an independent clause and a complete sentence. The clauses *nodding off all day* and *work another ten hours* do not meet the criteria for dependent clauses.

20. **(B)** Compound-complex sentences are composed of at least two independent clauses and one or more dependent clauses (see rationale for question 19). *The river flooded* is an example of an independent clause and a complete sentence. *When the river flooded* is an example of a dependent clause. In the correct answer, *if I were young* is the dependent clause, and the clauses beginning with *I think I would* and *I would want* are independent clauses and complete sentences. Option (A) is a simple sentence containing compound subjects and compound verbs. Option (C) is a simple sentence. Option (D) is a compound sentence with three independent clauses.

21. **(D)** The word *tropic* is capitalized when used with such names as the Tropic of Cancer or Capricorn. *Holy City* in option (A) should be capitalized. *Valley* in option (B) should not be capitalized, and *Eighty-Sixth Congress* in option (C) should be capitalized.

22. **(A)** *Brainstorming* is a conference or discussion technique used to gather information, create new ideas, encourage thinking, and problem solve. The remaining options are subsets of *brainstorming*.

23. **(A)** The root word *bibli-* means book. A bibliography is a listing of referenced or nonreferenced sources used in the process of researching. Simply put, it says where information came from and gives appropriate credit. The remaining options all contain some aspect of writing, but do not define the root word.

24. **(A)** The root word *strict* means bind or binding. A restriction places limitations, controls, or restraints on something. For example, in an adult community, there may be restrictions on children under the age of 18. They may be guests for a prescribed period of time but may not be permanent residents. Registered nurses are bound by restrictions; the law delineates what are acceptable and nonacceptable nursing practices. The remaining options do not meet the definition of the root word.

25. **(B)** The correct sentence should read, "The community hospital, having been supported by community donations for so long, had to revamp many of its practices when it became the county hospital." The dependent phrase beginning with *having been supported . . .* provides information about why the hospital had to change its practices. The remaining options are correctly punctuated.

26. **(D)** Use of *illusions* is incorrect; the word *allusions* should have been used. *Illusions* are deceptions or magic tricks. *Allusions* are suggestions or insinuations. The remaining options are correctly written.

27. **(B)** The logical answer is to develop an idea. While checking out books at the library and searching the Internet are subsumed in developing an idea, as written they are vague and nonspecific. A topical outline could not be written until the selected topic is identified and developed. The question asks for the first step in the writing process, not how that step was accomplished.

28. **(C)** A well-written paragraph is logical and sequenced, and one sentence leads the reader to the next. Option (C), the correct answer, provides all of these. As the paragraph progresses, the reader is introduced to Katrine:

- She is 56 years of age.
- She dreamed of writing a children's book for many, many years.
- She doubted she had the skill to write a book.
- She was encouraged to write by a friend of many years.
- She takes her friend's advice and begins to write.
- The beginnings of a manuscript exist.

All of the options contain the same information; the difference has to do with writing style.

Practice Test 3

Reading

1. Ⓐ Ⓑ Ⓒ Ⓓ
2. Ⓐ Ⓑ Ⓒ Ⓓ
3. Ⓐ Ⓑ Ⓒ Ⓓ
4. Ⓐ Ⓑ Ⓒ Ⓓ
5. Ⓐ Ⓑ Ⓒ Ⓓ
6. Ⓐ Ⓑ Ⓒ Ⓓ
7. Ⓐ Ⓑ Ⓒ Ⓓ
8. Ⓐ Ⓑ Ⓒ Ⓓ
9. Ⓐ Ⓑ Ⓒ Ⓓ
10. Ⓐ Ⓑ Ⓒ Ⓓ
11. Ⓐ Ⓑ Ⓒ Ⓓ
12. Ⓐ Ⓑ Ⓒ Ⓓ
13. Ⓐ Ⓑ Ⓒ Ⓓ
14. Ⓐ Ⓑ Ⓒ Ⓓ

15. Ⓐ Ⓑ Ⓒ Ⓓ
16. Ⓐ Ⓑ Ⓒ Ⓓ
17. Ⓐ Ⓑ Ⓒ Ⓓ
18. Ⓐ Ⓑ Ⓒ Ⓓ
19. Ⓐ Ⓑ Ⓒ Ⓓ
20. Ⓐ Ⓑ Ⓒ Ⓓ
21. Ⓐ Ⓑ Ⓒ Ⓓ
22. Ⓐ Ⓑ Ⓒ Ⓓ
23. Ⓐ Ⓑ Ⓒ Ⓓ
24. Ⓐ Ⓑ Ⓒ Ⓓ
25. Ⓐ Ⓑ Ⓒ Ⓓ
26. Ⓐ Ⓑ Ⓒ Ⓓ
27. Ⓐ Ⓑ Ⓒ Ⓓ
28. Ⓐ Ⓑ Ⓒ Ⓓ

29. Ⓐ Ⓑ Ⓒ Ⓓ
30. Ⓐ Ⓑ Ⓒ Ⓓ
31. Ⓐ Ⓑ Ⓒ Ⓓ
32. Ⓐ Ⓑ Ⓒ Ⓓ
33. Ⓐ Ⓑ Ⓒ Ⓓ
34. Ⓐ Ⓑ Ⓒ Ⓓ
35. Ⓐ Ⓑ Ⓒ Ⓓ
36. Ⓐ Ⓑ Ⓒ Ⓓ
37. Ⓐ Ⓑ Ⓒ Ⓓ
38. Ⓐ Ⓑ Ⓒ Ⓓ
39. Ⓐ Ⓑ Ⓒ Ⓓ
40. Ⓐ Ⓑ Ⓒ Ⓓ
41. Ⓐ Ⓑ Ⓒ Ⓓ
42. Ⓐ Ⓑ Ⓒ Ⓓ

43. Ⓐ Ⓑ Ⓒ Ⓓ
44. Ⓐ Ⓑ Ⓒ Ⓓ
45. Ⓐ Ⓑ Ⓒ Ⓓ
46. Ⓐ Ⓑ Ⓒ Ⓓ
47. Ⓐ Ⓑ Ⓒ Ⓓ
48. Ⓐ Ⓑ Ⓒ Ⓓ
49. Ⓐ Ⓑ Ⓒ Ⓓ
50. Ⓐ Ⓑ Ⓒ Ⓓ
51. Ⓐ Ⓑ Ⓒ Ⓓ
52. Ⓐ Ⓑ Ⓒ Ⓓ
53. Ⓐ Ⓑ Ⓒ Ⓓ

Mathematics

1. Ⓐ Ⓑ Ⓒ Ⓓ
2. Ⓐ Ⓑ Ⓒ Ⓓ
3. Ⓐ Ⓑ Ⓒ Ⓓ
4. Ⓐ Ⓑ Ⓒ Ⓓ
5. Ⓐ Ⓑ Ⓒ Ⓓ
6. Ⓐ Ⓑ Ⓒ Ⓓ
7. Ⓐ Ⓑ Ⓒ Ⓓ
8. Ⓐ Ⓑ Ⓒ Ⓓ
9. Ⓐ Ⓑ Ⓒ Ⓓ

10. Ⓐ Ⓑ Ⓒ Ⓓ
11. Ⓐ Ⓑ Ⓒ Ⓓ
12. Ⓐ Ⓑ Ⓒ Ⓓ
13. Ⓐ Ⓑ Ⓒ Ⓓ
14. Ⓐ Ⓑ Ⓒ Ⓓ
15. Ⓐ Ⓑ Ⓒ Ⓓ
16. Ⓐ Ⓑ Ⓒ Ⓓ
17. Ⓐ Ⓑ Ⓒ Ⓓ
18. Ⓐ Ⓑ Ⓒ Ⓓ

19. Ⓐ Ⓑ Ⓒ Ⓓ
20. Ⓐ Ⓑ Ⓒ Ⓓ
21. Ⓐ Ⓑ Ⓒ Ⓓ
22. Ⓐ Ⓑ Ⓒ Ⓓ
23. Ⓐ Ⓑ Ⓒ Ⓓ
24. Ⓐ Ⓑ Ⓒ Ⓓ
25. Ⓐ Ⓑ Ⓒ Ⓓ
26. Ⓐ Ⓑ Ⓒ Ⓓ
27. Ⓐ Ⓑ Ⓒ Ⓓ

28. Ⓐ Ⓑ Ⓒ Ⓓ
29. Ⓐ Ⓑ Ⓒ Ⓓ
30. Ⓐ Ⓑ Ⓒ Ⓓ
31. Ⓐ Ⓑ Ⓒ Ⓓ
32. Ⓐ Ⓑ Ⓒ Ⓓ
33. Ⓐ Ⓑ Ⓒ Ⓓ
34. Ⓐ Ⓑ Ⓒ Ⓓ
35. Ⓐ Ⓑ Ⓒ Ⓓ
36. Ⓐ Ⓑ Ⓒ Ⓓ

ANSWER SHEET
Practice Test 3

Science

1. Ⓐ Ⓑ Ⓒ Ⓓ
2. Ⓐ Ⓑ Ⓒ Ⓓ
3. Ⓐ Ⓑ Ⓒ Ⓓ
4. Ⓐ Ⓑ Ⓒ Ⓓ
5. Ⓐ Ⓑ Ⓒ Ⓓ
6. Ⓐ Ⓑ Ⓒ Ⓓ
7. Ⓐ Ⓑ Ⓒ Ⓓ
8. Ⓐ Ⓑ Ⓒ Ⓓ
9. Ⓐ Ⓑ Ⓒ Ⓓ
10. Ⓐ Ⓑ Ⓒ Ⓓ
11. Ⓐ Ⓑ Ⓒ Ⓓ
12. Ⓐ Ⓑ Ⓒ Ⓓ
13. Ⓐ Ⓑ Ⓒ Ⓓ
14. Ⓐ Ⓑ Ⓒ Ⓓ

15. Ⓐ Ⓑ Ⓒ Ⓓ
16. Ⓐ Ⓑ Ⓒ Ⓓ
17. Ⓐ Ⓑ Ⓒ Ⓓ
18. Ⓐ Ⓑ Ⓒ Ⓓ
19. Ⓐ Ⓑ Ⓒ Ⓓ
20. Ⓐ Ⓑ Ⓒ Ⓓ
21. Ⓐ Ⓑ Ⓒ Ⓓ
22. Ⓐ Ⓑ Ⓒ Ⓓ
23. Ⓐ Ⓑ Ⓒ Ⓓ
24. Ⓐ Ⓑ Ⓒ Ⓓ
25. Ⓐ Ⓑ Ⓒ Ⓓ
26. Ⓐ Ⓑ Ⓒ Ⓓ
27. Ⓐ Ⓑ Ⓒ Ⓓ
28. Ⓐ Ⓑ Ⓒ Ⓓ

29. Ⓐ Ⓑ Ⓒ Ⓓ
30. Ⓐ Ⓑ Ⓒ Ⓓ
31. Ⓐ Ⓑ Ⓒ Ⓓ
32. Ⓐ Ⓑ Ⓒ Ⓓ
33. Ⓐ Ⓑ Ⓒ Ⓓ
34. Ⓐ Ⓑ Ⓒ Ⓓ
35. Ⓐ Ⓑ Ⓒ Ⓓ
36. Ⓐ Ⓑ Ⓒ Ⓓ
37. Ⓐ Ⓑ Ⓒ Ⓓ
38. Ⓐ Ⓑ Ⓒ Ⓓ
39. Ⓐ Ⓑ Ⓒ Ⓓ
40. Ⓐ Ⓑ Ⓒ Ⓓ
41. Ⓐ Ⓑ Ⓒ Ⓓ
42. Ⓐ Ⓑ Ⓒ Ⓓ

43. Ⓐ Ⓑ Ⓒ Ⓓ
44. Ⓐ Ⓑ Ⓒ Ⓓ
45. Ⓐ Ⓑ Ⓒ Ⓓ
46. Ⓐ Ⓑ Ⓒ Ⓓ
47. Ⓐ Ⓑ Ⓒ Ⓓ
48. Ⓐ Ⓑ Ⓒ Ⓓ
49. Ⓐ Ⓑ Ⓒ Ⓓ
50. Ⓐ Ⓑ Ⓒ Ⓓ
51. Ⓐ Ⓑ Ⓒ Ⓓ
52. Ⓐ Ⓑ Ⓒ Ⓓ
53. Ⓐ Ⓑ Ⓒ Ⓓ

English and Language Usage

1. Ⓐ Ⓑ Ⓒ Ⓓ
2. Ⓐ Ⓑ Ⓒ Ⓓ
3. Ⓐ Ⓑ Ⓒ Ⓓ
4. Ⓐ Ⓑ Ⓒ Ⓓ
5. Ⓐ Ⓑ Ⓒ Ⓓ
6. Ⓐ Ⓑ Ⓒ Ⓓ
7. Ⓐ Ⓑ Ⓒ Ⓓ

8. Ⓐ Ⓑ Ⓒ Ⓓ
9. Ⓐ Ⓑ Ⓒ Ⓓ
10. Ⓐ Ⓑ Ⓒ Ⓓ
11. Ⓐ Ⓑ Ⓒ Ⓓ
12. Ⓐ Ⓑ Ⓒ Ⓓ
13. Ⓐ Ⓑ Ⓒ Ⓓ
14. Ⓐ Ⓑ Ⓒ Ⓓ

15. Ⓐ Ⓑ Ⓒ Ⓓ
16. Ⓐ Ⓑ Ⓒ Ⓓ
17. Ⓐ Ⓑ Ⓒ Ⓓ
18. Ⓐ Ⓑ Ⓒ Ⓓ
19. Ⓐ Ⓑ Ⓒ Ⓓ
20. Ⓐ Ⓑ Ⓒ Ⓓ
21. Ⓐ Ⓑ Ⓒ Ⓓ

22. Ⓐ Ⓑ Ⓒ Ⓓ
23. Ⓐ Ⓑ Ⓒ Ⓓ
24. Ⓐ Ⓑ Ⓒ Ⓓ
25. Ⓐ Ⓑ Ⓒ Ⓓ
26. Ⓐ Ⓑ Ⓒ Ⓓ
27. Ⓐ Ⓑ Ⓒ Ⓓ
28. Ⓐ Ⓑ Ⓒ Ⓓ

READING

NUMBER OF QUESTIONS: 53

TIME LIMIT: 64 MINUTES

Instructions: Read each question thoroughly. Select the single best answer. Mark your answer (A, B, C, or D) on the answer sheet provided for Practice Test 3.

Question 1 is based on the following two images.

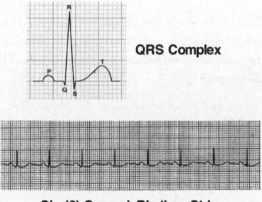

QRS Complex

Six (6) Second Rhythm Strip

1. The QRS complex is an electrical representation of one complete normal heartbeat. The rhythm strip is a series of normal heartbeats from an EKG (electrocardiogram) tracing. Determine the approximate heart rate for one (1) minute.

   (A) 60 beats/min
   (B) 80 beats/min
   (C) 90 beats/min
   (D) Not enough information is provided to determine the heart rate.

---

2. Sarah had wanted to sky dive since she was a teenager but never had the resources to do so. Now a strong, healthy adult with a sound, well-paying job, she is about to fulfill her dream. She'd taken the course from a licensed instructor at the jump school and practiced until she could do the procedures blindfolded. She was ready, or at least she thought she was, until she was four jumpers away from the plane's exit door. Everything was running smoothly, but something kept telling her that today was not the day to jump.

   What is the logical conclusion from reading this passage?

   (A) Sarah has had a premonition.
   (B) Sarah has pre-jump jitters.
   (C) Sarah is not psychologically prepared to jump today.
   (D) Sarah needs more practice to strengthen her resolve.

3. A politician tells his supporters that when elected he will lower the tax rate, bring more high-tech businesses to the city, upgrade the city's 911 system, and bring a level of prosperity the city hasn't enjoyed for over half a century.

   This statement is an example of a(n)

   (A) bias.
   (B) fact.
   (C) opinion.
   (D) stereotype.

Questions 4–6 are based on the following conversation between a father and his son who will soon graduate from high school.

Father: "James, I simply do not understand why you do not want to go to college. There's a perfectly good community college right here in the city where you could go for almost nothing. Have you forgotten the scholarship they offered would reduce your cost to around $100 per semester? And you could live at home to save money."

James: "No, I haven't forgotten, and we've talked about this before, Dad. I still think college is a waste of time and there are things I want to do, and it isn't more school!"

Father: "Yes, we've talked about this before, but as usual, you're weak on talking about the things you want to do. You've *balked* every time I asked. Let's get down to brass tacks here—tell me what it is you plan to do."

James: "Well, the first thing I want to do is get a car of my own. I've saved since I was old enough to get a job, and I've got almost $3,000 in the bank. I've found a Camaro at the Chevy house for a little over $26,000 and it's just three years old with low mileage and one owner. It's what I've always wanted. Then I want to move to Alaska and work on a fishing boat—those guys on TV make loads of money and most of them don't have college degrees. I figure I could get an off-road vehicle and travel around Alaska in the off-season. That way the Camaro wouldn't get beat up driving on dirt roads."

Father: "Whoa, son. Let's stop a minute and look at what you've just said. These things you want to do are admirable, but they're not realistic for someone with a high school education and no reliable source of income. You'd need a loan to buy the Camaro and you have no credit rating or a job so you can't make payments. Then there's car insurance—your age puts you in a higher bracket for insurance, and insurance on sports cars is high. You talk about moving to Alaska. How will you get there without money for transportation, food, gas, and lodging? Have you considered the distance from here in New Orleans to Alaska? It'll cost money just to get there. Where will the money come from to live in Alaska? Do you know how the cost of living in Alaska compares to New Orleans . . ."

James: "OK, Dad, stop already. You've made your point. There's a lot I hadn't thought of . . . ."

4. What type of reasoning is the father using when talking with his son about buying a car and moving to Alaska?

   (A) Assertion
   (B) Argument
   (C) Claim
   (D) Predictive

5. What does the father mean when he says "Let's get down to brass tacks here—tell me what it is you plan to do?"

   (A) Tacks made of brass are somehow involved.
   (B) The father is using jargon James will understand.
   (C) The phrase is a veiled threat.
   (D) The phrase is an idiom.

6. Based upon the conversation, what is an appropriate antonym for *balked*?

   (A) Acquiesced
   (B) Dodged
   (C) Hesitated
   (D) Resisted

Questions 7–9 are based on the following passage.

Lake Hope is a private recreation area located on a ranch in the mountains of Idaho. It offers all of the amenities including day activities, an information center with an ATM machine, overnight camping, bathroom/shower/laundry facilities, a combination gas station/grocery/restaurant, and a clinic for minor injuries. The area has been a favorite for outdoor enthusiasts for more than 60 years. While the area is open to the public, fees for admission are steep and rules are stringent. Lake Hope has always been family oriented. This year, however, a rowdy element has been negatively influencing area activities, causing a rise in complaints, vandalism, and serious injuries. The family owning Lake Hope has decided to implement a new policy making Lake Hope a drug-free recreational area since over 96 percent of problems have been directly associated with alcohol and other drug use. The owners have also decided to increase the security force, which is comprised of off-duty law enforcement officers, by 50 percent. Last, for the first time in its history, Lake Hope will permanently deny admission to individuals and/or groups deemed problematic.

7. What evidence is presented in the passage that suggests change needs to be made?

   (A) Increase in family-related complaints
   (B) High cost of admission
   (C) Lake Hope is a public area, not a private area.
   (D) Surge in negative activities

8. A local newspaper article maintains that the Lake Hope owners' actions are relevant to their situation. What does this newspaper statement mean? (The above passage is not the newspaper article.)

   (A) Actions are related to or connected to the situation.
   (B) Actions are trivial since the identified problems are common in all venues.
   (C) An exact description of all problems is needed to fully understand the newspaper's statement.
   (D) The newspaper statement cannot be fully understood unless the entire article is read.

9. What is the structure of the passage?

   (A) Chronicle
   (B) Explanatory
   (C) Influential
   (D) Vague

Questions 10–13 are based on the following chart.

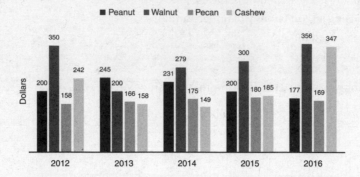

10. Select the presentation of the chart.

(A) Area
(B) Bar
(C) Column
(D) Line

11. Which nut brittle has been the best seller over time?

(A) Cashew
(B) Peanut
(C) Pecan
(D) Walnut

12. The steering committee has decided to offer only three types of nut brittle next year. Which nut brittle should be excluded?

(A) Cashew
(B) Peanut
(C) Pecan
(D) Walnut

13. Which of the following years had the best nut brittle sales?

(A) 2012
(B) 2013
(C) 2014
(D) 2015

14. Which of the following would employ a style guide?

    (A) A printer of books

    (B) A business card developer

    (C) A newspaper

    (D) A social club

15. All of the following are examples of secondary sources EXCEPT

    (A) a research paper written by you.

    (B) biographical sketches of Congressional Medal of Honor Awardees.

    (C) a commentary of state parks in Alaska.

    (D) an encyclopedia about nineteenth-century artwork.

Questions 16–19 are based on the following printed communication.

MEMO

To: All Employees of SoftwareCom, America

From: Thomas P. Hardling, Executive CEO, SoftwareCom, International

Date: March 16

Re: Realignment

As I am sure you all know, Crimson Mountain Tech and Hardling and Sons, Incorporated, merged into SoftwareCom, International, on March 13th of this year. While both companies have been strengthened by this merger, we recognize that duplication of services occurs when companies unite for the betterment of both. As a result, there will be a trimming of services over the next six months as SoftwareCom reorganizes. Realignment of employees will begin in approximately two weeks and will be companywide at all levels. SoftwareCom will cease using temporary employees on April 15th. All other employees will receive notification of their employment status with SoftwareCom at the end of their tier period. Please be aware that those employees continuing with SoftwareCom may or may not retain the same *position and/or grade level*. The following timeline has been developed.

Tier 1: Notification April 1st

- Less than five years' employment
- San Francisco and New York offices
- Work history

Tier 2: Notification May 15th

- Between five and nine years' employment
- Miami office
- Work history

Tier 3: Notification June 30th

- Between 10 and 19 years' employment
- Dallas, Miami, and New York offices
- Work history

Tier 4: Notification August 5th

- Greater than 20 years' of employment
- All U.S. offices
- Work history

Tier 5: Notification September 20th

- Employees not included in Tiers 1–4 regardless of employment time or location
- Work history

All terminated employees, except those released for problematic work history, may reapply for employment. There is no guarantee of rehire or appointment to previous *position or grade level* if rehired.

Please do not call Human Resources for clarification or additional information, as they will be following up and working with affected employees individually. Additional communications will be coming out weekly—be sure to check your company e-mail on a daily basis.

Thank you all for your cooperation with SoftwareCom, International.

16. What is the logical conclusion of reading this memo?

    (A) Employee rights will be violated.
    (B) Employees will be kept informed of company changes.
    (C) Many employees will be terminated for bogus reasons.
    (D) Employees will be terminated as a result of reorganization.

17. What is the nature of the information presented in the memo?

    (A) Conjecture
    (B) Implicit
    (C) Implied
    (D) Inferred

18. Is the information in the memo delineated?

    (A) No, information is not comprehensive.
    (B) No, information is not logical.
    (C) Yes, information is clearly and precisely stated.
    (D) Yes, information is presented in a topical fashion.

19. What does the term *position/grade level* imply?

    (A) They are federally mandated hiring practices based on modified versions of the Civil Rights Act of 1965 and 1969.
    (B) They are gender-related policies and procedures to ensure gender discrimination.
    (C) They are systems within an organization that make distinctions between employee positions and/or titles.
    (D) They have to do with the number of years in a position and the highest educational grade level achieved by an employee.

Question 20 is based on the following passage and map of the United States.

Nathan has a goal of visiting the capital of each state in the continental United States. He is plotting a road trip from his home in Austin, Texas, to Olympia, Washington, and plans on visiting the capital of each state he visits. He decides to take the westernmost route available in his travels.

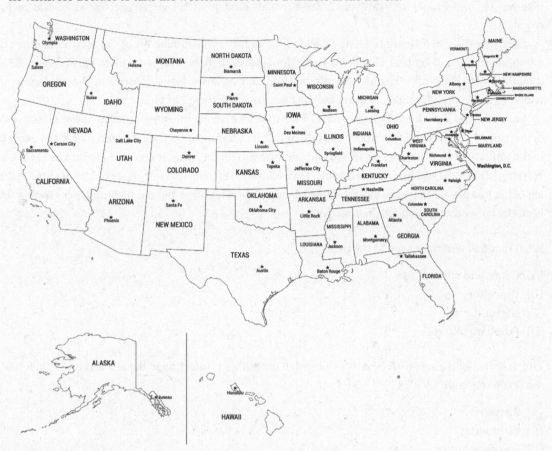

20. Select the correct order of capital cities Nathan will visit on his trip.

(A) Denver, Cheyenne, Boise, Salem, and Olympia
(B) Oklahoma City, Topeka, Lincoln, Pierre, Bismarck, Helena, and Olympia
(C) Santa Fe, Phoenix, Sacramento, Salem, and Olympia
(D) Santa Fe, Salt Lake City, Boise, and Olympia

Questions 21–25 are based on the following passage.

Denny decided to ride his bicycle to the recreation area to ride the mountain bike trials for the day. The weather forecast was hot and dry with a ten percent chance of afternoon thunderstorms so he left home with five sandwiches, one canteen of water, another filled with an energy drink, and a handful of energy bars. He also left a note telling his mother where he would be. Denny was a seasoned and safe mountain biker. He had earned merit badges teaching bicycle safety to elementary school children and mountain biking to a group of students who were forming a mountain biking club at the local high school. *Even with his safe practices and knowledge of mountain biking, Denny wasn't prepared for what he encountered after an incredibly fierce thunderstorm.*

The heavy rain had turned the trails into slippery, sliding mud and *potholes* filled with water, small pine branches, and other unseen hazards. His progress was slow. He fell several times, skinning his arms and legs. The last fall was the worst—he and his bike slid into a rock and tumbled headlong off the trail. Aside from more scraps and skins, he had a bad gash on his leg, he'd put a sizable dent into his helmet, and his bike was beyond simple trail-side repair. The tire had come off of the wheel, and the wheel was no longer circular.

After assessing his situation, Denny decided his best bet was to hike off of the mountain and call his parents to come and get him. He cut his T-shirt into pieces to make a pressure bandage for his leg. His first thought was to leave his bike and hike out, but he'd mowed lawns last summer and shoveled snow in the winter to have enough money to purchase the bike, and he just couldn't leave it.

Denny looked like a walking ball of mud by the time he reached the ranger station. It was closed because of inclement weather and the ranger had left. At first he was angry, then he realized that in his haste to get to the trails, he'd forgotten to sign in. No one knew he was on the trails. It was going to be a long walk home carrying his bicycle and his leg was hurting. He decided to rest, eat, and rehydrate before beginning the last leg of his journey. Denny was almost to the highway when he saw a big red pick-up truck coming toward him. His father drove a big red pick-up truck.

21. What mode of writing is used in the passage?

   (A) Cause and effect
   (B) Expository
   (C) Narrative
   (D) Problem/solution

22. Which of the following terms best identifies what the author is inferring in the last sentence (italicized) of the first paragraph?

   (A) Answer
   (B) Estimating
   (C) Foreshadowing
   (D) Result

23. What genre does the passage best fit into?

   (A) Adventure
   (B) Family and relationships
   (C) Humorous
   (D) Steampunk

24. Based on information given in the passage, what is a synonym for *pothole*?

   (A) Closing
   (B) Depression
   (C) Grade
   (D) Hill

25. What is meant by *Denny looked like a walking ball of mud* in the passage?

    (A) He was ball shaped.
    (B) He left a trail of dripping mud behind him.
    (C) He was covered in mud from head to foot.
    (D) He was a humorous-looking figure.

---

26. The mayor previously stated voting turnout would be light since the county usually reelected the incumbent. This statement is an example of

    (A) bias.
    (B) fact.
    (C) impartiality.
    (D) stereotype.

27. A chapter in a book on cells has the following subheadings: (a) The cell and its membranes; (b) Cell junctions; (c) Cell movement; and (d) Cell division. Which of the following subsections contains specific information on the average length of time for mitosis?

    (A) The cell and its membranes
    (B) Cell division
    (C) Cell junctions
    (D) Cell movement

28. Henry wants to find synonyms for the word *youth*. Which of the following would be his best source of information?

    (A) A word strategy book
    (B) A dictionary
    (C) An encyclopedia
    (D) A thesaurus

29. Ben exclaimed to his friend, "Man, I am in really deep doo-doo! Mrs. Strong caught me using a crib sheet on the math test."
    Select the best alternative wording for *I am in really deep doo-doo*.

    (A) I did a stupid thing.
    (B) I'm in trouble.
    (C) I'm on my way to detention.
    (D) I was discovered and can't get out of it.

30. The guides at the top of a page in a dictionary are *bushel* and *can*. Which of the following words are found on this page?

    (A) Burst
    (B) Bushwhack
    (C) Cancel
    (D) Cane

31. Dawn needs to earn a "B" in her creative writing course to take the advanced creative writing class next semester. She has submitted three writing assignments and received a "C" on each paper. Her creative writing teacher tells Dawn that her topic selections are excellent and her papers are grammatically correct, but she has one problem preventing her from receiving higher grades: her papers lack complexity and variability. Her writing abounds with simplistic phrases and words. Which of the following is the most logical for Dawn's teacher to suggest to improve her writing?

(A) *Robert's Rules of Order*
(B) *The Elements of Style*
(C) *The Oxford American Writer's Thesaurus*
(D) *Webster's New World College Dictionary*

32. Hanna is planning a three-week vacation through the mountain states. Which of the following states will not be included in her itinerary?

(A) Colorado
(B) Idaho
(C) Nebraska
(D) New Mexico

Questions 33–35 are based on the following passage and table.

Samantha is tired of physicians keeping her black ink pens when writing orders after seeing their patients. She decides to order pens that have her name on them to use at work. She searches the Internet and finds the following four companies who offer free shipping on all orders.

Pen Color	Good Write Pens	Wally's Scribbles	Mountain Pen Company	Reliable Ink
Black	$0.89/pen $40/50 pens $75/100 pens	$0.95/pen $45/50 pens $85/100 pens	$0.83/pen $35/50 pens $72/100 pens	$0.99/pen $95/100 pens
Blue	$0.95/pen $45/50 pens $90/100 pens	$1.00/pen $48/50 pens $90/100 pens	$0.76/pen $35/50 pens $60/100 pens	$0.85/pen $42/50 pens $80/100 pens
Red	$1.20/pen $40/50 pens $70/100 pens	$0.95/pen $45/50 pens $90/100 pens	$1.00/pen $43/50 pens $80/100 pens	$1.25/pen $58/50 pens $110/100 pens
Random color mix	$50/50 pens $95/100 pens	$40/50 pens $80/100 pens		

33. Which company offers the best price for black ink pens when bought individually?

(A) Good Write Pens
(B) Mountain Pen Company
(C) Reliable Ink
(D) Wally's Scribbles

34. Which company has the highest price for any individual color ink pen?

  (A) Good Write Pens
  (B) Mountain Pen Company
  (C) Reliable Ink
  (D) Wally's Scribbles

35. Samantha decides to purchase 50 red ink pens in addition to 100 black ink pens since she occasionally uses red ink at work. What companies should she buy from?

  (A) Good Write Pens and Wally's Scribbles
  (B) Good Write Pens and Mountain Pen company
  (C) Reliable Ink and Mountain Pen Company
  (D) Wally's Scribbles and Reliable Ink

Questions 36–39 are based on the following passage.

The following is the introduction from *The White Indian Boy: The Story of Uncle Nick Among the Shoshones*, by Elijah Nicholas Wilson. The book, published in 1910, is Wilson's autobiographical history of growing up in the 1800s in what is now Wyoming.

"The number of men and woman who played a part in the conquest and settlement of the Great West grows smaller year by year, and the passing of those plainsmen and mountaineers marks the close of an era in our national life. To put into permanent form, as has been done in the book, a pioneer's recollections of his early days, with their trials and adventures, is to make a certain contribution to history. Such a record shows us the courage, perseverance, and hardihood with which the foundations of the nation were laid, and to read it is to watch a state in the making. As a story of the days when Indian tribes still roamed the plains, this book will have for boys and girls all the interest of a tale of adventure. It is hoped that it will also give the reader a realization of the hardships and dangers so manfully faced by the settlers of the West and will implant in them a desire to prove themselves worthy successors to those builders of the nation."

36. What is the purpose of the above introduction to *The White Indian Boy*?

  (A) To announce the publication of the book
  (B) To explain why Wilson wrote the book
  (C) To get a potential reader's attention and present the subject and its limitations
  (D) To present a biographical sketch of pioneer life in the 1800s

37. The intended audience of *The White Indian Boy* is

  (A) children under the age of 13 or 14.
  (B) elderly individuals who grew to adulthood during the 1800s.
  (C) individuals from other countries interested in America's Great West.
  (D) individuals ranging from childhood through old age.

38. Why is *The White Indian Boy: The Story of Uncle Nick Among the Shoshones* italicized?

  (A) It accentuates the book is a narrative.
  (B) It is the title of the book.
  (C) It suggests the appropriate library location for placement.
  (D) It underscores the book is about a boy.

39. *The White Indian Boy: The Story of Uncle Nick Among the Shoshones* is an example of which of the following?

   (A) Bibliographical source
   (B) Biographical source
   (C) Nonverbal source
   (D) Primary source

---

40. Information on the back of a brochure said: *Queries should be sent to bnrw@runaway.com.* What is a *query*?

   (A) A command or decision
   (B) A question or inquiry
   (C) A repudiation or reply
   (D) A victory or agreement

41. Aidan was looking forward to taking a three-semester-hour course in marriage and family counseling until he discovered the course was offered as a five-day pass/fail course. What does the use of the slash (/) with pass/fail indicate in this sentence?

   (A) A slash indicates a choice such as peas/carrots, long route/short route, and red shoes/black shoes.
   (B) A slash indicates difference such as color/colour, honor/honour, and liter/litre.
   (C) A slash indicates an alternative such as up/down, male/female, and in/out.
   (D) A slash indicates a period of time such as 1898/1910, March/June, and 3:00 P.M./7:00 P.M.

Questions 42–44 are based on the following from the Dewey Decimal system.

200	Religion
201	Religious mythology, general classes of religion, interreligious relations and attitudes, social theology
202	Doctrines
203	Public worship and other practices
204	Religious experience, life, practice
205	Religious ethics
206	Leaders and organization
207	Missions and religious education
208	Sources
209	Sects and reform movements

42. Phil has decided to write his paper on the current guidelines and policies of the Roman Catholic Church. In which section of the Dewey decimal system is he most likely to find the information he needs?

   (A) Doctrines
   (B) Missions and religious education
   (C) Public worship and other practices
   (D) Religious ethics

43. Heidi is interested in offshoots of the Baptist Church. In which section should she begin her research?

(A) Leaders and organization

(B) Religious ethics

(C) Religious mythology, general classes of religion, interreligious relations and attitudes, social theology

(D) Sects and reform movements

44. Stephen is engaged to a woman who embraces the ancient religious philosophy of Taoism. He wants to learn more about her religious lifestyle. In what section of the Dewey decimal system should he begin?

(A) Missions and religious education

(B) Religious ethics

(C) Religious experience, life, practice

(D) Sources

Questions 45–50 are based on the following passage.

"As Speaker of this great legislative body, I tell you that this great state cannot endure another crisis! Twenty percent of our counties cannot pay for the gasoline to run their school bus service, and must ask parents to transport their children to and from school five days a week. Twenty-five percent of our counties have dropped their school meal programs—this means there are no meals for the underprivileged and the remaining students must bring their lunch if they wish to eat during the school day. Eighty-five percent of our schools have closed their athletic and after-school clubs and/or programs. Truancy has risen by 22 percent because nearly 100 percent of our schools have been forced to terminate their truancy officers. Over the past three years, the high school graduation rate has dropped by 12 percent a year across the state.

Fifteen percent of our counties have city and county employees who have not been paid in over 60 days. Seventy-two percent of our counties do not have the gasoline to keep their vehicles running, and law enforcement officers have ceased patrols and only respond to emergencies in many rural areas, and most other emergency services no longer exist. The state crime rate has risen by 32 percent in the last 20 months, and the jails are filled to capacity.

I could go on, but we'd be here for days. Our infrastructure is failing! It's time that we, as legislators who were elected by the people, address this problem that has been steadily growing for the past three years and act for the good of the people we serve. The time for *parsimonious* behavior is past. We've sat in this great chamber of integrity and done nothing but sit on a surplus of over $1 billion that we tell the people is saved for a rainy day. Well, that rainy day has about drowned us, and we need to do something!"

45. Which of the following is a concise summary of the passage?

(A) A lack of financial resources is the cause of the state's problems.

(B) Crisis has overwhelmed the infrastructure of a state, and the state's legislative body has the ability to intervene.

(C) Crisis in a state always causes problems that only elected officials can solve.

(D) The state's infrastructure has failed because of poor leadership and/or management at the state and local levels.

46. What is the crisis that has occurred in this state?

(A) The crisis is not given, only its negative results.

(B) The state's education program has collapsed.

(C) The state government has miscarried.

(D) The state has no financial resources.

47. Who is the Speaker addressing?

(A) Elected county policymakers
(B) Elected members of parliament
(C) Elected self-interest groups
(D) Elected state representatives

48. What is implied in the passage?

(A) The state's legislative body does not have the power or authority to intervene.
(B) The state's legislative body has the means to assist both the people and the state.
(C) The state's legislative body is not interested in the state's problems.
(D) The state's legislative body was unable to prevent the crisis.

49. What does the word *parsimonious* suggest about the legislators?

(A) They are out of touch with reality.
(B) They believe the counties should manage their resources in a more prudent fashion.
(C) They do not fully understand the needs of their constituents.
(D) They have been unwilling to spend money.

50. Which of the following best describes the mode of the passage?

(A) Argumentative/opinionated
(B) Problem/solution
(C) Cause/effect
(D) Compare/contrast

Question 51 is based on the following memo.

MEMO

To: Sharon Plides, Sophomore Class Coordinator

Marcus Thompson, Junior Class Coordinator

Phillip Swenson, Senior Class Coordinator

From: Molly Duncan, Vice Principal of Student Life

Date: August 5

RE: Student body president interviews

I am sending this memo as a follow-up to our meetings with the four students interested in serving as student body president for the upcoming academic year.

Marsha Johnsonstein: Three absences in last two years. GPA—3.7. President of Carthaginians, vice president of Volleyball Club, and member of Pep Squad. On time for interview. Professionally groomed and dressed. Had an acceptable working knowledge of duties of student body president and stated "my girls will always help when I need it." Saw no areas in need of improvement. Answered cell phone four times and talked with callers and responded to two text messages—stated "I just have to stay in touch with my girls."

Duncan MacMasters: Sixty-one absent days during sophomore year from motor vehicle accident that has left him wheelchair bound. Communication Club members videoed all courses and kept him up to date. Family members or friends delivered and returned homework assignments. GPA of 3.5 did not suffer during this time, current is 3.3. Member of Communication Club, student assistant to the coach for Gymnastics Club. On time for interview. Professionally groomed and dressed. Well prepared for interview. Excellent understanding of duties of student body president. Identified areas in need of improvement: staggering of lunch schedules, traffic congestion at end of school day, and better interface between students and security.

<u>Barbra Dunn</u>: Seventeen absent days during last school year with 14 truancies. History of truancy since seventh grade. GPA—2.05. Fifteen minutes late for interview. Did not state reason, just arrived late. Dressed casually in faded jeans, sandals, and halter top. No club affiliation. Stated, "I don't attend any of the sporting events—I don't like sports." Vague awareness of duties of student body president and stated, "If I get it, I'll learn what I need to do." Had no suggestions of needed improvements except covered parking should be provided for students to keep their cars cooler in hot weather.

<u>Honeysuckle Mimes</u>: Did not show for interview after calling and stating she would be approximately 30 minutes late. Presented at my office two days later requesting interview time. No reason given for failure to come to interview. No interview time given—told she did not meet criteria.

Please review my interview notes and let me know if any additions/deletions are necessary. The interview tapes are available, if needed. Formal file copies will be sent to you as soon as they are available.

51. Which of the following best describes the mode of the memo?

(A) Argument
(B) Expository
(C) Problem
(D) Opinion

Questions 52–53 are based on the following text and map.

You have been asked to develop written directions for the Buford family reunion picnic based on the map below. The directions and the map will be included in the packet sent to all individuals interested in attending the family reunion. County Road 117 leaving the small town of Bugtussle dead ends at Landers Lane. The family reunion will be held at picnic site C. The map is not drawn to scale.

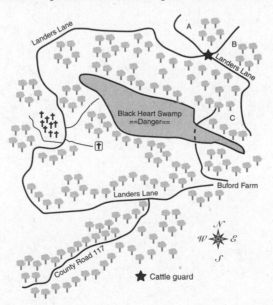

52. Select the most clearly written directions to the site of the Buford family reunion picnic.

(A) Take County Road 117 and turn left when it dead ends. Stay on Landers Lane until you reach picnic site C.

(B) Take County Road 117 east out of Bugtussle. The county road will dead end at Landers Lane. Turn west onto Landers Lane. You will stay on Landers Lane until you reach picnic site C. As you travel, you will pass Sweet Hope Community Church (on the right) and the Sweet Hope Cemetery (on the left). There are no other buildings on your route until you reach picnic site C. Continue on Landers Lane until you come to an intersection with a cattle guard. The pavement ends here. Cross the cattle guard and immediately turn right onto a gravel road. A short way down the road is a sign on your right identifying picnic site C.

(C) There are two possible routes to picnic site C. The shortest and most direct route is to take County Road 117 to Buford Farm. Take the dirt road around Buford Farm and then take the first north dirt road. You will come to Black Heart Swamp, which is usually dry during late summer. Make sure it's dry. Wet-looking places are probably quicksand. Cross the swamp and you will come out behind picnic site C. To take the longer route, take County Road 117 until it dead ends and turn left onto Landers Land and continue on it until reaching picnic site C.

(D) Take County Road 117 west to Landers Lane and turn right. Stay on this road until you reach the picnic site.

53. What part of the map suggests that hazards may exist?

(A) Lack of mile markers
(B) The word *Danger* under Black Heart Swamp label
(C) Traffic signs, such as stop signs and speed limit signs not indicated on the map
(D) Unpaved roads

MATHEMATICS

NUMBER OF QUESTIONS: 36

TIME LIMIT: 54 MINUTES

Instructions: Read each question thoroughly. Select the single best answer. Mark your answer (A, B, C, or D) on the answer sheet provided for Practice Test 3.

1. $10 \times 18.5 \div 34 =$ _____. Round your answer to the nearest tenth.

    (A) 4.6
    (B) 5.4
    (C) 8.0
    (D) 10.1

2. A gumball machine holds 200 candies. Fifteen percent of the candies are yellow, twenty percent are green, and seventeen percent are red. The remainder are multicolored. How many candies are multicolored?

    (A) 48
    (B) 52
    (C) 96
    (D) 104

3. What is the result when numbers are raised to the third power?

    (A) Cube
    (B) Even number
    (C) Odd number
    (D) Square

4. A nursing unit orders the following extra supplies because of a sudden census increase. What is the cost to the unit?

    > Cloth tape—4 boxes @ $30/box
    > Paper tape—6 boxes @ $55/box
    > NuGauze 1″—15 bottles @ $75/bottle
    > Alcohol swabs—30 boxes @ $15/box

    (A) $1,962
    (B) $2,025
    (C) $2,540
    (D) $2,750

5. Change $\frac{9}{5}$ to a mixed number.

    (A) $\frac{4}{5}$
    (B) $1\frac{1}{3}$
    (C) $1\frac{4}{5}$
    (D) 2

6. Solve the following equation. Round your answer to the nearest thousandth.

   23% of x = 25

   (A) 5.753
   (B) 57.006
   (C) 92.023
   (D) 108.696

7. Solve for x. Round your answer to the nearest hundredth.

   $$\frac{88}{x} = \frac{58}{100}$$

   (A) 51.04
   (B) 66.76
   (C) 144.39
   (D) 151.72

8. An amount b is equal to 5 plus 17 times 3 times 2 minus 4. Solve for b.

   (A) 103
   (B) 128
   (C) 152
   (D) 170

9. The sum of two numbers is 108. One number is 84. What is the first action after changing the sentences into an equation?

   (A) Addition
   (B) Division
   (C) Multiplication
   (D) Subtraction

10. What is the denominator in a fraction when 250 is the numerator and simplification of the fraction equals 50?

   (A) $\frac{1}{5}$
   (B) $\frac{3}{5}$
   (C) 5
   (D) 25

11. Determine the volume of a cube that has a side of 7.75 inches.

   (A) 60 cu in.
   (B) 146.75 cu in.
   (C) 232.74 cu in.
   (D) 465.48 cu in.

12. Arrange the following numbers from the least to the greatest.

    8   5.74   14   20.202   10.3   7.005

    (A) 5.74, 7.005, 8, 10.3, 14, 20.202
    (B) 5.74, 7.005, 10.3, 20.202, 8, 14
    (C) 8, 14, 10.3, 7.005, 20.202, 5.74
    (D) 20.202, 14, 10.3, 8, 7.005, 5.74

13. A sack of marbles contains 14 blue marbles out of a total of 150 marbles. What percentage of the marbles is blue?

    (A) 9.3%
    (B) 10%
    (C) 13.6%
    (D) 10.7%

14. Convert 0.6734 to a percent.

    (A) 6.734%
    (B) 67.34%
    (C) 673.4%
    (D) 6734%

15. Dividing a number such as $\frac{32}{8}$ is the same as multipling the denominator by _____ to yield the numerator.

    (A) $\frac{1}{4}$

    (B) $\frac{1}{2}$

    (C) 4
    (D) 8

16. A sound system was reduced from $1,500 to $1,300 in last week's printed advertisement. A midnight madness sale this weekend will give a 15% discount for each item over $500 in the store. What is the price of the sound system?

    (A) $1,075
    (B) $1,105
    (C) $1,286
    (D) $1,305

17. What action must be taken to reduce $\frac{40}{70}$ to its lowest terms?

    (A) Addition
    (B) Division
    (C) Multiplication
    (D) Subtraction

Questions 18–19 are based on the following table.

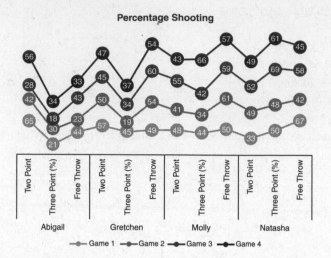

Percentage Shooting

18. Which player has the lowest three-point average in Game 1 and Game 4?

(A) Abigail

(B) Gretchen

(C) Molly

(D) Natasha

19. Which player has the highest three-point percentage in the four games?

(A) Abigail

(B) Gretchen

(C) Molly

(D) Natasha

20. Which of the following is a property or axiom of multiplication?

(A) $a(0) = a$

(B) $a - b = b - a$

(C) $a \times b = b \times a$

(D) $\dfrac{a}{b} = \dfrac{b}{a}$

21. In $\triangle ABC$, $\angle A$ is 25° less than the largest angle. $\angle B$ is 15° larger than $\angle A$. How many degrees are in $\angle C$? Let $\angle C = x$. (Draw a diagram to help set up the equation to determine the degrees in $\angle C$.)

(A) 63.33°

(B) 71.67°

(C) 88°

(D) 95.0°

22. Convert the following fraction to a percentage.

$$\frac{14}{6}$$

(A) 0.233%

(B) $2\frac{1}{3}$ %

(C) 23%

(D) 233%

23. Craig has decided he wants to be a physician's assistant (PA), but he has not done well in his classes all semester. He fears he may be dropped from the program because of his grades. He barely passed last semester and currently needs to earn a B (74–84) in each of his two PA courses to pass and stay in the program. He has one exam remaining in each course. Estimate Craig's final grade for each course, and determine if he will be dropped from the program. Assume the grades are equally weighted.

Course 1: 84, 65, 79, 53, 84, 80, 78, 77, 79, 80, 59, 70, 73, 82
Course 2: 86, 0, 57, 88, 49, 65, 45, 80, 76, 78, 73, 73, 80, 0

(A) It is likely Craig will remain in the PA program. Averaging the grades of the two classes will give him a low B average.

(B) It is likely Craig will remain in the PA program. Although he has a number of questionable grades, there is still enough time in the semester to bring his grade up if he applies himself.

(C) It is likely Craig will be dismissed from the PA program. His Course 1 grades are borderline. His Course 2 grades contain two grades of zero plus six other failing test grades out of a total of 14 grades.

(D) It is likely Craig will be dismissed from the PA program because of his grades. He will need to repeat the courses when readmitted to the program.

24. Hanna is baking pecan pies for her family reunion and needs 10 pounds of pecans. The market sells 4-pound bags of shelled pecans for $22.50/bag. How much will Hanna spend for pecans?

(A) $30.75

(B) $36.50

(C) $56.25

(D) $67.50

25. Select the correct mathematical statement for the following:

b pounds of beef is not equal to b kilograms of beef

(A) b lb $\approx b$ kg

(B) b lb $\neq b$ kg

(C) b lb $\geq b$ kg

(D) b lb $= b$ kg

26. Eric is over 30 days late in paying his monthly credit card balance. His minimum monthly payment has increased from $35.85/month to $52.50/month. What is the percent increase in his monthly payments?

(A) 31.71%

(B) 46.44%

(C) 50.24%

(D) 68.0%

27. Coaches in the Mountain State Football Conference are comparing weights of their most successful starting quarterbacks. Matt weighs 70.8 kilograms, Ben weighs 84.2 kilograms, Juan weighs 73 kilograms, and Eric weighs 86 kilograms. Which quarterback weighs the least in pounds?

   (A) Ben
   (B) Eric
   (C) Juan
   (D) Matt

Questions 28–30 are based on the following chart.

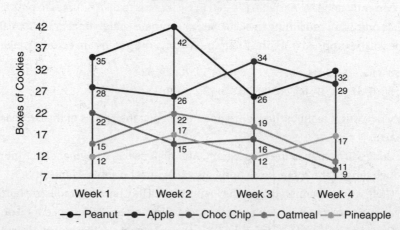

Easter Cookie Sales

28. What type of chart is used?

   (A) Area
   (B) Bar
   (C) Column
   (D) Line

29. What is the average number of whole boxes of cookies sold during Week 3?

   (A) 20 boxes
   (B) 21 boxes
   (C) 22 boxes
   (D) 23 boxes

30. Which type of cookie had the most level trend over the four-week period?

   (A) Apple
   (B) Oatmeal
   (C) Peanut
   (D) Pineapple

31. The demand for clay roof tiles has decreased. Eight thousand tiles per five-day work week are currently produced. The company has decided to reduce production to a four-day work week and produce six thousand five hundred tiles per week. What is the percent decrease in the number of tiles produced per week?

    (A) 18.75%
    (B) 23.42%
    (C) 46.76%
    (D) 76.33%

32. $36.34 \div 15 =$ _____. Round your answer to the nearest hundredth.

    (A) 2.40
    (B) 2.42
    (C) 2.44
    (D) 2.46

33. A number minus 80 is equal to 76. What is the number?

    (A) 16
    (B) 56
    (C) 156
    (D) 256

34. $(-44) \div (-22) =$

    (A) −2
    (B) 2
    (C) −22
    (D) 22

35. $\dfrac{7-(-5)}{-4} =$

    (A) −0.5
    (B) −3
    (C) 3
    (D) 8.75

36. What is the value of the expression $3x^2 + 2xy - 4y^3$ when $x = 5$ and $y = -2$?

    (A) 87
    (B) 99
    (C) 221
    (D) 231

SCIENCE

NUMBER OF QUESTIONS: 53

TIME LIMIT: 63 MINUTES

Instructions: Read each question thoroughly. Select the single best answer. Mark your answer (A, B, C, or D) on the answer sheet provided for Practice Test 3.

1. Positive feedback occurs during which of the following?

   (A) Balancing calcium
   (B) Blood clotting
   (C) Maintaining temperature
   (D) Regulating glucose

2. The heart wall consists of three layers. These layers, from the inside out, are

   (A) endocardium, myocardium, and epicardium.
   (B) epicardium, endocardium, and myocardium.
   (C) myocardium, epicardium, and endocardium.
   (D) The heart wall actually has four layers. The outermost layer is the pericardium.

3. Which of the following is a false statement regarding the spleen?

   (A) Asplenic individuals without spleens display an increased risk for certain types of bacterial infections.
   (B) In the fetus, the spleen is an important location for hemostasis.
   (C) The splenic artery delivers blood to the spleen where it is filtered by the red pulp.
   (D) The white pulp regions of the spleen contain lymphatic.

4. All of the following are examples of chemical reactions EXCEPT

   (A) melting an ice cube.
   (B) metabolic pathways in a human cell.
   (C) mixing baking soda and vinegar.
   (D) rusting of an iron fence.

Questions 5-7 are based on the following passage.

A pharmaceutical company has been researching a new drug to lower blood sugar levels in individuals who have had Type 2 diabetes for 10 to 15 years. The beginning A1C provides an individual baseline prior to the start of taking the trial drug with an additional A1C every three months for a one-year period. The A1C measures blood sugar levels over a three-month period. Nondiabetic A1C levels are below 5.7, and for individuals with long-standing diabetes, they are around 7 or 8.

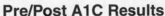
Pre/Post A1C Results

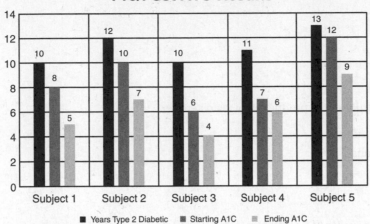

Years Type 2 Diabetic ■ Starting A1C ■ Ending A1C

5. What stage of research is presented in the passage and chart?

(A) Analyzing evidence
(B) Conducting additional experiments
(C) Drawing a logical conclusion
(D) Information collection

6. The chart provides various sets of information. What is the correct name for this information?

(A) Assumptions
(B) Data
(C) Empiric
(D) Notes

7. Based on the information presented in the chart, do the results of the study suggest a new treatment for blood sugar control for individuals with Type 1 diabetes for 10 to 15 years?

(A) No, the cost of the new medicine for diabetic individuals figures into the decision.
(B) No, individuals with Type 1 diabetes were not included in the study.
(C) Yes, based on the results the medication could be helpful for individuals who periodically develop elevated blood sugar.
(D) Yes, the results of the study support the conclusion that the medication would help diabetics with blood sugar control regardless of diabetic type and/or length of time with the disease.

8. Propane, a hydrocarbon fuel classified as an alkane, has many everyday uses. What is the molecular formula of propane?

(A) C_2H_6
(B) C_3H_8
(C) C_4H_{10}
(D) CH_4

9. The _____ is intermediate to the ovaries.

   (A) bladder
   (B) uterus
   (C) vagina
   (D) vulva

10. The _____ stimulates the production of testosterone.

   (A) adrenal medulla
   (B) hypothalamus
   (C) male testes
   (D) thalamus

11. What is the relationship between trace elements and the human body?

   (A) The human body cannot achieve optimal developmental and metabolic functioning without trace elements.
   (B) There is no relationship. Trace elements are found in the environment but do not affect human well-being.
   (C) Trace elements are found in certain muscle cells and assist with coordinated movement.
   (D) Trace elements assist with regulation of the external functions of the parasympathetic nervous system.

12. Which of the following would you use to change 500 centimeters to meters using ratio and proportion?

   (A) 10 cm = 1 m :: 500 cm = x m
   (B) 10 cm = 1 m :: x m = 500 cm
   (C) 100 cm = 1 m :: 500 cm = x m
   (D) 100 cm = 1 m :: x m = 500 cm

13. Skeletal muscle terms *flexor*, *extensor*, *abductor*, and *adductor* are terms that indicate which of the following types of movement?

   (A) Action
   (B) Circular
   (C) Parallel
   (D) Pennate

14. The sympathetic and parasympathetic systems are part of the

   (A) afferent system.
   (B) central nervous system.
   (C) peripheral nervous system.
   (D) special senses system.

15. The reticular activating system (RAS) is responsible for all of the following EXCEPT

   (A) filtering out unimportant sensory information.
   (B) maintaining alertness.
   (C) maintaining muscle tone.
   (D) maintaining wakefulness.

16. The majority of hormone production is regulated by which of the following?

    (A) Antagonistic hormones
    (B) Hemopoiesis
    (C) Negative feedback systems
    (D) Posterior pituitary

17. In which of the following type of solutions are the concentrations of solutes equal, and water does not move into or out of the cell?

    (A) Diffusion
    (B) Endocytosis
    (C) Exocytosis
    (D) Isotonic

18. Plasma (blood plasma) is approximately ____ % water.

    (A) 55
    (B) 70
    (C) 90
    (D) 100

19. Which of the four classes of macromolecules has structural and energy storage functions?

    (A) Carbohydrates
    (B) Lipids
    (C) Nucleic acids
    (D) Proteins

20. All of the following are characteristics of the human body EXCEPT

    (A) conductivity.
    (B) growth.
    (C) movement.
    (D) rationality.

21. An individual with damage to the hypoglossal nerve will exhibit which of the following?

    (A) Impaired or absent gag reflex
    (B) Difficulty speaking
    (C) Drooping of the eyelids
    (D) Inability to walk a straight line

22. Which of the following are antagonistic hormones?

    (A) Adrenaline and epinephrine
    (B) Calcium and thyroid hormone
    (C) Glucagon and insulin
    (D) Sodium and potassium

23. Which of the following substances found in plasma is the result of protein breakdown?

   (A) Bilirubin
   (B) Cholesterol
   (C) Creatinine
   (D) Urea

24. Systolic pressure is highest in the

   (A) aorta.
   (B) arteries.
   (C) arterioles.
   (D) vena cava.

25. Which of the following organs furnishes a hormonal mechanism for the management of blood pressure by controlling blood volume?

   (A) Brainstem
   (B) Heart
   (C) Kidney
   (D) Lungs

26. What is the largest lymphatic organ in the human body?

   (A) Liver
   (B) Lymph nodes
   (C) Spleen
   (D) Thymus

27. An individual wants to determine the measurement of a thin, flat disc that will fit in the palm of a two-year-old's hand. The most appropriate unit of measurement is

   (A) centimeters.
   (B) decimeters.
   (C) meters.
   (D) millimeters.

28. Willis, age 42 and retired, has severe chronic problems with his knee and hip joints. Which of the following occupations has the potential to lead to these orthopedic problems?

   (A) College athletic director
   (B) Professional football player
   (C) Professional poker player
   (D) Swimming coach

29. A muscle acting as a prime mover has an opposition muscle called a(n)

   (A) antagonist.
   (B) assistant.
   (C) protagonist.
   (D) supporter.

30. What muscle in the temple can be felt when the jaws are clenched?

    (A) Buccinator
    (B) Semimembranosus
    (C) Temporalis
    (D) Zygomaticus

31. Which of the following transmits nerve impulses from the brain or spinal cord to an effector?

    (A) Affecter
    (B) Motor neuron
    (C) Receptor
    (D) Sensory neuron

32. _____ are collections of lymph node tissue located after or behind the epithelial lining of the oral cavity.

    (A) Eustachian tubes
    (B) Perilymph
    (C) Salivary glands
    (D) Tonsils

33. The Krebs cycle (citric acid cycle) takes place in the _____ of the cell.

    (A) cytoplasm
    (B) mitochondrion
    (C) nucleus
    (D) plastids

34. Where does general reabsorption occur in the kidney?

    (A) Ascending limb of the loop of Henle
    (B) Descending limb of the loop of Henle
    (C) Proximal convoluted tubules
    (D) Renal cortex

35. All of the following are considered excretory organs EXCEPT

    (A) the intestines.
    (B) the liver.
    (C) the lungs.
    (D) the urinary bladder.

36. The ovaries contain numerous clusters of cells called

    (A) follicles.
    (B) fertilized ovum.
    (C) flagella.
    (D) oocytes.

37. Acids and bases can be termed as weak or strong. What do these terms indicate?

    (A) During a chemical reaction, a strong substance becomes weak and a weak substance becomes strong.
    (B) How well the acid or base conducts electricity in solution
    (C) Strong or weak acids or bases are determined by the type of chemical reaction (combustion, decomposition, replacement, or synthesis).
    (D) The potency or fragility of covalent bonds of acids or bases in solution

38. How many pairs of ribs does an adult human have?

    (A) 6
    (B) 8
    (C) 10
    (D) 12

39. The movement of a substance from an area of high concentration to an area of low concentration is known as

    (A) active reorganization.
    (B) active transport.
    (C) diffusion.
    (D) endocytosis.

40. What structure and its cell contents is key to cellular reproduction?

    (A) Cytoplasm
    (B) Endoplasmic reticulum
    (C) Mitochondria
    (D) Nucleus

41. Select the most appropriate word for the following.

    _____ is the fundamental physical and functional component of heredity.

    (A) Deoxyribonucleic acid (DNA)
    (B) Ribonucleic acid (RNA)
    (C) The codon
    (D) The gene

42. What is the purpose of the serous membranes?

    (A) It improves stretching.
    (B) It furnishes support.
    (C) It lubricates organs.
    (D) It provides organ continuity.

43. Which of the following has the highest degree of vascularization and innervation in the integument?

    (A) Dermis
    (B) Epidermis
    (C) Sensory receptors
    (D) Superfacial fascia

44. Which of the following is an example of a short bone?

   (A) Patella
   (B) Metatarsals in the hip
   (C) Tarsals in the ankles and carpals in the wrists
   (D) Ulna

45. Select the best/logical statement.

   (A) The overall purpose of the brain is coordination of nerves.
   (B) The overall purpose of the brain is organizing and processing.
   (C) The overall purpose of the brain is regulation of two highly specialized and antagonistic hemispheres.
   (D) The overall purpose of the brain is coordination of motor activity and balance.

46. The target organ of prolactin is

   (A) the female mammary glands.
   (B) the ovarian follicles.
   (C) the placenta.
   (D) the uterus.

47. What trace element is necessary for normal functioning of the thyroid?

   (A) Copper
   (B) Iodine
   (C) Manganese
   (D) Zinc

48. Total body water is approximately 63 percent intracellular and 37 percent extracellular fluid. Select one of the differences in these two fluid compartments.

   (A) Sodium ions make up approximately 90% of cations in extracellular fluid.
   (B) Potassium is the major cation in extracellular fluid, followed by calcium.
   (C) Intracellular fluid contains lymph and interstitial fluid; extracellular fluid does not.
   (D) Transcellular fluid is found in both intracellular and extracellular fluid.

49. Based on information presented in the Periodic Table of Elements (page 53), the electrons per shell for krypton (Kr) are

   (A) 2, 8, 13, 1.
   (B) 2, 8, 18, 3.
   (C) 2, 8, 18, 6.
   (D) 2, 8, 18, 8.

Questions 50–53 refer to the following chart.

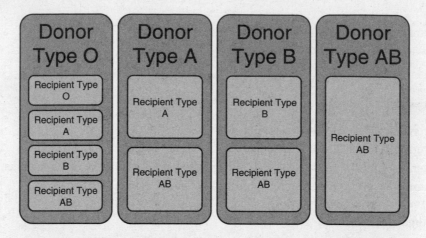

Blood Donors and Blood Recipients

50. Group O is considered the

    (A) universal donor.
    (B) universal recipient.
    (C) donor for group AB only.
    (D) donor for group O only.

51. You have group AB blood. The recipient of your blood must have

    (A) group A blood.
    (B) group AB blood.
    (C) group B blood.
    (D) group O blood.

52. A recipient with group A blood can receive blood from which of the following donor groups?

    (A) Individuals from any of the groups
    (B) Individuals from group A only
    (C) Individuals from group A and O
    (D) Individuals from group B and AB

53. Which of the following blood groups is considered a universal recipient?

    (A) Group A
    (B) Group AB
    (C) Group B
    (D) Group O

> **Instructions:** Read each question thoroughly. Select the single best answer. Mark your answer (A, B, C, or D) on the answer sheet provided for Practice Test 3.

1. Select the correct spelling when adding the suffix *-able* to the word *move*.

   (A) Movable
   (B) Moveable
   (C) Move-able
   (D) Move able

2. Select the sentence with correct subject-verb agreement.

   (A) A few in the audience were hecklers.
   (B) He say no one has the right to tell him what to do.
   (C) Linda walk to the park every morning to exercise her dog.
   (D) Sam believe he would be successful if he worked hard.

3. Select the homograph that has the same spelling but different meaning.

   (A) Address: where a person lives or a scolding
   (B) Bow: a weapon or a pair of tied loops
   (C) Buffet: a self-service food bar or moving air
   (D) Wave: a hand greeting or type of metal

4. Select an appropriate synonym for the italicized word in the following sentence.

   The child *balked* when his mother scolded him for his unruly behavior.

   (A) Consented
   (B) Continued
   (C) Hesitated
   (D) Persevered

5. Select the most appropriate meaning of the root word italicized in the following sentence.

   With great whooping and hollering, the youth rammed the ac*celer*ator to the floorboard when the light changed to green.

   (A) Measure
   (B) Near
   (C) Rapid
   (D) Speed

6. Select the incorrectly punctuated sentence.

   (A) The judge asked "Ladies and gentlemen of the jury, have you reached a verdict?"
   (B) The organization that provided the financial assistance remains unknown.
   (C) "Why did you take the blue ribbon, Pete?"
   (D) In his anger and without thinking, the man slammed his fist into the wall and broke three of his four knuckles.

7. Select the incorrectly spelled word.

   (A) Corregeted
   (B) Heritage
   (C) Marital
   (D) Patient

8. Select the sentence using an incorrect word.

   (A) Alex admitted he had always had trouble deciding when to use affect and effect.
   (B) "Alright, I'll do it," the confused youth said.
   (C) I lost Harper's book—it was in my backpack and must have fallen out when I took a tumble on my bike.
   (D) The teacher asked her students if any of them knew what the word *ipsilateral* meant.

9. Select the meaning of the slang term italicized in the following sentence.

   During the sixties, *woodies* were popular with surfers in California.

   (A) A hairstyle cut short in the back and sides with extra length in the front.
   (B) A wooden shoe or clog that leaves unique tracks in the sand.
   (C) Surfboards having the coarseness or appearance of wood.
   (D) Station wagons with wood or fabricated wood panels or siding on the outside of the body of the car.

10. Select the correctly punctuated sentence.

   (A) Concession prices at the local theater, are so high they encourage sneaking food in to have something to eat, during the movie.
   (B) Mason, had a growth spurt over the summer, and was now, the tallest boy in his class.
   (C) Residents, were unsure how to take the new boarder; since she stayed shut up in her room during the evening hours.
   (D) I attended the memorial service because I thought it was the proper thing to do.

11. Select the sentence using an incorrect word.

   (A) By the end of the day, only cookies with strange names and colors remained.
   (B) His mother said, "Take the flowers over to me."
   (C) I hate taking tests because they rarely demonstrate what I really know.
   (D) Todd received a notice from the bank that his account was overdrawn.

12. Which of the following is a complex sentence?

    (A) Attendees of the family reunion were treated to a day of food, fun, and frivolity.
    (B) J. H. Westerling, in the U.S. Senate for 24 years, lost the election to a nonpolitician because he believed he was a shoe-in.
    (C) Patrick, Eugene, and Frank volunteered to work with the local literacy program.
    (D) Michael called all of Jed's friends to come to his surprise birthday party, Mary planned on baking the cake, and Philip was trying to find out what Jed wanted for his birthday.

13. Analyze the parts of the following word to determine its correct meaning.

    Autocratic

    (A) Auto = citizen, cratic = government. Government by the people and elected rulers.
    (B) Auto = rule, cratic = government. A ruler with power over the government.
    (C) Auto = same, cratic = criticize. A form of self-analysis.
    (D) Auto = self, cratic = rule or power. An individual with unlimited power or influence.

14. Select the sentence written in an informal language or tone.

    (A) Rod and Michael wouldn't admit it, but secretly they wanted to date a cougar.
    (B) The bride feared being late for the ceremony and had five alarm clocks set for seven o'clock the next morning.
    (C) The campers walked miles through a mosquito-infested, humid swamp and were exhausted when they finally reached the ancient ruins.
    (D) Tom's parents never understood his passion for long-distance running, but his brothers did.

15. Select an appropriate synonym for the italicized word in the following sentence.

    No one in their right mind would have attempted to ford the *swollen* river.

    (A) Compressing
    (B) Declining
    (C) Rising
    (D) Shrinking

16. Select the most appropriate meaning of the root word italicized in the following sentence.

    At the age of eight, Marion surprised her parents when she told them she wanted to be a *mort*ician when she grew up.

    (A) Change
    (B) Dealer
    (C) Death
    (D) Helper

17. Select the most appropriate meaning of the root word italicized in the following sentence.

    A con*junct*ion is a part of speech.

    (A) Cut
    (B) Include
    (C) Join
    (D) Strengthen

18. Select the incorrectly punctuated sentence.

    (A) Because of the fracas at last year's prom Frank's repeated requests to be included on this year's prom planning committee have been ignored.
    (B) Of the children who entered paintings at the county fair, six won white ribbons, three won red ribbons, two won blue ribbons, and one received an honorable mention.
    (C) Sarah, who broke her leg skiing a week before the spring semester started, didn't miss a single day of school.
    (D) What were we supposed to do when they didn't call or show up?

19. Select the incorrectly spelled word.

    (A) Abandoned
    (B) Confectionery
    (C) Contenence
    (D) Tyranny

20. Select the correctly worded sentence.

    (A) He wanted to purchase the DVD, but he had all ready spent his allowance for the month.
    (B) Jamison was proud to accept the honor on behalf of his mother.
    (C) Members of last year's championship basketball team had allusions of grandeur until they lost to the worst team in the conference by 55 points.
    (D) The owner of the company promised to divide his wealth between his wife and three sons.

21. Select the incorrectly punctuated sentence.

    (A) Bill has worked for the city for ten years, and his wife, Cindy, has worked for the county for seven years.
    (B) Lost Victory who won the Kentucky Derby sired four Preakness winners.
    (C) Lyle trains at the local gym; he frequently invites the press to come and watch him work out.
    (D) The medication is guaranteed to cure childhood cancer.

22. Select the incorrectly punctuated sentence.

    (A) Even though he was severely injured in the accident, he was able to pull himself out of the car and crawl to the side of the road.
    (B) No, I cannot endorse the mayor for reelection.
    (C) They could tell by his accent he was from the South.
    (D) Vince told his friends that "he would meet them at the trail head."

23. Select the most appropriate meaning of the root word italicized in the following sentence.

    Leadership in the primitive society was *matri*lineal before the introduction of organized religion in the early 1800s.

    (A) Material
    (B) Mother
    (C) Multi
    (D) Nomad

24. Select the incorrectly punctuated sentence.

   (A) Brent thought skipping school was a brilliant idea—provided he didn't get caught.
   (B) Mary Johnson who runs 25 miles a week can outrun any boy at the school.
   (C) The sunset was a brilliant pink and orange the night before the thunderstorm.
   (D) When did the parents first notice their children were missing?

25. All of the following are elements of the writing process EXCEPT

   (A) brainstorming.
   (B) organizing.
   (C) revising.
   (D) writing.

26. Select the sentence using a conjunction.

   (A) In addition to the contributions from community businesses, the local high school football team volunteered to serve as drivers.
   (B) The admissions committee discovered that many of their fall applicants came from out of state.
   (C) The club met last evening and decided to sell cookies at the homecoming fair in the fall.
   (D) The child had been waiting for his ride since school was dismissed.

27. A _____ is a punctuation mark used to show a break, pause, or interruption in a sentence.

   (A) colon
   (B) comma
   (C) dash
   (D) period

28. Select the incorrectly spelled word.

   (A) Accommodate
   (B) Beleive
   (C) Chauffeur
   (D) Moribund

ANSWER KEY
Practice Test 3

Reading

1.	B	15.	D	29.	B	43.	D
2.	A	16.	D	30.	B	44.	C
3.	C	17.	B	31.	C	45.	B
4.	B	18.	C	32.	C	46.	A
5.	D	19.	C	33.	B	47.	D
6.	A	20.	C	34.	C	48.	B
7.	D	21.	C	35.	B	49.	D
8.	A	22.	C	36.	C	50.	B
9.	B	23.	A	37.	D	51.	B
10.	C	24.	B	38.	B	52.	B
11.	D	25.	C	39.	D	53.	B
12.	C	26.	A	40.	B		
13.	A	27.	B	41.	C		
14.	C	28.	D	42.	A		

Mathematics

1.	B	10.	C	19.	D	28.	D
2.	C	11.	D	20.	C	29.	C
3.	A	12.	A	21.	B	30.	D
4.	B	13.	A	22.	D	31.	A
5.	C	14.	B	23.	C	32.	B
6.	D	15.	C	24.	D	33.	C
7.	D	16.	B	25.	B	34.	B
8.	A	17.	B	26.	B	35.	B
9.	D	18.	A	27.	D	36.	A

ANSWER KEY
Practice Test 3

Science

1.	B	15.	C	29.	A	43.	A
2.	A	16.	C	30.	C	44.	C
3.	B	17.	D	31.	B	45.	B
4.	A	18.	C	32.	D	46.	A
5.	C	19.	A	33.	B	47.	B
6.	B	20.	D	34.	C	48.	A
7.	B	21.	B	35.	D	49.	D
8.	B	22.	C	36.	A	50.	A
9.	B	23.	D	37.	B	51.	B
10.	B	24.	A	38.	D	52.	C
11.	A	25.	C	39.	C	53.	B
12.	C	26.	C	40.	D		
13.	A	27.	D	41.	D		
14.	C	28.	B	42.	C		

English and Language Usage

1.	A	8.	B	15.	C	22.	D
2.	A	9.	D	16.	C	23.	B
3.	B	10.	D	17.	C	24.	B
4.	C	11.	B	18.	A	25.	A
5.	D	12.	B	19.	C	26.	C
6.	A	13.	D	20.	B	27.	B
7.	A	14.	A	21.	B	28.	B

ANSWER EXPLANATIONS

Reading

1. **(B)** To correctly answer this question, information from the two images and the stem (question) must be combined. Having assessed the images and information in the stem, it can be concluded: (1) the QRS complex represents one normal heartbeat; (2) the rhythm strip indicates the number of normal heartbeats during a six-second period; (3) one minute or sixty seconds is equal to ten six-second intervals; (4) there are eight QRS complexes in the six-second rhythm strip; and (5) the answer is an approximation, not the exact number of heartbeats per minute. The question can be answered by using the above information, and the answer can be determined via two methods. The first, and simplest, method is to count the tallest spike in each QRS complex in the rhythm strip and multiply the number by 10 (8 spikes $\times$ 10 seconds = 80 beats per minute). The second method is to use a ratio and proportion equation (8 spikes = 6 seconds $::$ x spikes = 60 seconds), where the answer also equals 80.

2. **(A)** A *premonition* is a warning or foreboding; an intuition of a future, customarily undesirable occurrence. There is nothing to suggest that Sarah is nervous or frightened. There is nothing to suggest that Sarah is not mentally or emotionally prepared for the jump. Nothing suggests that she needs more practice.

3. **(C)** *Opinions* are typically beliefs or viewpoints that do not have a sound foundation. The four things the politician says he will do if elected are not facts and cannot be guaranteed. A *bias* is a preconceived or unreasonable inclination. *Stereotypes* are concepts or images that have had special meaning given to them. An example of an American stereotype is girls are not good at math or sports, and men who like the color pink are not real men.

4. **(B)** An argument is not always verbal opposition. It is also a discussion addressing different points of view or a reasoning process. The father is pointing out money-related matters his son has not considered. The father is not asserting, claiming, or predicting.

5. **(D)** *Brass tacks* is an idiom or expression meaning to pay attention, focus, or concentrate. The father is not using jargon. Jargon is language unique to a group or profession, or speech/writing that has no meaning. The use of the phrase has nothing to do with tacks made of brass, and it is not a veiled threat.

6. **(A)** *Acquiesced* is an antonym for *balked*. As used in the sentence, it means pulling back or stopping short. *Acquiesce* means to yield or comply. The remaining options are synonyms for *balk*.

7. **(D)** A surge in negative activities has brought about the need for change. While Lake Hope has a family orientation, there is nothing in the passage that states that the complaints are family related. If you selected this answer, you probably made an assumption. The cost of admission is not an issue. Lake Hope is a private recreational area, not a public one.

8. **(A)** The key to correctly answering this question is the word *relevant*, and recognizing the relationship between negative activity and policy. The word *relevant* suggests one thing has an influence or connection with another thing. In this case, the increase in negative activities has had an influence on, or a connection to, the actions taken by the Lake Hope owners to stem the situation. The remaining options do not apply.

9. **(B)** The passage is explanatory in nature. It gives an overview of Lake Hope as a recreation area and explains how it has changed over the course of a summer. It further presents what action the family has taken or will take to keep Lake Hope family friendly. It may, at first, appear to be a chronology, but it is not because it explains why the owners of Lake Hope took the actions they did.

10. **(C)** The chart is a column chart. This type of chart presents data in a column or vertical fashion. Bar charts, on the other hand, present data in horizontal bars.

11. **(D)** Walnut brittle has been the best seller over time. It has been the best or highest seller in four of the five years.

12. **(C)** Pecan brittle has been the lowest seller for three of the five years, and the second lowest seller for two of the five years.

13. **(A)** Based on the four available options, the best year for nut brittle sales was 2012 with $950 in sales. The remaining years ranged from $769 to $865. The best seller for any year can be estimated since an exact amount was not asked for.

14. **(C)** Style guides, sometimes referred to as style manuals, establish standards for design and writing papers, books, essays, and other documents. They are used in academia, professional organizations, or disciplinary fields, and establish consistency within documents. Examples of style guides are *AP (Associated Press) Stylebook*, *The Chicago Manual of Style*, *MLA (Modern Language Association) Handbook*, and *APA (American Psychological Association) Handbook*. A printer of books prints books and nothing more. A business card developer would not employ a style guide since business cards are unique to the business or individual. Social clubs do not employ style guides.

15. **(D)** An encyclopedia on nineteenth-century artwork is a tertiary source. The other options are secondary sources.

16. **(D)** This question can be easily missed if the reader makes assumptions about information in the memo. The most logical conclusion is employees will be terminated due to reorganization secondary to the merger. Violation of rights and termination for bogus reasons is opinion. Keeping employees apprised of company changes is only one element found in the memo.

17. **(B)** The memo indicates a definite action not open to question. The memo does not speculate, suggest, or suppose.

18. **(C)** Knowing the definition of *delineated* is key to correctly answering the question. Information in the memo is clear and precise—it provides who, where, what, why, and when. The memo is well configured. The remaining options do not support the definition of *delineated*.

19. **(C)** Position or grade-level policies were developed to avert or reduce discrimination in the workplace. They may serve as guidelines for promotion within an organization and may also address such factors as gender, ethnicity, criteria for hiring or firing, and criteria for promotion or demotion. There were no Civil Rights Acts of 1965 and 1969; the act was implemented in 1964. While position/grade-level policies may address gender, they also address much more, and may also include time in position and educational preparation for a specific level. These policies typically work to reduce discrimination. Position/grade-level policies may have specific educational and years-in-position requirements, but these are two of many components that may be included.

20. **(C)** The westernmost route includes traveling through the states of New Mexico (Santa Fe), Arizona (Phoenix), California (Sacramento), Oregon (Salem), and Washington (Olympia). The remaining options are not the westernmost route.

21. **(C)** The passage is a narrative and tells the story of Denny's adventures on a particular day. Cause and effect, expounding, and problem solving do not fit the criteria for the passage.

22. **(C)** *Foreshadowing* is an indication or warning of something to come. Synonyms for foreshadowing are *adumbrative* and *prefiguration*. Foreshadowing is frequently used in literary pieces where the author gives readers a hint of a change in the plot or direction of a story.

The remaining options are not suggestive of foreshadowing—they do not suggest something to come.

23. **(A)** The most appropriate genre is adventure. The passage relates an experience. The passage does not address family or relationships. It is not a humorous passage or steampunk (subsystems of fantasy and science fiction).

24. **(B)** In this instance, a *pothole* is a hole or depression in the trail caused by excessive use or weather. They may also be referred to as chuckholes or ruts. The remaining options are antonyms for pothole.

25. **(C)** The correct answer is an example of *personification*, which gives human qualities to something nonhuman—in this case, suggesting mud balls can walk and Denny resembled or looked like one as he walked. There is nothing in the passage to suggest Denny is ball shaped. He may have been dripping mud behind him as he walked, but the passage does not tell the reader this. Denny may have been humorous looking, but the question asks for the meaning of the phrase, not what he looked like.

26. **(A)** The mayor's statement is *biased, prejudiced, opinionated,* or *preconceived*. The use of the word *usually* rejects a statement as a fact. *Usual* indicates something that is probable by reasoning or prior experience. *Impartiality* and *stereotype* are not supportive of the statement.

27. **(B)** Being able to correctly define *mitosis* is the key to correctly answering the question. Mitosis is a process of cell division. The remaining options would not be found in the subheading of cell division.

28. **(D)** A thesaurus identifies synonyms and antonyms. The word *strategy* is vague—does it mean spelling, grammatical use, or some other strategy? Dictionaries do not always provide synonyms or antonyms, and encyclopedias typically do not provide synonyms or antonyms.

29. **(B)** There are two slang terms that must be understood to correctly identify an alternative phrase for *I am in really deep doo-doo*. A *crib* or *crib sheet* is a cheat sheet. Ben was caught cheating on a math test by his teacher, and he is now in trouble. The remaining options all relate to Ben's cheating, but do not support the notion that *deep doo-doo* means trouble.

30. **(B)** *Bushwhack* is the only word found between the words *bushel* and *can*. The remaining words come before or after *bushel* and *can*.

31. **(C)** *The Oxford American Writer's Thesaurus* is the logical selection. *Robert's Rules of Order* is a guide for conducting meetings and discussions efficiently and impartially. *The Elements of Style* is a guide for writing grammatically correct papers and documents. *Webster's New World College Dictionary* provides meanings of words, but may or may not provide antonyms and synonyms.

32. **(C)** Nebraska is not considered one of the mountain states. It is referred to as a plains state since it is located in the Central Plains. The remaining options are considered mountain states.

33. **(B)** Comparing each company's price for individual black pens reveals the Mountain Pen Company has the lowest price at $0.83/pen. The remaining companies' prices are higher.

34. **(C)** Reliable Ink has the prices for red pens at $1.25/pen, $58/50 pens, and $110/200 pens. The remaining companies are lower across the board.

35. **(B)** Good Write Pens has the lowest price for red pens at $40/50 pens. Mountain Pen Company has the lowest price for black pens at $72/100 pens. The remaining companies have higher prices.

36. **(C)** An introduction to a literary work introduces the (potential) reader to what the work has to offer. It's an attempt to persuade an individual or individuals into purchasing and/

or reading it. The introduction is not a notification of publication and does not indicate why Wilson wrote the book, and the book is not a biography. It is an autobiography.

37. **(D)** While the introduction mentions boys and girls, it does not specify the book is written for children. The word *reader* is used, suggesting the book is appropriate for individuals ranging from childhood through old age. Options (A), (B), and (C) are subsystems of option (D).

38. **(B)** Underlining or italicizing *The White Indian Boy: The Story of Uncle Nick Among the Shoshone* indicates the title of the book. Underlining or italicizing does not suggest the book is a narrative, does not indicate the placement or location of the book in a library, and does not indicate that the book is about a boy.

39. **(D)** *The White Indian Boy* is a primary source. It was written by the author and tells the story of his growing up in 1800s Wyoming. The remaining options do not meet the criteria for a primary source.

40. **(B)** *Queries* are questions or requests for information. Queries may also be comments about something. In the question, readers of the brochure are told that queries will be addressed and an e-mail address is provided. The remaining options are not definitions for queries.

41. **(C)** Each of the options indicates an appropriate use of a slash (/). However, the question asks specifically what the slash means in terms of a pass/fail grade in a course. Pass/fail is an alternative and are opposites as are up/down, male/female, and in/out. The remaining options do not support the use of a slash indicated in the sentence.

42. **(A)** Information on policies and guidelines for a religious denomination would be found in the Religion section in the subsystem of Doctrines. Synonyms of doctrines include principles, dogmas, rules, guidelines, or sets of guidelines. This information would not be found in the other subsections of Religion.

43. **(D)** As used in the question, a *sect* is a branching off from a church. Offshoots from religious groups still hold the fundamental beliefs of the church but have strong disagreement regarding specific beliefs. The subsystem of *Sects and religious reform movements* is the logical place to find the needed information.

44. **(C)** The most appropriate choice is the Religious experience, life, practice in the Religion section. Stephen is interested in his fiancée's religious lifestyle and practice. The remaining options would not focus on this.

45. **(B)** The Speaker of a legislative body provides numerous examples of problems in the state, and also points out that the legislators have the means to correct or alleviate the problem. There is nothing to suggest that the state has a financial resource problem. The use of *always* negates option (C) as being a correct answer. There is nothing to suggest that the infrastructure has failed because of poor leadership.

46. **(A)** One way to address this question is to treat it as true/false and determine which option is the truest. The cause of the crisis is not presented, but its negative consequences are. This is the most logical option. The state's education program is in danger of collapse, but it has not totally collapsed. Nothing suggests that the state government has miscarried. The state has financial resources.

47. **(D)** The Speaker is addressing elected state representatives. Speakers are presiding officers of legislative bodies. Throughout the passage there are statements or clues that assist in determining the correct answer—the last paragraph is the most specific. Based on the passage, the Speaker is not addressing county officials or self-interest groups. Parliament is not a legislative body in the United States.

48. **(B)** The passage implies the state's legislative body has the means to assist the state as well as the people of the state. Nothing in the passage suggests that the legislative body does not have

authority or power to intervene, is disinterested in the problems of the state, or was unable to prevent the crisis. These options are nothing more than speculation.

49. **(D)** *Parsimonious* means stingy or unnecessarily thrifty. Scrooge, in *A Christmas Carol*, is parsimonious. Synonyms for parsimonious are *ungenerous*, *tightfisted*, *penny-pinching*, or *cheap*.

50. **(B)** The mode of the passage is best described as *problem/solution*. The Speaker announces that the state cannot endure another crisis and proceeds to give numerous facts about what has been going on in the state—he presents the problem. He then points out that the legislators were elected by the people of the state and have been parsimonious in their actions. He reminds them that they have the means to alleviate and, perhaps, solve the state's problem. The remaining options do not support the mode of the passage.

51. **(B)** *Expository* means to set forth in detail or explain. The memo expounds on the student interviews and provides readers with information to compare with their own notes from the interviews. The memo is not an argument, problem, or opinion.

52. **(B)** This option is comprehensive and provides vital information to get to picnic site C. The written description specifies going east out of Bugtussle and turning west onto Landers Lane. It also indicates two structures—a church and a cemetery—that will be passed. It points out a lack of structures or sites past the church/cemetery. The cattle guard is of importance because it has to be crossed, and after the cattle guard the road is unpaved. The reader is specifically instructed to make a right turn after crossing the cattle guard and to proceed on a gravel road until the picnic site C sign indicates the destination has been reached. The remaining options are poor or incorrect, or potentially place individuals in harm's way.

53. **(B)** The inclusion of the word *danger* indicates potential hazards. Traffic signs or other information are typically not included on maps, and the presence of an unpaved road does not necessarily indicate a possible hazard; it merely indicates a change in road surface.

Mathematics

1. **(B)** The rules of operation must be followed to calculate the correct answer. Multiply 10×18.5, and then divide by 34.

$$10 \times 18.5 \div 34 = 10 \times \frac{18.5}{34} \times \frac{185}{34} = 5.44 = 5.4$$

2. **(C)** The question asks for the number of multicolored candies in the machine. Other colors of candies are given in percentages. The numbers of these candies must be determined—the number should be less than 200.

$15\% = 0.15 \times 200 = 30$ yellow	$100\% - 52\% = 48\%$ multicolored
$20\% = 0.20 \times 200 = 40$ green	$48\% = 0.48 \times 200 = 96$ multicolored
$17\% = 0.17 \times 200 = 34$ red	$30 + 40 + 34 + 96 = 200$ candies

3. **(A)** Cube is the term used when a number is raised to the third power ($a \times a \times a$ or a^3). Square is the term used when a number is raised to the second power ($a \times a$ or a^2). Cubed and squared numbers can be even or odd.

4. **(B)**

$$4 \text{ boxes @ } \$30/\text{box} = \$120$$

$$6 \text{ boxes @ } \$55/\text{box} = \$330$$

$$15 \text{ bottles @ } \$75/\text{bottle} = \$1,125$$

$$30 \text{ boxes @ } \$15/\text{box} = \$450$$

$$\$120 + \$330 + \$1,125 + \$450 = \$2,025$$

5. **(C)** Five can be divided into 9 one time with 4 remaining, or $1\frac{4}{5}$.

6. **(D)**

$$23\% \text{ of } x = 25$$
$$0.23x = 25$$
$$x = 108.6956 = 108.696$$

7. **(D)** Cross multiply to solve the problem.

$$\frac{88}{x} = \frac{58}{100} \qquad\qquad \frac{88}{x} = \frac{58}{100}$$

$$58x = 8,800 \qquad\qquad \frac{88}{151.72} = \frac{58}{100}$$

$$x = 151.72 \qquad\qquad 0.58 = 0.58$$

8. **(A)** The first action is to change the sentence into an equation, and then solve the equation. The rules or order of operations must be followed to correctly solve the problem. Many have the mistaken idea that a lack of parentheses in an equation changes the manner in which the problem is solved. It does not. Parentheses were added to the equation below for clarification—the addition of parentheses does not change the order of calculations. After multiplication is complete, 5 is added to 102, and 4 is subtracted from 107, equaling 103.

$$b = 5 + 17 \times 3 \times 2 - 4$$
$$b = 5 + (17 \times 3 \times 2) - 4$$
$$b = 5 + 102 - 4$$
$$b = 107 - 4$$
$$b = 103$$

9. **(D)** After the sentences are changed into an equation, 84 is *subtracted* from each side of the equation, leaving x equal to 24.

$$84 + x = 108$$
$$84 - 84 + x = 108 - 84$$
$$x = 24$$

10. **(C)** In a fraction, the top number is the numerator and the bottom number is the denominator or n/d. Convert the sentence into an equation and solve for d.

$$\frac{n}{d} = \frac{250}{d} = 50$$
$$250 = 50d$$
$$5 = d$$

11. **(D)** The formula for the volume of a cube is Volume = (length of a side)^3

$$s = 7.75 \text{ in.}$$
$$V = s^3 = 7.75 \times 7.75 \times 7.75 = 465.48 \text{ cu in.}$$

12. **(A)** This problem is easier to solve than it looks. Since each whole number is not in direct sequence with another, drop everything to the right of the decimal. This leaves 8, 5, 14, 20, 10, and 7, which can easily be arranged from smallest to largest.

13. **(A)** Ratio and proportion can be used to solve the problem.

$$150 \text{ marbles} = 100\% :: 14 \text{ marbles} = x\%$$

$$150 = 100 :: 14 = x$$

$$150x = 14$$

$$x = 9.3\%$$

14. **(B)** A decimal number is changed to a percent by moving the decimal point two places to the right. A percentage is changed to a decimal number by moving the decimal two places to the left.

$$0.6734 = 67.34\%$$

15. **(C)** Dividing the numerator by the denominator is the same as multiplying the answer by the denominator and will give you the original numerator.

$$\frac{32}{8} = 4 \text{ and } 4 \times 8 = 32$$

16. **(B)** The current selling price for the sound system is $1,300. A 15% discount will be given during the midnight madness sale since the system sells for over $500.

$$\$1,300 \times 15\% = 1,300 \times 0.15 = \$195$$

$$\$1,300 - \$195 = \$1,105$$

17. **(B)** The fraction must be divided to reduce it to lowest terms. Ten is the largest number that can be divided into both terms.

$$\frac{40}{70} = \frac{40 \div 10}{70 \div 10} = \frac{4}{7}$$

18. **(A)** [*This chart is more difficult to read because it does not follow the classic chart format. There are no horizontal lines on this chart (horizontal lines are usually something measureable such as money, days, or years, and are a range of numbers from low to high). In this case, the reader must look at the legend to determine what the uneven horizontal information means—on this chart it represents percentages in four different basketball games. Percentages are provided in the shaded circles along each line. The vertical information is also in a different format. It consists of four categories—each the name of a basketball player. There are three subcategories above the names of each player. Subcategories are two-point, three-point, and free-throw percentages.*] Abigail has the lowest three-point average in the first and fourth game at 27.5 percent. Gretchen's average is 41 percent, Molly's is 55 percent, and Natasha's is 55.5 percent. The average for each player is determined by adding the three-point percentage scores of the first and fourth games and dividing by two. The answer to this question can be determined by looking at the player with the two lowest three-point percentages of Games 1 and 4. Abigail has the lowest percentage average in Games 1 and 4. The remaining players have higher averages in Games 1 and 4.

19. **(D)** The italicized information in brackets in question 18 also applies here. Natasha has the highest three-point percentage in the four games. Her highest percentage is in Game 3 and is 69 percent, Abigail is 34 percent (Game 4), Molly 66 percent (Game 4), and Gretchen

45 percent (Game 1). This question asked for the highest percentage of three-points in all of the games, not an average.

20. **(C)** The commutative property of multiplication indicates that order does not make any difference. For example, let $a = 4$ and $b = 5$.

$$
\begin{array}{ll}
a(0) = a & 4(0) \neq 4 \\
a - b = b - a & 4 - 5 \neq 5 - 4 \\
a \times b = b \times a & 4 \times 5 = 5 \times 4 \\
\dfrac{a}{b} = \dfrac{b}{a} & \dfrac{4}{5} \neq \dfrac{5}{4}
\end{array}
$$

21. **(B)** The problem appears to be more difficult than it is. Each component or angle must be addressed separately and logically. The total degrees in a triangle is 180. If $\angle C = x$, then $\angle A = x - 25°$, and $\angle B = x - 25° + 15°$. One key to correctly determining $\angle C$ rests on how you interpreted angle B for your equation. Angle C is the unknown. Angle A is straightforward; it is 25 degrees less than the largest angle. Angle B is 15 degrees larger than angle A ($x - 25°$), which makes $\angle B = x - 25° + 15°$. In considering the angles, angle A is smaller than angle B, which is smaller than angle C.

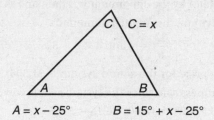

$$A = x - 25° \qquad B = 15° + x - 25°$$

$$\angle A = x - 25° \quad \angle B = x - 25° + 15° \quad \angle C = x°$$
$$\angle A + \angle B + \angle C = 180°$$
$$x + (x - 25) + (x - 25 + 15) = 180$$
$$x + (x - 25) + (x - 10) = 180$$
$$3x - 35 = 180$$
$$3x = 215$$
$$x = 71.67°$$

$$\angle A = x - 25 = 71.667 - 25 = 46.67°$$
$$\angle B = x - 25 + 15 = 71.667 - 25 + 15 = 61.67°$$
$$\angle C = 71.667°$$

$$\angle A + \angle B + \angle C = 180°$$
$$46.67 + 61.67 + 71.667 = 180.007° = 180°$$
$$180° = 180°$$

22. **(D)** To change a fraction to a percent, change the fraction into a decimal, and move the decimal point two places to the right.

$$\frac{14}{6} = 2\frac{1}{3} \text{ or } 2.33 = 233\%$$

23. **(C)** There are numerous methods for approximating or estimating. The goal is to find a number that is close to the actual number. One method is to compare the grades in the two courses since Craig has to have a minimum average of 74 percent (not rounded) in *each* course. He has nine passing and five failing grades in Course 1. He is probably borderline in this course and could pass or fail the course depending on how he does on the one remaining test. In Course 2, he has six passing and eight failing grades. Having two grades of zero included in the eight failing grades heavily suggests Craig is currently failing this course. There are not enough points available for him to pass this course.

Rounding up or down is the second method. Of the fourteen grades in Course 1, five are below 74 percent and failing, and nine are within the B range and passing. The majority of the grades are passing in Course 1, with the highest grade rounded down to 80 and lowest rounded down to 50. An estimate of the course grade is below 74 percent, but an exact calculation would have to be performed to determine the exact grade. Of the Course 2 grades, eight are below 74 percent with two of these zeroes, and six are in the B range. Rounding puts the highest grade at a 90 and the lowest at a zero. An estimate suggests failure of the course with a course grade of below 70. In all likelihood, Craig will be dismissed from the PA program.

A third method is to look at the course with the lowest grades since Craig must pass both courses to remain in the PA program. The second course has the lowest grades with the majority of test grades in the failing range and the highest test grade a low B. Based on this, he will fail this course and be dropped from the program.

The information provided speaks only of being dropped from the PA program. It does not address readmission.

24. **(D)** It is important to notice pecans are only sold in 4-pound bags. There is nothing to suggest that a partial bag could be purchased. She will have to buy more pecans than she needs—three 4-lb bags of pecans.

$$3 \text{ bags of nuts} \times \$22.50 = 3 \times 22.50 = \$67.50$$

25. **(B)** Understanding mathematical symbols is key to correctly answering the question. The amount of beef and the systems of measurement are not an issue because the sentence simply says that two unlike amounts of beef are not equal to each other. The mathematical symbol $\neq$ means *not equal to*. The symbol $\approx$ means *approximately equal to*, and $\geq$ means *equal to or greater than*.

26. **(B)** The formula for percentage change is used to obtain the correct answer.

$$\text{Original payment} = \$35.85 \qquad \text{New payment} = \$52.50$$

$$\text{Percent change (PC)} = \frac{\text{change}}{\text{starting point}}$$

$$PC = \frac{52.50 - 35.85}{35.85}$$

$$PC = \frac{16.65}{35.85}$$

$$PC = 0.4644 = 46.44\% \text{ increase}$$

27. **(D)** Weight must be converted from kilograms to pounds. One kilogram is equal to 2.2 pounds. It is not necessary to determine the weight in pounds for each player since the question asks for the quarterback with the lowest weight. Matt weighs the lowest in kilograms. The lowest kilogram weight is also the lowest pound weight.

28. **(D)** Chart data are presented in a line format.

29. **(C)** The key to the correct answer is *whole boxes* of cookies. To determine the average number of boxes of cookies sold in the third week, the numbers of boxes for each type of cookie are added together and divided by the number of types of cookies. The answer must be taken to the next higher number since 21.4 is equal to 21 whole boxes plus four-tenths of an additional box or 22 boxes.

$$\frac{107}{5} = 21.4 = 22 \text{ boxes}$$

30. **(D)** Pineapple cookies had the most even or level trend over the four-week period, with weekly box sales of 12, 17, 12, and 17. The remaining options had trends with greater variances.

31. **(A)** The formula for percentage change is used to obtain the correct answer.

Original # weekly tiles = 8,000   New # of weekly tiles = 6,500

$$\text{Percent change (PC)} = \frac{\text{change}}{\text{starting point}}$$

$$PC = \frac{8,000 - 6,500}{8,000}$$

$$PC = \frac{1,500}{8,000}$$

$$PC = 0.1875 = 18.75\%$$

32. **(B)**

$$\frac{36.34}{15} = 2.4227 = 2.42$$

33. **(C)**

$$x - 80 = 76$$
$$x = 76 + 80$$
$$x = 156$$

34. **(B)** When dividing a negative number into a negative number, the product is a positive number.

35. **(B)**

$$\frac{7 - (-5)}{-4} = \frac{12}{-4} = -3$$

36. **(A)**

$$x = 5 \qquad y = -2$$
$$3x^2 + 2xy - 4y^3 =$$
$$3(5 \cdot 5) + 2(5)(-2) - 4(-8) =$$
$$75 + (-20) + 32 =$$
$$107 - 20 = 87$$

Science

1. **(B)** Positive and negative feedback systems are opposites, but both work to maintain homeostasis or balance in the body. Positive systems enhance and are self-amplifying—an action intensifies a condition and drives it beyond its normal limits. Hemostasis activates with injury to blood vessels. The following is a simplified description of blood clotting. Damaged cells at the site of injury release substances causing a chain reaction that attracts platelets to the site and clotting begins. Platelets release additional substances which accelerate clotting. A clot forms at the injury site and the clotting mechanism stops. The remaining options are examples of negative feedback. Negative feedback works to return the body back to its original or ideal state. Negative systems inhibit.

2. **(A)** The endocardium (innermost layer) is an endothelial lining, the myocardium (middle layer) is a muscle layer, and the epicardium (outermost layer) is a visceral layer. The pericardium is a sack that surrounds the heart and is not a part of the heart wall.

3. **(B)** In the fetus, the spleen is an important location of hematopoiesis or hemopoiesis, not hemostasis which is the process of clotting blood. The spleen has two main components—the red pulp and the white pulp. Asplenic individuals (those without spleens) are at greater risk of bacterial infection because of splenic absence (white pulp). The white pulp is considered part of the immune system and is the infection-fighting lymphatic area of the spleen where white cells are produced. The red pulp of the spleen filters blood and removes abnormal, old, and damaged red blood cells, cellular waste, pathogens, and bacteria.

4. **(A)** Melting of an ice cube is an example of a physical change. The ice cube changed from a solid state to a melted or liquefied state. There was no change in the matter. The remaining options are examples of a chemical change in which a new substance is formed.

5. **(C)** The information presented in the passage and on the chart suggests making a conclusion. The chart title includes the word *results*. The chart gives the values for the number of years as a Type 2 diabetic and the starting and ending A1C for each of the five participants. Analysis has been completed. Nothing suggests additional experiments are necessary, and the information has already been collected.

6. **(B)** Information collected in preparation for, during, or after a study is referred to as *data*. *Assumptions* are guesses, conjectures, or notions. Something *empiric* is practical or based on experience. *Notes* are explanations, observations, or clarifications.

7. **(B)** The key to answering this question correctly is thoroughly reading the stem which introduces information that has nothing to do with the study. Specific criteria are given for inclusion in the study—individuals had to have had Type 2 diabetes for 10 years to 15 years. Type 1 diabetes and Type 2 diabetes are not the same thing and are treated differently. Cost of a medication is not a factor, and all nondiabetics periodically have elevated blood sugar, but the body is able to adjust without outside intervention.

8. **(B)** Alkanes have single bonds between carbon atoms. As hydrocarbons, they are composed solely of hydrogen and carbon. CH_4 is methane, C_2H_6 is ethane, and C_4H_{10} is butane.

9. **(B)** The word *intermediate* means between. Of the options, only the uterus lies between the ovaries. The remaining structures lie below the uterus.

10. **(B)** Levels of testosterone are regulated by the negative feedback system of the pituitary gland which is stimulated by the hypothalamus. The remaining options do not stimulate testosterone production.

11. **(A)** Trace elements, such as iodine and cobalt, are required for physiological functioning and biochemical processes in organisms. The remaining options are incorrect.

12. **(C)** This question may be more difficult and requires thinking outside of the box. There is no need to determine the answer because the question does not ask for this. Each of the options is already in a ratio and proportion format, so this is not an issue. The issue is correctly setting up the equation. Options (A) and (B) can be discarded as incorrect because 100 centimeters is equal to 1 meter, *not* 10 centimeters equal to 1 meter. Option (D) can also be discarded because the equation is set up incorrectly. Ratio and proportion equations are balanced:

$$\text{centimeters} = \text{meters} :: \text{centimeters} = \text{meters}$$
$$\text{or}$$
$$\text{meters} = \text{centimeters} :: \text{meters} = \text{centimeters}$$

Option (C) is the only possible answer.

13. **(A)** Skeletal muscles are named based on specific characteristics such as shape, origin, insertion, location, and size. Action is a type of muscle movement produced or generated by a muscle. Flexor and extensor are opposites, as are abductor and adductor. The remaining options are types of muscle fascicles.

14. **(C)** The nervous system is divided into the central nervous system (composed of the brain and spinal cord) and peripheral nervous system (composed of the cranial nerves and spinal cord). Peripheral nervous system ⇒ autonomic nervous system ⇒ parasympathetic and sympathetic systems. Options (A) and (D) are subsystems of the peripheral nervous system.

15. **(C)** While maintaining muscle tone is part of the reticular formation, it is not a component of the reticular activating system (RAS). The remaining options are functions of the RAS.

16. **(C)** Negative feedback systems repair or correct deviations from normal homeostasis. Their actions cease when the deviation has been corrected. The nervous system and components of the endocrine system continually monitor the conditions of the body, and hormones are released when a deviation is found. Antagonistic hormones work within the negative feedback system. Hemopoiesis is the process that produces blood elements. The posterior pituitary produces vasopressin and oxytocin.

17. **(D)** Having an understanding of prefixes and suffixes can aid in correctly answering the question. Diffusion has to do with flowing or dispersion and should be dismissed as an incorrect answer. The prefixes *endo-* and *exo-* are opposites with *endo-* meaning inside or within, and *exo-* meaning outside. The suffix *–osis* means condition of something. Endocytosis and exocytosis can also be dismissed. The prefix *iso-* means equal and isotonic becomes the logical answer. Isotonic solutions are characterized by equal osmotic pressures.

18. **(C)** Blood is composed of formed cellular elements and plasma. Red blood cells, white blood cells, and platelets comprise the formed elements and are approximately 45 percent of blood volume. Plasma, approximately 55 percent of blood volume, is the clear straw or yellowish fluid part of blood. It is approximately 90 percent water, 8 percent protein plus electrolytes, waste products, oxygen and carbon dioxide, and nutrients.

19. **(A)** Of the four types of macromolecules, carbohydrates have structural and energy storage functions. Lipids, also known as fats, store energy. They have little or no liking or attraction to water and help separate aqueous solutions. DNA and various types of RNA are nucleic acids that carry genetic information. Proteins are highly varied organic molecules necessary in the diet of nonphotosynthesizing organisms.

20. **(D)** Rationality is not a characteristic of the human body. It is the mental state or ability to use logical reasoning in everyday life. The remaining options are characteristics of the human body.

21. **(B)** An individual with damage to the hypoglossal nerve (12th cranial nerve) will have difficulty with the tongue muscles and speaking. Impaired or absent gag reflex exhibits prob-

lems with the vagus nerve (10th cranial nerve), drooping eyelids can be seen with oculomotor nerve (3rd cranial nerve) problems, and problems with balance can be seen with auditory or vestibulocochlear nerve (8th cranial nerve) problems.

22. **(C)** Hormones are chemical controllers in the body. Antagonistic hormones have opposing outcomes or effects on the body. Glucagon and insulin work in opposition in the body. Glucagon increases blood glucose levels, while insulin decreases blood glucose levels. Adrenaline and epinephrine are the same thing, with epinephrine being the technically accepted term. Calcium is an element, not a hormone. Sodium and potassium are electrolytes, not hormones.

23. **(D)** Urea, a waste product, is a nitrogen-containing substance normally cleared from the blood via the kidneys and urine. Urea is toxic to the body and is produced in the liver during the process of converting amino acids to energy-supplying compounds. Other waste products are bilirubin from the breakdown of hemoglobin, and creatinine from the breakdown of creatine phosphate. Cholesterol is found in all animal tissues, predominantly the brain, spinal cord, and adipose tissues. It is a detoxifier in the blood and the precursor of many steroids.

24. **(A)** Blood pressure is the force of blood against the inner walls of blood vessels and varies throughout the body. Systolic pressure is highest in the aorta as oxygenated blood leaves the heart. The pressure falls as blood moves through the arterial system, to the venous system where the pressure falls to its lowest. Pressure is near zero in the vena cava.

25. **(C)** The renin-angiotensin-aldosterone system (RAAS) in the kidneys is responsible for regulating the body's blood pressure. The antidiuretic hormone, ADH or vasopressin, released from the posterior pituitary is included in this progression. In a complex process, the RAAS acts on the kidney tubules where it influences the rate of water reabsorption, thereby controlling blood pressure. The remaining options cannot perform this function.

26. **(C)** The spleen is the largest lymphatic organ in the human body. The liver is not a lymphatic organ. Of the organ components of the lymphatic system, the spleen is larger than lymph nodes and the thymus.

27. **(D)** The most *precise* measurement can be obtained using millimeters. While the diameter might be measured in centimeters, the height of the disc cannot. Centimeters, decimeters, and meters will not give the preciseness of millimeters.

28. **(B)** Professional football is a contact sport. Professional football players typically retire young and have numerous orthopedic problems. Of the options, this is the only logical answer. There is a high probability that Willis' orthopedic problems are related to his career history. The remaining careers typically do not have such problems at such a young age.

29. **(A)** Muscles are defined as agonist, antagonist, synergist, and fixator. Prime movers are agonist muscles that initiate the beginning of movement. Antagonist muscles oppose the prime mover muscle by controlling the motion and/or slowing it down. The remaining options are antonyms of antagonist.

30. **(C)** Four muscles control the movement of the mandible: the lateral pterygoid, medial pterygoid, masseter, and temporalis. The temporalis muscle can be felt in the temple when the mandible is clenched or closed. The buccinator and zygomaticus muscles have to do with facial expression, and the semimembranosus muscle is in the lower leg.

31. **(B)** Motor neurons transmit from the brain or spinal cord to an effector. Affecter is not an anatomic term. Receptors exist within the human body, but the word is nonspecific because it does not specify its type. Sensory neurons transmit impulses from the receptor to the brain or spinal cord.

32. **(D)** The stem is the definition of tonsils. Eustachian tubes connect the pharynx and middle ears. Perilymph is one of the two types of fluid found in the cochlear canals of the ear. Salivary glands are found in the mouth and secrete the enzyme amylase.

33. **(B)** The Krebs cycle is a multistep cellular, aerobic, metabolic process occurring in the mitochondria of a cell after glycolysis. The Krebs cycle does not occur in the cytoplasm or nucleus, and plastids are found in plant cells, not animal cells.

34. **(C)** Reabsorption takes place in the proximal convoluted tubules. Reabsorption occurs by osmosis (water), active transport (glucose, amino acids, sodium, and other ions), and diffusion (chloride). The ascending loop of Henle reabsorbs sodium by active transport, and the descending loop of Henle reabsorbs sodium via diffusion. The renal cortex is not involved in reabsorption.

35. **(D)** While the urinary system excretes urine, the urinary bladder is a holding structure, not an organ or organ system. The epithelial cells lining the intestines excrete iron and calcium salts and release water. The liver excretes bilirubin. The lungs excrete carbon dioxide and water vapor.

36. **(A)** Follicles are clusters of cells found in the ovaries. They contain an immature egg and play a part in the menstrual cycle. A fertilized egg would not be found in the ovary, an oocyte is an immature egg, and flagella are the lash-like "tails" that provide movement in sperm cells.

37. **(B)** Strong acids and bases release numerous ions in a reaction and are strong conductors of electricity. Weak acids and bases are the opposite. They release few ions and are poor conductors of electricity. The remaining options are incorrect.

38. **(D)** The human adult has 12 pairs of ribs. All of the ribs attach to the vertebrae. The first seven pairs of ribs articulate directly to the sternum and are called true ribs. The remaining five ribs do not directly connect to the sternum and are called false ribs.

39. **(C)** The stem of the question is the definition of diffusion. Active transport moves substances across a membrane from a lower to a higher concentration. With endocytosis, the membrane engulfs the substance and pulls it into the cell. Active reorganization is not a physiologic term.

40. **(D)** The nucleus is key to cellular reproduction. It is contained within the nuclear envelope which separates the nucleus from the cytoplasm. The nuclear envelope assists with regulation of what enters and leaves the nucleus. Chromosomes, consisting of DNA and other proteins, are located in the nucleus. Cytoplasm is fluid-like matter forming the basis of a cell. Organelles are found in the cytoplasm. The endoplasmic reticulum is located in the cytoplasm and is involved with protein and membrane synthesis. Mitochondria, also found in the cytoplasm, are the powerhouses of the cell.

41. **(D)** Gene is the word defined in the stem. DNA is located in the chromosomes of the gene. Codons are found in messenger RNA.

42. **(C)** Serous membranes cover the surfaces of organs located in the ventral cavity and line body cavities. These membranes lubricate or grease the organs and permit frictionless movement. The remainder of options are functions of connective tissue.

43. **(A)** The dermis (second major layer of the skin) is the most highly innervated and vascularized component of the integumentary system. The epidermis safeguards underlying tissues. Sensory receptors provide for touch, temperature, pain, and other things. The superfacial fascia stores fat.

44. **(C)** Short bones are basically cube-shaped and provide stability and a limited amount of movement. The patella is a sesamoid bone. The metatarsals and ulna are long bones. There are no metatarsals in the hip.

45. **(B)** The brain is the organizing and processing center of the nervous system. The brain receives impulses from the nerves via the spinal cord, interrupts these impulses, and transmits responses back to the appropriate sensory organs, glands, or muscles. The spinal cord coordinates nerve coordination. The option regarding regulation of two antagonistic hemispheres in the brain is incorrect—the brain does not regulate these hemispheres, and they are

not antagonistic in nature. The cerebellum, one component of the brain, coordinates organs of balance for motor activities.

46. **(A)** The pituitary hormone, prolactin, stimulates milk production in the mammary glands of the female after birth. The ovaries, placenta, and uterus are not affected by prolactin.

47. **(B)** Iodine is necessary for triiodothyronine and thyroxine production. Deficiencies can cause goiter, and in pregnancy deficiencies can cause permanent brain damage in newborns. Copper, essential for many body functions, prevents cell damage and is an enzyme factor in energy production, and the formation of connective tissues, erythrocytes, and bone. Manganese is essential in enzyme formation and activation, wound healing, and bone development. Zinc is involved in immune functioning, coagulation of blood, and normal growth and development.

48. **(A)** In terms of ion concentration in intracellular and extracellular fluids, the extracellular fluid has the highest concentration of sodium and chloride ions and bicarbonate. The intracellular fluid has the highest concentration of potassium, manganese, and phosphate. Extracellular fluid contains transcellular fluid, lymph, interstitial fluid, and plasma; intracellular does not.

49. **(D)** The atomic number of an element is equal to the number of electrons in an element. Electrons per shell for krypton (Kr) are 2, 8, 18, 8; for chromium (Cr) 2, 8, 13, 1; for gallium (Ga) 2, 8, 18, 3; and for selenium (Se) 2, 8, 18, 6.

50. **(A)** Group O is considered a universal donor because type or group O blood can be given to individuals of each of the remaining blood group.

51. **(B)** As a group AB donor, your blood can only be given to a group AB recipient.

52. **(C)** Group A blood recipients can only receive blood from donor group A or O blood grouping.

53. **(B)** Group AB is considered a universal recipient because it can receive blood from any donor blood grouping.

English and Language Usage

1. **(A)** The correct spelling is *movable*. The remaining options are incorrect.

2. **(A)** Subject and verb are in agreement. Correct agreement for the incorrect options follows:
   - He said no one has the right to tell him what to do.
   - Linda walked to the park every morning to exercise her dog.
   - Sam believed he would be successful if he worked hard.

3. **(B)** A homograph is a word that has the same spelling as another but has a different meaning. Homographs can also be spelled the same and have different pronunciation. *Address* is not a scolding, *buffet* is not fast-moving air, and *wave* is not a type of metal.

4. **(C)** The word *balk* has numerous definitions including to stop short, refuse to go forward, a sudden reversal, or a term in baseball. A synonym of *balked* or stopping short is *hesitate* or *hesitated*. The remaining options are antonyms of *balked*.

5. **(D)** The root word *celer* means speed. *Accelerators* are pushed or manipulated to decrease or increase speed. The remaining options are incorrect.

6. **(A)** Correctly punctuated, the sentence should read: *The judge asked, "Ladies and gentlemen of the jury, have you reached a verdict?"* The remaining sentences are correct.

7. **(A)** *Corrugated* is the correct spelling, not *corregeted*. The remaining options are spelled correctly.

8. **(B)** The incorrect term *alright* is spelled incorrectly for formal writing and is often confused with *all right*, the correct term. *All right* signifies agreement, something satisfactory, or appropriate. The remaining sentences are correct.

9. **(D)** *Woodies* are station wagons with wood or simulated wood paneling on the outside body of the car. Originally meant as utility vehicles, and unpopular in the fifties, woodies came into vogue in the sixties with the surfer craze. Woodies could be bought cheaply and were long enough to carry the long surfboards of the day. The remaining options are incorrect.

10. **(D)** The correct sentence does not require punctuation within the sentence, only at the end of the sentence. The remaining options should be punctuated as follows:
   - Concession prices at the local theater are so high they encourage sneaking food in to have something to eat during the movie.
   - Mason had a growth spurt over the summer and was now the tallest boy in his class.
   - Residents were unsure how to take the new boarder since she stayed shut up in her room during the evening hours.

11. **(B)** In the majority of instances, *take* is action going away from the speaker where *bring* is action moving in the direction of the speaker. The sentence should read: *His mother said, "Bring the flowers over to me."* The remainder of the options have correct usage of words.

12. **(B)** Complex sentences are composed of an independent clause (or sentence) joined to one or more dependent clauses by a subordinating conjunction. *J. H. Westerling, in the U.S. Senate for 24 years, lost the election to a nonpolitician* is the independent clause, *because* is the subordinating conjunction, and *because he believed he was a shoe-in* is the dependent clause. Options (A) and (C) are simple sentences, and option (D) is a compound sentence.

13. **(D)** *Autocratic* is a form of ruling where the people have no voice in their government and may have little say over their daily lives. An autocratic ruler is one who rules with absolute power and authority. Adolf Hitler was an autocratic ruler. The remaining options are incorrect.

14. **(A)** The use of the word *cougar* is a slang term for an older woman dating a younger man. Slang terms are frequently found in informal writing and speech. The remaining options are written in a formal tone or language.

15. **(C)** *Swollen* means enlarged or puffed-up. *Rising* is a synonym for swollen. The remaining options are antonyms of swollen.

16. **(C)** The root word *mort* means death. Morticians take care of the dead; they are undertakers. The remaining options do not support the definition.

17. **(C)** The word *junct* means join. A conjunction is a word that joins independent and dependent clauses or phrases together. The remaining options do not satisfy the definition of *junct*.

18. **(A)** The sentence is a complex sentence. A comma is needed when the dependent clause comes first. No comma is needed when the independent clause is first. *Because of the fracas at last year's prom, Frank's repeated requests to be included on this year's prom planning committee have been ignored* is correctly punctuated. The remaining options are correctly punctuated.

19. **(C)** *Countenance* is the correct spelling, not *contenence*. The remaining options are spelled correctly.

20. **(B)** *Accept* is the correct word to use in the sentence. The correct word in option (A) should have been *already*, meaning the action occurred in the past, and has nothing to do with *all ready*, which means prepared. *Allusions*, in option (C), is an indirect reference or a hint. The correct word is *delusions* meaning attitudes, opinions, or false beliefs. *Between* is incorrect in option (D) and is used when referring to two things. The sentence would have been correct if it read, *Divide his wealth among his wife and three sons.* The correct word should have been *among*, which is used for three or more.

21. **(B)** Correctly punctuated, the sentence reads, *Lost Victory, who won the Kentucky Derby, sired four Preakness winners.* The clause, *who won the Kentucky Derby*, is not essential to the sen-

tence and can be removed without changing the intent or meaning of the sentence. Commas are used to set off nonessential clauses. The remaining options are correctly punctuated.

22. **(D)** The following is correctly punctuated: *Vince told his friends that he would meet them at the trail head.* The sentence is not a direct quote and does not require quotation marks. The remaining options are correct.

23. **(B)** The root word *matri* means mother. *Matrilineal* means descending or handed down via the female line. The remaining options are incorrect.

24. **(B)** *Mary Johnson, who runs 25 miles a week, can outrun any boy at the school* is correctly punctuated. The clause, *who runs 25 miles a week,* is not essential to the sentence and can be removed without changing the intent or meaning of the sentence. Commas are used to set off nonessential clauses. The remaining options are correctly punctuated.

25. **(A)** Brainstorming, if used, comes prior to the writing process. The elements of the writing process are planning, organizing, writing, and editing and revising.

26. **(C)** Conjunctions are used in writing to tie words and clauses (phrases) together. The word *and* is a joining word or conjunction. The remaining options contain prepositions (*in addition to, many, from,* and *since*).

27. **(B)** The stem of the question is the definition of *comma*. It is an interruption or pause. A colon creates or introduces a list, series, or statement. A dash indicates a sudden change in thought, explanation, or definition. A period terminates a statement. Periods are placed at the end of a sentence.

28. **(B)** The correct spelling is *believe*. The remaining options are correctly spelled.

Practice Test 4

ANSWER SHEET
Practice Test 4

Reading

1. Ⓐ Ⓑ Ⓒ Ⓓ
2. Ⓐ Ⓑ Ⓒ Ⓓ
3. Ⓐ Ⓑ Ⓒ Ⓓ
4. Ⓐ Ⓑ Ⓒ Ⓓ
5. Ⓐ Ⓑ Ⓒ Ⓓ
6. Ⓐ Ⓑ Ⓒ Ⓓ
7. Ⓐ Ⓑ Ⓒ Ⓓ
8. Ⓐ Ⓑ Ⓒ Ⓓ
9. Ⓐ Ⓑ Ⓒ Ⓓ
10. Ⓐ Ⓑ Ⓒ Ⓓ
11. Ⓐ Ⓑ Ⓒ Ⓓ
12. Ⓐ Ⓑ Ⓒ Ⓓ
13. Ⓐ Ⓑ Ⓒ Ⓓ
14. Ⓐ Ⓑ Ⓒ Ⓓ

15. Ⓐ Ⓑ Ⓒ Ⓓ
16. Ⓐ Ⓑ Ⓒ Ⓓ
17. Ⓐ Ⓑ Ⓒ Ⓓ
18. Ⓐ Ⓑ Ⓒ Ⓓ
19. Ⓐ Ⓑ Ⓒ Ⓓ
20. Ⓐ Ⓑ Ⓒ Ⓓ
21. Ⓐ Ⓑ Ⓒ Ⓓ
22. Ⓐ Ⓑ Ⓒ Ⓓ
23. Ⓐ Ⓑ Ⓒ Ⓓ
24. Ⓐ Ⓑ Ⓒ Ⓓ
25. Ⓐ Ⓑ Ⓒ Ⓓ
26. Ⓐ Ⓑ Ⓒ Ⓓ
27. Ⓐ Ⓑ Ⓒ Ⓓ
28. Ⓐ Ⓑ Ⓒ Ⓓ

29. Ⓐ Ⓑ Ⓒ Ⓓ
30. Ⓐ Ⓑ Ⓒ Ⓓ
31. Ⓐ Ⓑ Ⓒ Ⓓ
32. Ⓐ Ⓑ Ⓒ Ⓓ
33. Ⓐ Ⓑ Ⓒ Ⓓ
34. Ⓐ Ⓑ Ⓒ Ⓓ
35. Ⓐ Ⓑ Ⓒ Ⓓ
36. Ⓐ Ⓑ Ⓒ Ⓓ
37. Ⓐ Ⓑ Ⓒ Ⓓ
38. Ⓐ Ⓑ Ⓒ Ⓓ
39. Ⓐ Ⓑ Ⓒ Ⓓ
40. Ⓐ Ⓑ Ⓒ Ⓓ
41. Ⓐ Ⓑ Ⓒ Ⓓ
42. Ⓐ Ⓑ Ⓒ Ⓓ

43. Ⓐ Ⓑ Ⓒ Ⓓ
44. Ⓐ Ⓑ Ⓒ Ⓓ
45. Ⓐ Ⓑ Ⓒ Ⓓ
46. Ⓐ Ⓑ Ⓒ Ⓓ
47. Ⓐ Ⓑ Ⓒ Ⓓ
48. Ⓐ Ⓑ Ⓒ Ⓓ
49. Ⓐ Ⓑ Ⓒ Ⓓ
50. Ⓐ Ⓑ Ⓒ Ⓓ
51. Ⓐ Ⓑ Ⓒ Ⓓ
52. Ⓐ Ⓑ Ⓒ Ⓓ
53. Ⓐ Ⓑ Ⓒ Ⓓ

Mathematics

1. Ⓐ Ⓑ Ⓒ Ⓓ
2. Ⓐ Ⓑ Ⓒ Ⓓ
3. Ⓐ Ⓑ Ⓒ Ⓓ
4. Ⓐ Ⓑ Ⓒ Ⓓ
5. Ⓐ Ⓑ Ⓒ Ⓓ
6. Ⓐ Ⓑ Ⓒ Ⓓ
7. Ⓐ Ⓑ Ⓒ Ⓓ
8. Ⓐ Ⓑ Ⓒ Ⓓ
9. Ⓐ Ⓑ Ⓒ Ⓓ

10. Ⓐ Ⓑ Ⓒ Ⓓ
11. Ⓐ Ⓑ Ⓒ Ⓓ
12. Ⓐ Ⓑ Ⓒ Ⓓ
13. Ⓐ Ⓑ Ⓒ Ⓓ
14. Ⓐ Ⓑ Ⓒ Ⓓ
15. Ⓐ Ⓑ Ⓒ Ⓓ
16. Ⓐ Ⓑ Ⓒ Ⓓ
17. Ⓐ Ⓑ Ⓒ Ⓓ
18. Ⓐ Ⓑ Ⓒ Ⓓ

19. Ⓐ Ⓑ Ⓒ Ⓓ
20. Ⓐ Ⓑ Ⓒ Ⓓ
21. Ⓐ Ⓑ Ⓒ Ⓓ
22. Ⓐ Ⓑ Ⓒ Ⓓ
23. Ⓐ Ⓑ Ⓒ Ⓓ
24. Ⓐ Ⓑ Ⓒ Ⓓ
25. Ⓐ Ⓑ Ⓒ Ⓓ
26. Ⓐ Ⓑ Ⓒ Ⓓ
27. Ⓐ Ⓑ Ⓒ Ⓓ

28. Ⓐ Ⓑ Ⓒ Ⓓ
29. Ⓐ Ⓑ Ⓒ Ⓓ
30. Ⓐ Ⓑ Ⓒ Ⓓ
31. Ⓐ Ⓑ Ⓒ Ⓓ
32. Ⓐ Ⓑ Ⓒ Ⓓ
33. Ⓐ Ⓑ Ⓒ Ⓓ
34. Ⓐ Ⓑ Ⓒ Ⓓ
35. Ⓐ Ⓑ Ⓒ Ⓓ
36. Ⓐ Ⓑ Ⓒ Ⓓ

ANSWER SHEET
Practice Test 4

Science

1. Ⓐ Ⓑ Ⓒ Ⓓ
2. Ⓐ Ⓑ Ⓒ Ⓓ
3. Ⓐ Ⓑ Ⓒ Ⓓ
4. Ⓐ Ⓑ Ⓒ Ⓓ
5. Ⓐ Ⓑ Ⓒ Ⓓ
6. Ⓐ Ⓑ Ⓒ Ⓓ
7. Ⓐ Ⓑ Ⓒ Ⓓ
8. Ⓐ Ⓑ Ⓒ Ⓓ
9. Ⓐ Ⓑ Ⓒ Ⓓ
10. Ⓐ Ⓑ Ⓒ Ⓓ
11. Ⓐ Ⓑ Ⓒ Ⓓ
12. Ⓐ Ⓑ Ⓒ Ⓓ
13. Ⓐ Ⓑ Ⓒ Ⓓ
14. Ⓐ Ⓑ Ⓒ Ⓓ

15. Ⓐ Ⓑ Ⓒ Ⓓ
16. Ⓐ Ⓑ Ⓒ Ⓓ
17. Ⓐ Ⓑ Ⓒ Ⓓ
18. Ⓐ Ⓑ Ⓒ Ⓓ
19. Ⓐ Ⓑ Ⓒ Ⓓ
20. Ⓐ Ⓑ Ⓒ Ⓓ
21. Ⓐ Ⓑ Ⓒ Ⓓ
22. Ⓐ Ⓑ Ⓒ Ⓓ
23. Ⓐ Ⓑ Ⓒ Ⓓ
24. Ⓐ Ⓑ Ⓒ Ⓓ
25. Ⓐ Ⓑ Ⓒ Ⓓ
26. Ⓐ Ⓑ Ⓒ Ⓓ
27. Ⓐ Ⓑ Ⓒ Ⓓ
28. Ⓐ Ⓑ Ⓒ Ⓓ

29. Ⓐ Ⓑ Ⓒ Ⓓ
30. Ⓐ Ⓑ Ⓒ Ⓓ
31. Ⓐ Ⓑ Ⓒ Ⓓ
32. Ⓐ Ⓑ Ⓒ Ⓓ
33. Ⓐ Ⓑ Ⓒ Ⓓ
34. Ⓐ Ⓑ Ⓒ Ⓓ
35. Ⓐ Ⓑ Ⓒ Ⓓ
36. Ⓐ Ⓑ Ⓒ Ⓓ
37. Ⓐ Ⓑ Ⓒ Ⓓ
38. Ⓐ Ⓑ Ⓒ Ⓓ
39. Ⓐ Ⓑ Ⓒ Ⓓ
40. Ⓐ Ⓑ Ⓒ Ⓓ
41. Ⓐ Ⓑ Ⓒ Ⓓ
42. Ⓐ Ⓑ Ⓒ Ⓓ

43. Ⓐ Ⓑ Ⓒ Ⓓ
44. Ⓐ Ⓑ Ⓒ Ⓓ
45. Ⓐ Ⓑ Ⓒ Ⓓ
46. Ⓐ Ⓑ Ⓒ Ⓓ
47. Ⓐ Ⓑ Ⓒ Ⓓ
48. Ⓐ Ⓑ Ⓒ Ⓓ
49. Ⓐ Ⓑ Ⓒ Ⓓ
50. Ⓐ Ⓑ Ⓒ Ⓓ
51. Ⓐ Ⓑ Ⓒ Ⓓ
52. Ⓐ Ⓑ Ⓒ Ⓓ
53. Ⓐ Ⓑ Ⓒ Ⓓ

English and Language Usage

1. Ⓐ Ⓑ Ⓒ Ⓓ
2. Ⓐ Ⓑ Ⓒ Ⓓ
3. Ⓐ Ⓑ Ⓒ Ⓓ
4. Ⓐ Ⓑ Ⓒ Ⓓ
5. Ⓐ Ⓑ Ⓒ Ⓓ
6. Ⓐ Ⓑ Ⓒ Ⓓ
7. Ⓐ Ⓑ Ⓒ Ⓓ

8. Ⓐ Ⓑ Ⓒ Ⓓ
9. Ⓐ Ⓑ Ⓒ Ⓓ
10. Ⓐ Ⓑ Ⓒ Ⓓ
11. Ⓐ Ⓑ Ⓒ Ⓓ
12. Ⓐ Ⓑ Ⓒ Ⓓ
13. Ⓐ Ⓑ Ⓒ Ⓓ
14. Ⓐ Ⓑ Ⓒ Ⓓ

15. Ⓐ Ⓑ Ⓒ Ⓓ
16. Ⓐ Ⓑ Ⓒ Ⓓ
17. Ⓐ Ⓑ Ⓒ Ⓓ
18. Ⓐ Ⓑ Ⓒ Ⓓ
19. Ⓐ Ⓑ Ⓒ Ⓓ
20. Ⓐ Ⓑ Ⓒ Ⓓ
21. Ⓐ Ⓑ Ⓒ Ⓓ

22. Ⓐ Ⓑ Ⓒ Ⓓ
23. Ⓐ Ⓑ Ⓒ Ⓓ
24. Ⓐ Ⓑ Ⓒ Ⓓ
25. Ⓐ Ⓑ Ⓒ Ⓓ
26. Ⓐ Ⓑ Ⓒ Ⓓ
27. Ⓐ Ⓑ Ⓒ Ⓓ
28. Ⓐ Ⓑ Ⓒ Ⓓ

READING

NUMBER OF QUESTIONS: 53

TIME LIMIT: 64 MINUTES

Instructions: Read each question thoroughly. Select the single best answer. Mark your answer (A, B, C, or D) on the answer sheet provided for Practice Test 4.

Questions 1–2 are based on the following heart and blood pressure monitor.

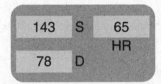

1. What is the heart rate?

   (A) 65 beats per hour
   (B) 65 beats per minute
   (C) 65 beats per second
   (D) 65 beats per 24 hours

2. What is the systolic blood pressure?

   (A) 78
   (B) 95.3
   (C) 110.5
   (D) 143

3. Austin joins the Navy to see the world. Halfway through his period of enlistment a regional conflict develops into a war. His ship is sent to a war-torn area where he is killed in action.

   The organization of events in this passage is

   (A) dissimilar.
   (B) individual.
   (C) isolated.
   (D) sequential.

Questions 4–6 are based on the following chart.

HPER 3713

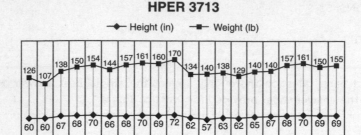

4. Of the 20 students with height/weight information on the chart, which student is both the tallest and heaviest?

(A) #4
(B) #9
(C) #10
(D) #18

5. How many students on the chart weigh less than 150 pounds?

(A) 10
(B) 12
(C) 14
(D) 16

6. How many students are 5-feet tall or taller?

(A) 7
(B) 12
(C) 15
(D) 19

Questions 7–11 are based on the following letter appearing in the *Letters to the Editor* section of a small-town newspaper.

If you have been following the local news, you are aware of the escalating vandalism that has been running rampant in the rural areas of our county for the last six months. It started off with simple Halloween pranks and has grown more dangerous and costly as time has progressed. Last Wednesday, Tom Parker's barn burned down as the result of several bales of hay near the barn being torched. Livestock were safely removed, but the barn and its contents were totally destroyed.

Based on the nature of the vandalism, Sheriff Brander and his deputies say the perpetrators are most likely juveniles, but they have not found enough evidence to be sure. Sheriff Brander stated that 43 individual acts of vandalism have occurred in the past six months. Based on a review of this year's budget, the Sheriff's Department does not have the money or manpower to constantly patrol a county as large as ours.

It's time the good folks of this county start to take responsibility and look into where their children are after the sun goes down. This vandalism is the work of a gang of boys, not just one or two. Teachers, what are your students whispering in the hallways? Students, when are you going to *step up* and help law enforcement put an end to this problem?

7. Who is the author's anticipated audience?

    (A) Individuals residing in the rural areas of the county
    (B) Individuals reading the editorial section of the newspaper
    (C) County law enforcement
    (D) Newspaper subscribers

8. What is the tone of the piece?

    (A) Appeasement
    (B) Hostility
    (C) Pleasantry
    (D) Vexation

9. What, in the passage, demonstrates the writer is biased?

    (A) Lack of money and manpower in the Sheriff's Department
    (B) Rampant vandalism in the county
    (C) Vandalism is the work of a gang of boys.
    (D) Vandals are most likely juveniles.

10. What is the writer's intent in the letter to the editor of the newspaper?

    (A) Education
    (B) Information
    (C) Narration
    (D) Persuasion

11. What does the idiom *step up* in the last sentence suggest?

    (A) Betray their peers involved with the vandalism
    (B) Exacerbate the vandalism problem
    (C) Have a responsibility or obligation to help solve the vandalism problem
    (D) Provoke individuals involved with the vandalism

12. What is the meaning of the italicized word in the following sentence?

    It didn't seem to matter to Sue Ann that her *recalcitrant* behavior had suspended her from school for the third time this year.

    (A) Adaptable
    (B) Manageable
    (C) Practicable
    (D) Noncompliant

13. What does the italicized abbreviation in the following sentence mean?

    Moises was diagnosed with pet dandruff allergy when he was four years old, but as an adult he found he still had problems with long-haired dogs as opposed to short-haired dogs (*e.g.,* Dachshund, Chihuahua, Ibizan Hound, Fox Terrier, and Doberman).

    (A) For example
    (B) In addition to
    (C) Instead of
    (D) That is

Questions 14–16 are based on the following passage and chart.

The coach of four 20-km runners of the Prairie Tornado Running Club is conducting an informal study to try to determine if there is a correlation between training hours per week and finish position in a race. Mavis and CeCe are female runners, and Tom and Randall are male runners. All four of the runners are married, have young families, and work 40 hours a week. There are three 20-km races each running season.

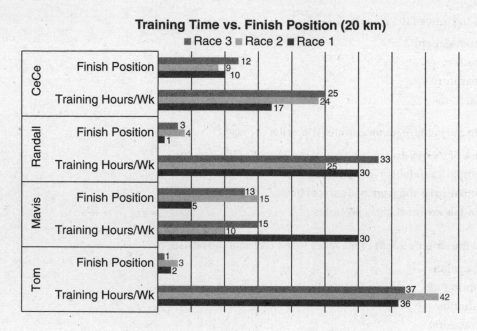

14. In what position did Randall finish in the first race?

(A) First
(B) Fourth
(C) Second
(D) Third

15. Which runner had the highest number of training hours for the second race?

(A) CeCe
(B) Mavis
(C) Randall
(D) Tom

16. What could the coach have done to make the study more precise?

(A) Define what is meant by "training hours"
(B) Hire a professional trainer to work with the four runners
(C) Increase the number of 20 km races in the study
(D) Use either female or male participants but not both

Questions 17–19 are based on the passage and descendant chart of Abner Johnson.

Abner Johnson—whose birth date is unknown and who died in 1840—and his family were early settlers of America. Abner was married three times and outlived his wives and many of his children.

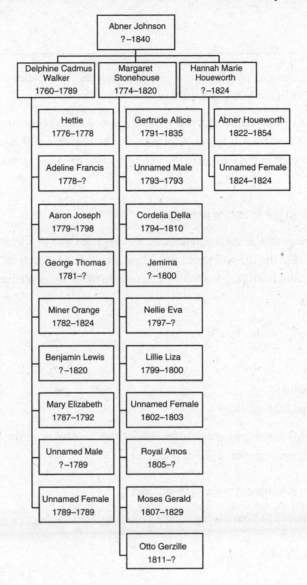

17. What is the name of Abner's second wife?

(A) Gertrude Alice Johnson

(B) Hannah Marie Houeworth

(C) Hettie Johnson

(D) Margaret Stonehouse

18. Abner Johnson had a total of _____ son(s).

(A) five

(B) four

(C) seven

(D) ten

19. Of Abner's living children, in what year was the first male born?

(A) 1778
(B) 1779
(C) 1782
(D) 1822

---

20. Which of the following is not a reliable reference source for a scholarly paper on advances in the treatment of Gaucher's disease in the past 100 years?

(A) A Gaucher's disease research site that offers disease specific medicine for purchase
(B) An out-of-print medical book containing information on Gaucher's disease with a 1922 copyright
(C) A medical journal such as the *Journal of the American Medical Association*
(D) MedlinePlus

Questions 21–23 are based on the following passage.

John is a *sucker* for magazine advertisements and has been known to spend $200 to $300 a month on substandard merchandise that he will never use. He is presently planning on purchasing a flashlight for $50 plus tax, shipping, and handling. The following are from the magazine advertisement:

- All sales are final
- Compact enough to fit in a backpack
- Durable
- Lifetime guarantee
- Strongest light available
- Used by professional organizations

John approaches you, his best friend, about his potential purchase because you have previously *chided* him on his lack of thorough investigation with his purchases.

21. What does the word *sucker* suggest in the first sentence?

(A) John is a laughingstock or joke.
(B) John is eager to please.
(C) John is easily conned or deceived.
(D) John is solicitous.

22. Not wanting to embarrass John and make him feel imprudent, you try to turn the situation into a positive moment. Which of the following would be most helpful for John?

(A) Knowing if the magazine is reputable
(B) Knowing who the flashlight manufacturer is
(C) Knowing the total cost of the purchase
(D) Knowing the type of batteries the flashlight uses and if the flashlight bulb is replaceable

23. What is a synonym for *chided* in the last sentence of the passage?

(A) Complimented
(B) Eulogized
(C) Extolled
(D) Nagged

Questions 24–25 are based on the following passage.

Some say that Angela is *bullheaded* and refuses to learn from her mistakes because she does not believe she has ever been wrong. She wants to be a nurse anesthetist but has not been able to gain admittance to any bachelor's level nursing program because she has not passed the entrance exams. Angela minimally meets the requirements for each nursing program she has applied to, and the problem, as she sees it, is the various entrance tests do not test what she believes is important for admittance to a nursing program and subsequent admission to a nurse anesthetist program.

24. Angela's probability of achieving her goal of becoming a nurse anesthetist is

    (A) good if she repeats her borderline courses.
    (B) highly improbable.
    (C) Not enough information is provided to answer this question.
    (D) probable.

25. Which of the following is a definition for *bullheaded* in the first sentence of the passage?

    (A) A person who has little common sense.
    (B) A person who is adamantly opinionated and refuses to consider other possibilities.
    (C) A person who is hesitant to consider other possibilities and is supportive of freedom of choice.
    (D) A person who will compromise when all else fails.

---

26. Use the following instructions to change SECRET into another word.

    1. Drop the S and add a B.
    2. Move the second E to after the T.
    3. Drop the CR and add HA.
    4. Drop the T and add V.

    The new word is

    (A) becr.
    (B) becrave.
    (C) behave.
    (D) secrets.

27. The guides at the top of a dictionary page are *zamindari* and *zoetrope*. Which of the following words are found on this page?

    (A) Zabajone
    (B) Zetetics
    (C) Zugzwang
    (D) Zyzzyvas

Questions 28–30 are based on the following e-mail.

To: All library card holders of Flat Rock County Library
From: Marcia Wintstet, Head Librarian, Flat Rock County Library
Date: April 5

As of the library's yearly audit, it was found that library cards for one-third of patrons have been inactive for the last five or more years. Library card status may be checked online at *www.flatrocklib.org/patrons/cardstatus*. Cards inactive for five or more years will be deactivated on June 1st if one of the following is not done:

- Contact the library via e-mail at *library10@flatrockco.org* stating you would like to keep your card status active. Include the number of the library card, your current name and home address, telephone number, and e-mail address in the e-mail. A new library card will be available for pickup at the library within three to four weeks.
- Come to the library and fill out a new library card form if you have lost your library card. A new card will be available for pickup within three to four weeks.

If you no longer wish to have a library card with Flat Rock County Library, no action is required.

28. What type of communication is the e-mail?

(A) Cause and affect
(B) Exclamatory and rhetorical
(C) Information and technical
(D) Structural and persuasive

29. Who is the intended audience of the e-mail?

(A) All library card holders of the library
(B) Individuals who currently use their library card on a regular basis
(C) Library card holders who have fines they have not paid
(D) Library card holders who have not used their library card in five or more years

30. What is a synonym for the word *patron* in the first sentence of the e-mail message?

(A) Advocate
(B) Customer
(C) Detractor
(D) End user

Questions 31–35 are based on the following passage.

A Simple Sepsis Fact Sheet

- **Definition**
  - Sepsis is a potentially lethal complication of infection somewhere in the body.
  - The death rate from sepsis can be as high as 50 percent.
- **Etiology**
  - An individual cannot develop sepsis without first having a serious infection.
    - Infections can be brought about by many different microbes. The most frequent causes are bacteria, fungi, and viruses.
  - Sepsis develops as a result of chemicals released by the immune system to combat the infection that instigate widespread inflammation.
- **Risk factors**
  - Any individual with a serious infection may develop sepsis.
  - Individuals most at risk
    - Sustained severe trauma such as burns and physical trauma
    - Chronic illnesses such as diabetes, AIDS, cancer, respiratory, liver, and kidney disease
    - Weakened immune systems
    - Infants, children, and the elderly
- **Symptoms**
  - Hypothermia or hyperthermia
  - Increased respiratory rate
  - Increased heart rate
  - Difficulty breathing
  - Chills/shaking
  - Rash
  - Changes in mental status such as confusion and/or disorientation
  - Drop in blood pressure
  - Inability of body organs to function properly
  - Decrease in urinary output
- **Diagnosis by health care provider**
  - Medical/surgical history
  - Physical assessment
  - Blood tests
    - Complete blood count
    - Arterial blood gases
    - Kidney function
  - Wound, urine, sputum, and blood cultures
  - Radiologic studies such as X-ray, CT scan, and MRI
- **Treatment**
  - Hospital admission usually to intensive care unit
  - Broad spectrum antibiotics (never started until after cultures have been drawn)
- **Focus on prevention of infection**
  - Receiving recommended vaccinations against preventable diseases
  - Removal of urinary catheters and intravenous lines when no longer needed
  - Good hand washing
  - Do not self-medicate with antibiotics.

31. What is the purpose of a fact sheet?

   (A) To entertain
   (B) To inform
   (C) To persuade
   (D) To provide instruction

32. What kind of condition is sepsis?

   (A) Primary
   (B) Secondary
   (C) Both primary and secondary
   (D) Neither primary nor secondary

33. What body system brings about sepsis?

   (A) Any organ system in the body
   (B) The cardiovascular or respiratory system
   (C) The immune system
   (D) The organ system with the infection

34. What does hyperthermia suggest?

   (A) An individual's temperatures cannot be determined.
   (B) An individual's temperature is decreased.
   (C) An individual's temperature is elevated.
   (D) An individual's temperature is normal.

35. A health care provider orders blood cultures for a patient recently diagnosed with sepsis. What is inferred when the fact sheet states, *Broad spectrum antibiotics (never started until after cultures have been drawn)*?

   (A) Antibiotics administered prior to the drawing of blood can adversely affect the culture results.
   (B) Antibiotics administered prior to the drawing of blood can encourage the growth of infectious microbes.
   (C) Infectious aerobic microbes will be more susceptible to antibiotics after the cultures have been drawn.
   (D) Infectious anaerobic microbes will be more susceptible to antibiotics after the cultures have been drawn.

36. What are the following poll results suggestive of?

   ■ Thirty-eight percent of males preferred chocolate ice cream; 63 percent of females preferred vanilla ice cream.
   ■ Males as well as females state that coloring hair was acceptable in most circumstances.
   ■ Three percent of males and females had juvenile records, with 97 percent having no experience with the judicial system.
   ■ In spite of gender differences, the majority of students prefer summer sports to winter ones.

   (A) Cause and effect
   (B) Compare and contrast
   (C) None of the above
   (D) Problem and solution

37. What is the figurative device used in the following sentence?

   Getting Marty to take a nap is as difficult as nailing jelly to a tree.

   (A) Alliteration
   (B) Metaphor
   (C) Non-sequitur
   (D) Simile

38. The topic of Kally's research paper for her literature course is the poetry of James Kavanaugh. Which of the following would be the best source of information?

   (A) A poetry journal
   (B) An anthology
   (C) An autobiography
   (D) An encyclopedia

39. As the chairperson for a hiring committee, you receive a letter of recommendation for an individual applying for the position of journalistic director for the department. The letter speaks highly of the applicant and his accomplishments. From a previously submitted résumé, you know the applicant is 28 years old, received his bachelor's degree in journalism five years ago, and has been one of two reporters for the *Swankway Bulletin*, a weekly publication for a village of 1,200 people, for four and a half years, and has no publications outside of the *Swankway Bulletin*.

   Which of the following from the letter of recommendation would you fact check?

   (A) Four short stories submitted to local writing club annual prize writing contest
   (B) Nobel Prize for Journalism finalist
   (C) Represents field of journalism at local high school career day
   (D) *Swankway Bulletin* reporter of the month for eight consecutive months

40. Using the five shapes below, follow the directions to form a new shape.

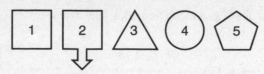

- Join the top of Shape 2 to the bottom of Shape 1.
- Attach Shape 3 to the center of the left side of Shape 1.
- Attach Shape 4 to the uppermost right corner of Shape 1.
- Attach the topmost peak of Shape 5 to the bottommost part of Shape 2.

Select the new shape.

(A)

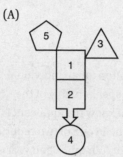

(B)

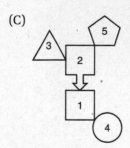

(C)

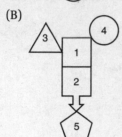

(D)

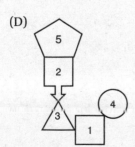

Questions 41–43 are based on the following passage and table.

Oliver Bates, aged 77, is considering a number of local house-painting contractors to repair and paint the exterior of his wood-framed home. He researched the following contractors.

Contractor	Ratings (Five stars highest)	Labor, Repair, Material, & Supply Cost	Time Estimate	Paint Cost	Coats of Paint	Paint Warranty
Smith Bros.*	★★★★★	$1200/day (2 men)	5 days (9 hr days)	$216/5 gal × 2**	1	Limited lifetime
Pine Mountain	★★★★	$1400/day (2 men + apprentice)	5–6 days (9 hr days)	$198/5 gal × 2	1	Limited lifetime
Jones & Walker	★	$780/day (2 full-time college students) (labor only, no repair)	6 to 8 weekends (weekends only, 5–6 hr days)	Buyer is responsible for obtaining all supplies, materials, and other items for painting. Buyer is also responsible for cleaning items after each work day.		
Abbotts	★★	$558/day (1 man)	12 to 16 days (8 hr days)	$95.99/5 gal × 5	2	1 year

*All work 100% guaranteed for 5 years

**Owner preselected paint and price is included in supply/material cost

41. Estimate the amount Jones & Walker would receive to paint the house.

   (A) $6,000 to $8,500
   (B) $7,800 to $10,000
   (C) $9,600 to $12,800
   (D) $11,500 to $14,000

42. Which of the following companies has the best offer?

   (A) Abbotts
   (B) Jones & Walker
   (C) Pine Mountain
   (D) Smith Bros.

43. Which of the following companies would be the costliest to the homeowner?

   (A) Abbotts
   (B) Jones & Walker
   (C) Pine Mountain
   (D) Smith Bros.

Questions 44–47 are based on the following passage and diagram.

Anxiety is a response to an actual or perceived stressor. The stressor causing the anxiety may be challenging, harmful, or threatening. Anxiety is not necessarily a bad thing. A small amount contests and motivates. Responses to stressors are subjective. For example, if I am afraid of snakes, and you have snakes as pets and handle them on a daily basis, our responses to being around snakes will be different—my anxiety level will be much different from yours. In nursing, subjective information comes from and is unique to the patient. Subjective data may or may not be evident to others. Objective data is the opposite of subjective data. The following diagram presents increasing levels of anxiety and their effects.

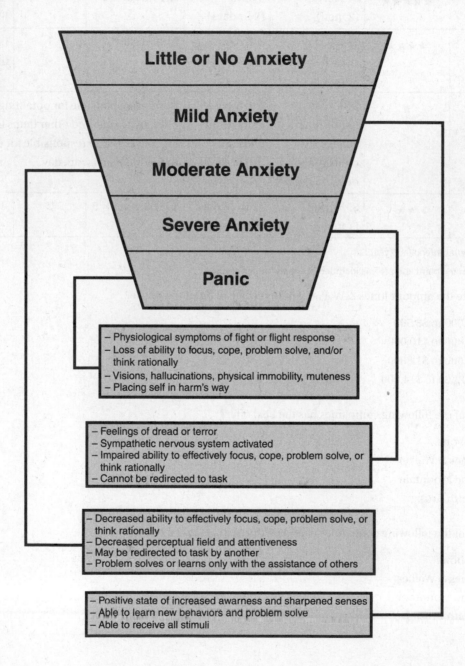

44. What are objective data as opposed to subjective data?

    (A) Objective data always include biological variables.
    (B) Objective data can be observed, seen, or known by others.
    (C) Objective data influence age and developmental maturity or both.
    (D) Objective data are a learned coping response.

45. Robin and Fara are hiking in the woods and come upon a swarm of bees. Robin is allergic to bees and panics. What is the best action for Fara to take?

    (A) Attempt to scatter the bees
    (B) Leave Robin and go for help
    (C) Stay with Robin and support her
    (D) Use a loud, authoritative voice when talking to Robin

46. Peter and Paula's parents have gone to a Christmas party and left them alone without a babysitter for the first time. They decide to watch psychological thrillers on television and, by the end of the second movie, they are convinced that danger lurks in every dark shadow in the house. Upon returning home, Peter and Paula's parents find their children have every light in the house turned on. What level of anxiety have Peter and Paula demonstrated?

    (A) Mild anxiety
    (B) Moderate anxiety
    (C) Panic
    (D) Severe anxiety

47. Markus has suffered from an anxiety disorder since he was trapped in his car for 20 hours after the car went over an embankment and plunged 35 feet into a ravine. He has been in therapy to treat his anxiety for the past several months. Which of the following would be the most positive outcome for Markus?

    (A) He accepts, but cannot identify or articulate, his reactions to anxiety.
    (B) He demonstrates use of coping mechanisms approximately 45 percent of the time.
    (C) He has received a promotion at work since he began therapy.
    (D) He actively participates in his ongoing treatment program.

Question 48 refers to the following advertisement.

Mr. and Mrs. Jackson have a small guest house with an attached garage at the rear of their property. They place the following ad in their town newspaper for a single female college student.

Female Renter Wanted

Single, nonsmoking, nondrinking female, junior or senior university student.

Freestanding furnished guest house at back of property with attached garage and private entrance. One bedroom, one bath, kitchen with dining area, and large living area. Updated appliances and furnishings, freshly painted. Central air conditioning and heating.

First and last month's rent, plus $1,000 deposit due upon signing.

$950/month payable on first day of every month. Includes utilities. $50/day late fee. $100 charge for bad checks.

Internet/cable/telephone available at your cost.

Walking distance to university and strip mall with laundry services, small grocery, and drug store.

No loud parties, loud music, or sleepovers.

Call for interview at 555-555-5555.

---

48. The response to the ad has been good. The list has been narrowed to four senior students. Which of the following has the highest probability of renting the guest house?

(A) Annalee, a sophomore university student, who admits she has trouble handling money and generally moves when she is unable to pay the rent. She becomes evasive if asked if she smokes or drinks, and states she lives for the weekends to party.

(B) Frannie, a junior university student, who smokes and drinks but states she will not smoke or drink in the house. She will be readmitted this semester after a one-year suspension for underage drinking in university housing and destruction of university property.

(C) Jini, a senior university student, who does not smoke or drink. She works 20 hours a week at one job and six to ten hours as a hospital sitter. She does not have an automobile and rides a bicycle around town.

(D) Priscilla, a senior university student, who rented from Mr. and Mrs. Jackson two years ago. She was evicted after renting for three months because of an altercation with her boyfriend who kicked in the door of the guest house, drove his car through the garage door, and threatened to burn the house down if Mr. Jackson called the police. He was subsequently arrested and paid over $9,000 for repairs. Priscilla states she and the boyfriend have been engaged for six months and do not fight as often as they used to.

Questions 49–51 are based on the following map of Saudi Arabia.

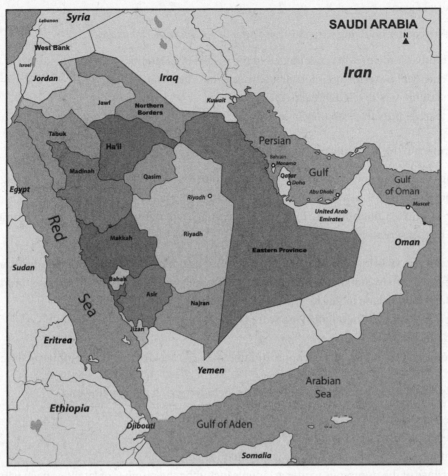

$\dfrac{1"}{4} = 200$ km

49. The western boundary of Saudi Arabia is

   (A) Iraq.
   (B) the Persian Gulf.
   (C) the Red Sea.
   (D) Yemen.

50. The largest area in Saudi Arabia is

   (A) Asir.
   (B) Bahah.
   (C) the Eastern Province.
   (D) the Northern borders.

51. Jawf is closest to

   (A) Jizan.
   (B) Qasim.
   (C) Sudan.
   (D) the West Bank.

52. At the end of the lesson, the teacher said to the class, "A number of you haven't been paying attention, and today's lesson provides the foundation for the next several lessons. I hope you understand you will see this material again."

What is the teacher implying when he says *you will see this material again*?

(A) Inattentive students will not understand the next several lessons.
(B) The class will be tested on information from today's lesson.
(C) The statement is a veiled threat to the class.
(D) The teacher is joking with the class.

Question 53 refers to the following passage.

A geography class has completed studying transportion routes in the United States and is beginning a study of transportation routes of "our neighbors to the north." Angela's presentation assignment is the Coquihalla Highway in British Columbia. The following is a partial list of information that she is planning to incorporate into her presentation.

- Southern part of British Columbia Highway 5 running north-south through Cascade Mountains
- It is approximately 200-km long and runs north from Hope to Kamloops, British Columbia.
- Two-lane to four-lane highway
- Highest elevation is Coquihalla Pass at 1,244 m
- Speed limit 120 km/hr
- Dangerous winter highway with approximately 400–500 accidents and numerous fatalities each winter

53. Angela's presentation would be enhanced if she included which of the following?

(A) American system of measurement
(B) British Columbia is in Canada.
(C) Summer and winter recreation areas around the highway
(D) The cause of the numerous winter accidents including the number of fatalities each winter

MATHEMATICS

NUMBER OF QUESTIONS: 36

TIME LIMIT: 54 MINUTES

> **Instructions:** Read each question thoroughly. Select the single best answer. Mark your answer (A, B, C, or D) on the answer sheet provided for Practice Test 4.

1. Evaluate $a^3 + 5a - 4$, if $a = 4$.

   (A) 8
   (B) 80
   (C) 621
   (D) 1,292

2. A man needs to buy a custom-made ladder to access the second-story windows of his house. The windows are 16 feet above the ground, and the closest he can get a ladder to the house is 10 feet. To the nearest foot, how long of a ladder does the man need to purchase?

   (A) 16 ft
   (B) 19 ft
   (C) 21 ft
   (D) 24 ft

3. What is the numerator in a fraction where 29 is the denominator and simplification of the fraction equals 50?

   (A) 5.4
   (B) 80
   (C) 784
   (D) 1,450

4. 57 minus 18 times 7 minus 3 times 4 equals x. Solve for x.

   (A) −47
   (B) −81
   (C) 261
   (D) 624

5. $\sqrt{(50)(2)} =$

   (A) 10
   (B) 25
   (C) 100
   (D) 10,000

6. The Belson quadruplets are saving money for summer camp. They need $255 per person plus $25 spending money per person for each of the four weeks of camp. They also want an additional $200 for buying gifts for family members. They currently have $875. What percentage of money do they still need? Round your answer to the nearest whole number.

(A) 38%
(B) 46%
(C) 60%
(D) 63%

7. Add the following: 879 + 654.021 + 16.42 + 105.87 + 10

(A) 1,664.512
(B) 1,665.311
(C) 1,665.527
(D) 1,666.307

8. Solve for x.

$$x + 22(10 - 7) = 6x + 14$$

(A) 0.212
(B) 7.32
(C) 10.4
(D) 60

9. Determine the value of x.

$$|2 - 3x| - 2 \geq 4$$

(A) $x \leq -1.33$ or $x \geq 2.67$
(B) $x \leq -2.33$ or $x \geq 3.67$
(C) $x \leq -3.33$ or $x \geq 4.67$
(D) $x \leq -4.33$ or $x \geq 5.67$

10. The cost for materials has increased the cost of production to $6,210. The additional cost is being passed on to the customer. The original cost of the items was $5,400. What is the percentage change of the cost of the item?

(A) 1.15%
(B) 11.5%
(C) 15%
(D) 1,150%

11. A woman is preparing to paint the walls in several rooms in her home. How many square feet will she be painting based on the following room dimensions?

- Rooms 1 and 5: 15 feet (l) by 13 feet (w) by 12 feet (h)
- Room 2: 12 feet (l) by 14 feet (w) by 10 feet (h)
- Rooms 3 and 4: 12 feet (l) by 12 feet (w) by 9 feet (h)

(A) 1,580 sq ft
(B) 1,620 sq ft
(C) 2,728 sq ft
(D) 5,316 sq ft

12. Grandfather Jones has a unique method of contributing to his grandchildren's college fund that begins when the child is in the first grade and ends when the child graduates from high school. He contributes a certain amount of money based on the grade earned as follows: $25 for each A, $15 for each B, and $5 for each C. He subtracts $25 for each D earned, and any failing grade cancels contributions for a six-week period. His oldest grandchild, Abigail, has the following grades for her junior year in high school.

$$A = 26 \ B = 20 \ C = 8 \ D = 0 \ F = 0$$

What amount will her grandfather contribute to her college fund?

(A) $40
(B) $300
(C) $750
(D) $990

13. Select the equation that demonstrates the associative property or axiom of addition.

(A) $(xy) + z = (yz) + x$
(B) $(x + y) + z = (x + z) + y$
(C) $x + x + y = z + z + x$
(D) $x + y - z = x + z - y$

14. The number 8 is in which place value in 4,753.9821?

(A) Billions
(B) Hundredths
(C) Ones
(D) Tenths

15. Samuel is four times as old as Marcy. The sum of their ages is 19 years. How old is Samuel?

(A) 3.8 years
(B) 5.75 years
(C) 10 years
(D) 15.2 years

16. One angle in a triangle is 56 degrees. A second angle is 12 degrees larger than the third angle. How many degrees are in each of the remaining angles? Let x equal the unknown angle.

(A) Second angle = 50°, third angle = 74°
(B) Second angle = 68°, third angle = 56°
(C) Second angle = 74°, third angle = 50°
(D) Second angle = 118°, third angle = 6°

17. The length of a rectangle is six inches more than the width. What is the length and width of the rectangle if the perimeter is 26 inches?

(A) Length = 6.5", width = 0.5"
(B) Length = 9.5", width = 3.5"
(C) Length = 13", width = 1"
(D) Length = 19", width = 7"

18. Select the unequal pair.

   (A) $\frac{3}{10}$, 0.3

   (B) $\frac{14}{5}$, 2.8

   (C) $\frac{7}{2}$, 3.5

   (D) $\frac{1}{8}$, 0.143

19. The sum of four consecutive odd numbers is 344. What is the largest number?

   (A) 85
   (B) 87
   (C) 89
   (D) 91

20. Tom buys 15 cat eye marbles for $22.50. How many cat eye marbles can he buy for $33.00?

   (A) 18
   (B) 22
   (C) 33
   (D) 40

21. Solve for y in the following equation.

   $$15(y + 7) - 3(5 + 25 \div 5) = 100$$

   (A) $\frac{5}{15}$ or 0.3333

   (B) $\frac{5}{3}$ or 1.6667

   (C) $\frac{46}{20}$ or 2.3

   (D) $\frac{33}{12}$ or 2.75

22. Solve the following. Round your answer to the nearest whole number.

   $$78.3207 \div 0.00715$$

   (A) 78
   (B) 1,095
   (C) 10,954
   (D) 15,320

23. Multiply the following.

   $$(5x + 2y)(2x + 6y)$$

   (A) $7x + 11y + 22$
   (B) $10x^2 + 34xy + 12y^2$
   (C) $120x^2y^2$
   (D) $10x^3 + 3xy + 8y$

24. What is the arithmetic mean of the following numbers? Round your answer to the nearest hundredth.

32, 45, 45, 67, 23, 17, 8

(A) 27.43
(B) 33.86
(C) 39.50
(D) 42.09

25. Marti's bus leaves at 10:00 A.M. It will take her an hour and 45 minutes to get out of bed, shower, and dress. Breakfast will take an hour to prepare and eat. It will take 30 minutes to recheck her suitcase, and her mother will take her to the bus station, 65 minutes from her house, where she must check in 45 minutes before her bus leaves. What time does Marti need to set her alarm for while allowing an additional 20 minutes for unexpected delays?

(A) 4:10 A.M.
(B) 4:25 A.M.
(C) 4:35 A.M.
(D) 4:55 A.M.

Questions 26–28 are based on the following diagram.

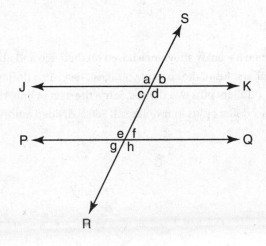

26. Select the true statement.

(A) $\overline{JK} \perp \overline{PQ}$

(B) $\overline{JK} \not\equiv \overline{PQ}$

(C) $\overline{JK} \therefore \overline{PQ}$

(D) $\overline{JK} \parallel \overline{PQ}$

27. If $\angle c = 50°$, what is the sum of $\angle c$ and $\angle b$?

(A) 100°
(B) 130°
(C) 150°
(D) 180°

28. Angles e and f form a straight line and are adjacent angles. They are also supplementary. What is the sum of $\angle g + \angle h$?

(A) 90°
(B) 130°
(C) 150°
(D) 180°

_____

29. Solve for y in the following equation.

$$\frac{4}{5}y - 15 + 7 = 52$$

(A) 48
(B) 57
(C) 62
(D) 75

30. The Martin children are given a weekly allowance based on their age and ability. David, the youngest, receives an amount of x dollars; John, the second youngest, receives x dollars plus one dollar; Gaius, the middle child, receives x dollars plus two dollars; Jerry, the next in line, receives x dollars plus three dollars; and Hank receives x dollars plus four dollars. If $50 is divided among the children, how much will the oldest child receive?

(A) $12
(B) $13
(C) $14
(D) $15

31. $\dfrac{4(11+7)+(2^3-15)}{3^3+7} =$

(A) 1.3
(B) 1.9
(C) 2.4
(D) 5.1

32. $\dfrac{34}{12} \cdot \dfrac{15}{7} \cdot \dfrac{10}{20} =$

(A) 3.00
(B) 3.04
(C) 3.07
(D) 3.90

33. What is MDCCCXXXIX?

    (A) 1,635
    (B) 1,735
    (C) 1,839
    (D) 2,241

34. How many centimeters are in 15 inches? Round your answer to the nearest tenth.

    (A) 22
    (B) 30
    (C) 32.7
    (D) 38.1

Question 35 is based on the following chart.

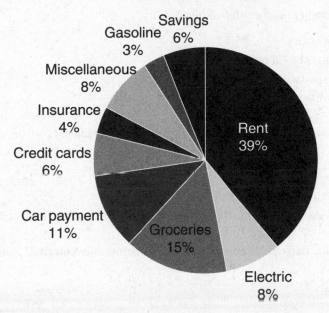

Monthly Budget

35. The monthly budget totals $3,255.00. What is the monthly dollar amount budgeted for gasoline and insurance?

    (A) $227.85
    (B) $245.22
    (C) $250.14
    (D) $267.23

36. Simplify the following equation.

    $$10 + 10 \times 10 + 10 =$$

    (A) 40
    (B) 120
    (C) 210
    (D) 400

SCIENCE

NUMBER OF QUESTIONS: 53

TIME LIMIT: 63 MINUTES

Instructions: Read each question thoroughly. Select the single best answer. Mark your answer (A, B, C, or D) on the answer sheet provided for Practice Test 4.

1. As a biological process, evolution is best defined as

   (A) change in living things over time.
   (B) comparison of animals and plants.
   (C) gradual wear down of mountain ranges to plains.
   (D) sea creatures becoming land creatures.

2. Baroreceptors are sensory neurons that monitor

   (A) arterial blood pressure.
   (B) arterial and venous blood pressure.
   (C) fight or flight response.
   (D) venous blood pressure.

3. The principal effect of the follicle stimulating hormone (FSH) in males is

   (A) follicle growth.
   (B) induction of spermatogenesis.
   (C) production of male sex characteristics.
   (D) The follicle stimulating hormone (FSH) is a female hormone and is not found in males.

4. Based on the following diagram, how many valence electrons does chlorine ($_{17}$Cl) have?

   $$_{17}\text{Cl} = \overset{\text{nucleus}}{\bullet} \ ) 2 \ ) 8 \ ) 7$$

   (A) 2
   (B) 8
   (C) 7
   (D) 17

5. Antibodies are _____ that are released from _____ by _____.

   (A) amino acids, cytotoxic cells, macrophages
   (B) antigens, macrophages, agglutination
   (C) proteins, lymphoid tissue, B cells
   (D) T lymphocytes, memory cells, suppressor cells

6. One function of the right ventricle is to ·

   (A) prevent backflow of blood into the right atrium.
   (B) pump blood into the pulmonary circulation.
   (C) serve as a holding chamber for arterial blood.
   (D) stimulate filling of the left ventricle.

7. The longitudinal fissure separates the left and right cerebral hemispheres in the brain. Which of the following best describes a fissure?

   (A) A deep groove
   (B) A shallow furrow
   (C) A shallow ridge
   (D) An elevated ridge

8. The group of muscles referred to as the hamstrings are composed of all of the following EXCEPT

   (A) adductor magnus.
   (B) biceps femoris.
   (C) semimembranosus.
   (D) semitendinosus.

9. Carbonated water is formed when

   (A) aluminum is added to heated hydrogen.
   (B) carbon dioxide is dissolved in water.
   (C) hydrogen is dissolved in a weakly acidic solution.
   (D) water and a chronotropic solution are amalgamated under pressure.

10. Which of the following is a freely movable joint that characterizes most of the joints in the human body?

    (A) Articulated
    (B) Synovial
    (C) Cartilaginous
    (D) Fibrous

11. The purpose of cell adhesion proteins (ground substances secreted by connective tissue cells) is to

    (A) hold or fasten connective tissue together.
    (B) provide firmness or inflexibility to ground substances.
    (C) provide vascularity or vascular assistance.
    (D) support or buttress osteoblasts and osteocytes.

12. Which of the following occurs during metaphase I of meiosis?

    (A) Chromosomes reach the poles.
    (B) Homologous pairs of chromosomes spread across the metaphase plate.
    (C) Nuclear envelope disappears and the spindle develops.
    (D) Daughter cells are formed.

13. Based on information presented in the Periodic Table of Elements (page 53), how many neutrons are there in a magnesium (Mg) atom?

    (A) 10
    (B) 12
    (C) 14
    (D) 16

14. Which of the following is a living unit?

   (A) A cell
   (B) A gland
   (C) A pore
   (D) A ribosome

15. Isotopes of elements differ in their number of

   (A) atomic number.
   (B) energy.
   (C) neutrons.
   (D) particles.

16. Select the option that depicts the correct anatomical relationship between two parts of the human body.

   (A) The cuboid bone is superior to the calcaneus bone.
   (B) The cuneiform bone is lateral to the navicular bone.
   (C) The phalanges are distal to the metatarsals.
   (D) The talus bone is superior to the malleolus of the tibia.

17. The central nervous system is composed of the

   (A) autonomic nervous system.
   (B) brain and spinal cord.
   (C) brainstem, cerebellum, and cerebral hemispheres.
   (D) nerves that branch from the spine.

18. All of the following are part of the axial skeleton EXCEPT

   (A) mandible.
   (B) true ribs.
   (C) parietal bone.
   (D) femur.

19. Atomic structure includes all of the following EXCEPT

   (A) electrons arranged in shells or orbitals.
   (B) the majority of the mass of an atom is in the nucleus.
   (C) positive protons and negative neutrons.
   (D) subatomic particles.

20. Which of the following is a true statement regarding compounds and mixtures?

   (A) Mixtures are amalgamations of two or more compounds; compounds are a combination of two different elements.
   (B) Compounds are not chemically bonded; mixtures form chemical bonds.
   (C) Mixtures are in precise proportion by mass; compounds are substances that interact together by weight.
   (D) Compounds can be separated by physical means; mixtures cannot.

Questions 21–22 are based on the following passage and diagram.

Referred pain occurs when a nerve is irritated or injured. Referred pain may be felt at one site when the actual site of pain is in a different location.

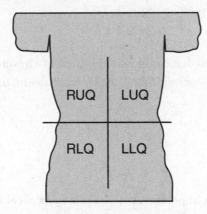

21. In which of the following quadrants would an individual most likely experience left ureteral colic?

(A) Left lower quadrant
(B) Left upper quadrant
(C) Midline of quadrants at the umbilicus
(D) Right and left lower quadrants

22. An individual experiencing pain in the superior right upper quadrant near the midline may be experiencing pain from the

(A) appendix.
(B) colon.
(C) liver.
(D) pancreas.

23. An individual had colon surgery and has no bowel sounds (indicators of a functioning bowel) after surgery. What needs to occur for the individual to have a functioning bowel?

(A) Activation of the reflex arc
(B) Bowel movement
(C) Hyperpolarization of colon cells
(D) Peristalsis

24. Somatostatin is

(A) a growth hormone inhibitor.
(B) an amino acid derivative hormone.
(C) an enhancer of dopamine.
(D) an inhibitor of dopamine.

25. The production of sperm is regulated by all of the following EXCEPT

   (A) follicle stimulating hormone (FSH).
   (B) gonadotropin releasing hormone (GnRH).
   (C) human chorionic gonadotropin hormone (hCG).
   (D) luteinizing hormone (LH).

26. An individual with type AB blood donates blood to be given to a hospitalized friend who needs a blood transfusion. What type of blood does the friend, the blood recipient, have?

   (A) Type A
   (B) Type AB
   (C) Type B
   (D) Type O

27. All of the following are elements important in the life processes of cells EXCEPT

   (A) barium (Ba).
   (B) carbon (C).
   (C) iron (Fe).
   (D) magnesium (Mg).

28. Based on the Periodic Table of Elements (page 53), fluorine (F) has nine protons in its nucleus. How many electrons does fluorine (F) have?

   (A) 2
   (B) 7
   (C) 9
   (D) 12

29. Organic compounds contain

   (A) ammonia and chlorine.
   (B) carbon and hydrogen.
   (C) carbon monoxide and nitrogen monoxide.
   (D) hydrochloric acid and sodium hydroxide.

30. _____ is the term used when a fragment of a broken chromosome attaches to a completed chromosome.

   (A) Crossing over
   (B) Linkage
   (C) Replication
   (D) Transcription

31. All of the following are nonspecific barriers that provide specific defenses against invaders through the skin or openings in the body EXCEPT

(A) cilia.
(B) interferons.
(C) skin.
(D) symbiotic bacteria.

32. What is the origin of the nerve impulses that stimulate contraction of the diaphragm and external intercostal muscles?

(A) The apneustic area
(B) The Hering–Breuer area
(C) The medullary inspiratory center
(D) The pheumotaxic area

33. Starch, a carbohydrate, is an example of a

(A) disaccharide.
(B) monosaccharide.
(C) polysaccharide.
(D) trisaccharide.

34. All of the following are examples of passive transport EXCEPT

(A) diffusion.
(B) osmosis.
(C) dialysis.
(D) receptor-mediated endocytosis.

35. Epithelial tissues are classified by cell shape and number of cell layers. Which of the following cell shapes range from flat to tall and can extend or compress to accommodate body movement?

(A) Columnar cells
(B) Cuboidal cells
(C) Squamous cells
(D) Transitional cells

36. _____ is a conventional tool for measuring liquid volume.

(A) The digital balance
(B) The graduated cylinder
(C) The hydrometer
(D) The pan balance

37. Joseph-Louis Gay-Lussac made discoveries about volume and the mass of gas. Considering the Gay-Lussac constant given below, select the supportive graph.

$$\frac{P_1}{T_1} = \frac{P_2}{T_2} = \frac{P_3}{T_3} K \quad (\text{a constant})$$

(A)
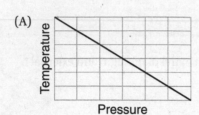

(B)
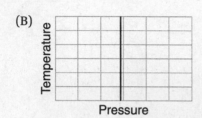

(C)
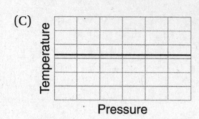

(D)
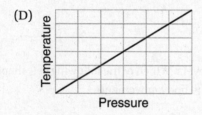

38. _____ are foreign substances or living things that cause immune system responses.

(A) Antigens
(B) Neutrophils
(C) Phagocytes
(D) Stem cells

39. HIV affects the

(A) reproductive system.
(B) immune system.
(C) nervous system.
(D) respiratory system.

40. Which of the following organs is located in the superior reaches of the left upper quadrant and lies inferior to the diaphragm?

(A) Adrenal gland
(B) Appendix
(C) Liver
(D) Spleen

41. The pulse is a pressure wave in the arteries. What creates this wave form?

(A) Backflow of systolic pressure in the venous system
(B) Blood pushed by the left ventricle through the arteries as the heart contracts and relaxes
(C) Epinephrine or norepinephrine induced positive feedback in the cerebral cortex
(D) Negative feedback in the aortic bodies

42. The brain and spinal cord are surrounded by three protective layers of membranes commonly referred to as the meninges. From the inside out, the three layers are the

(A) arachnoid, pia mater, and subarachnoid.
(B) arachnoid, subarachnoid, and pia mater.
(C) dura, pia mater, and subarachnoid.
(D) pia mater, arachnoid, and dura.

43. The eye contains two fluid-filled cavities: the _____ and the _____.

(A) aqueous cavity, vitreous cavity
(B) posterior cavity, anterior cavity
(C) pupil, iris
(D) retinal, choroid

44. The foremost region of hearing in the brain is

(A) in the cerebellar peduncles of the cerebellum.
(B) in the cortex of the temporal lobe of the cerebrum.
(C) in the frontal lobe of the dominant hemisphere.
(D) in the sensory elaboration portion of the occipital lobe.

45. _____ is an example of a nonsteroidal hormone.

(A) Amines such as cortisol
(B) Glycoproteins such as prolactin
(C) Peptides such as oxytocin
(D) Proteins such as estrogen

46. Which of the following glands are located on the superior aspect of each kidney?

(A) Adrenal glands
(B) Apocrine glands
(C) Olfactory glands
(D) Thymus glands

47. Which of the following is a researchable hypothesis?

(A) Gender is a predictor of intolerance.

(B) Oranges come from pear trees.

(C) When offered all four types of edible leaves found in their natural habitat, black bearded monkeys will prefer leaf B.

(D) Which interest group contributes most to American Society for Prevention to Animals?

Questions 48–49 are based on the following graphic.

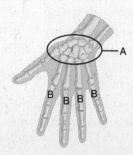

48. Bones in the circled area A are the

(A) carpal bones.

(B) proximal phalanxes.

(C) radials.

(D) ulna.

49. Bones labeled as B are called

(A) distal phalanxes.

(B) metacarpals.

(C) middle phalanxes.

(D) proximal phalanxes.

50. The _____ nerve is the largest single nerve in the human body, running from the sacral plexus and down each side of the lower spine through the buttock down the back of the thigh and extending down to the posterior aspect of the foot.

(A) common peroneal

(B) sciatic

(C) spinal accessory

(D) tibial

51. Cerebral spinal fluid is formed by

(A) plasma filtering from a network of capillaries in the choroid plexus in the first and second ventricles in the brain.

(B) plasma filtering from a network of capillaries in the choroid plexus in the first and fifth ventricles in the brain.

(C) plasma filtering from a network of capillaries in the choroid plexus in the fourth and fifth ventricles in the brain.

(D) plasma filtering from a network of capillaries in the choroid plexus in the third and fourth ventricles in the brain.

52. Strong base + Strong acid =

(A) Acidic sodium dioxide
(B) Alkaline sodium chlorine
(C) Hyperosmolar salt
(D) Neutral salt

53. Bonds attach atoms of molecules and compounds together. An ionic bond forms when

(A) a metallic atom transfers an electron to a nonmetal atom.
(B) covalent bonds achieve full valence.
(C) metallic atoms share covalent electrons.
(D) nonmetal atoms share covalent electrons.

ENGLISH AND LANGUAGE USAGE

NUMBER OF QUESTIONS: 53

TIME LIMIT: 64 MINUTES

> **Instructions:** Read each question thoroughly. Select the single best answer. Mark your answer (A, B, C, or D) on the answer sheet provided for Practice Test 4.

1. "Sit!" is an example of a sentence giving a command or directive. What is the subject of the sentence?

    (A) Command
    (B) Sit
    (C) There is no subject in the sentence.
    (D) You

2. Select the incorrectly punctuated sentence.

    (A) Atticus read five books over the summer and qualified for the third-grade reader's award.
    (B) Sandra, Thomas, and Evelyn each wanted to attend the workshop, but they only had enough money for one of them to attend.
    (C) The city council voted on the following measures parking at the city zoo, repainting fire hydrants east of Baker Avenue and increasing security at varsity home games.
    (D) Tom had never had a paying job before, and he was looking forward to opening a savings account at the bank when he received his first check.

3. Select the sentence using the correct action word.

    (A) For as long as anyone could remember, Mr. Hanson had always wore a bow tie.
    (B) The family would not have gone to see the movie on a school night if they had knew how long the movie was.
    (C) The swimmer had swum the channel in record time.
    (D) Three of the soccer players admitted they had draw the graffiti on the stadium walls.

4. Which of the following sentences contains an interrogative pronoun?

    (A) Do you understand why he refused to attend class?
    (B) He ran all the way home?
    (C) Where are the magazines I left on this table?
    (D) Whose jacket was left on the bus?

5. Select the sentence containing an incorrectly spelled word.

    (A) Marsha was the most mischievious child ever enrolled at the day care facility.
    (B) Most remembered Lance as being a facetious short story writer in his teen years, and now he was a published author.
    (C) The expensive ukulele he had always wanted was finally on sale at a price he could afford.
    (D) The pushy salesperson lied to John when he said the tent would easily accommodate five adults.

6. Select the meaning of the italicized word in the following sentence.

> Pete is such a *knucklehead*. The other day he walked into the self-serve gas station and asked to have ethyl wait on him.

(A) A lazy person
(B) A repulsive person
(C) A stupid person
(D) An important person

7. Select the sentence with incorrect subject-verb agreement.

(A) A large lizard darted across the trail and frightened the hikers.
(B) None of the jokes told by the student was funny.
(C) The city council, as well as many of the attending townspeople, does not realize the importance of after-school programs for latch-key children.
(D) The puppies were born on the first day of summer.

8. Select the sentence incorrectly using either *accept* or *except*.

(A) The judges made an exception and allowed John to enter the race since he would be 18 years old two days before the day of the race.
(B) The manager told Tina her work was acceptable but still needed improvement.
(C) The politician told his constituents he would not accept the nomination for vice president of the political organization.
(D) The winner of the lottery graciously excepted his prize.

9. Which of the following is the correct plural form of the word *vita*?

(A) Vitae
(B) Vitas
(C) Vitase
(D) Vitus

10. Which of the following represents an incorrect usage of double quotation marks?

(A) Margaret, having raised six robust boys to adulthood by herself, did not support the notion of "suffer the little ones" when she attended the theater.
(B) Matthew glared at his son when he entered the room and said, "Sit down and don't say a word."
(C) The reading was over when the author said, "The village in the mist was never seen again, but on quiet summer nights the sounds of music and singing could be heard coming from the glen."
(D) The representative of the company said, "That all of the defective products would be replaced by the company without charge to the customer."

11. Which of the following sentences demonstrates correct use of capitalization?

(A) An accident closed the golden gate bridge during rush hour.
(B) Mark always ordered French Fries with his bowl of chili.
(C) The continuation of the Monarchy was assured with the birth of a son.
(D) The most frequent site that visitors want to see is the Egyptian pyramids.

12. Select the punctuation that marks the end of a declarative sentence.

(A) A comma
(B) A period
(C) A question mark
(D) An exclamation point

13. The following is an example of a _____ sentence.

The children ran for the house, but the skunk ran ahead of them and blocked the door.

(A) complex
(B) compound-complex
(C) compound
(D) simple

14. Select the correctly spelled word.

(A) Exhortation
(B) Happyness
(C) Pagent
(D) Talcom

15. Select the prepositional phrase in the following sentence.

The children ran around the mulberry bush.

(A) around the mulberry bush
(B) bush
(C) mulberry bush
(D) ran around the mulberry bush

16. Identify the direct object in the following sentence.

Marion offered a workshop on how to do origami last winter.

(A) offered
(B) origami
(C) winter
(D) workshop

17. Identify the subject in the following sentence.

After striking out during the championship game, Jeff threw his bat at the umpire and was ejected from the game.

(A) championship game
(B) Jeff
(C) striking out
(D) umpire

18. The following is an example of a _____ sentence.

>   Jason forgot to walk his brother home from school this afternoon.

   (A) complex
   (B) compound
   (C) simple-complex
   (D) simple

19. Select the sentence with correct subject-verb agreement.

   (A) Aaron break the vase when he ran into the table.
   (B) Mary told her friend, "I knowed it was him when I saw his picture on the news."
   (C) Neither of the ex-wives nor his children attended the funeral.
   (D) Shanna drug her suitcases up three flights of stairs because the elevator wasn't working.

20. Select the verb in the following sentence.

>   After the bus departed for Omaha, Marsh discovered he had left his jacket, as well as his sack of sandwiches, in the lobby of the terminal.

   (A) departed
   (B) discovered
   (C) left
   (D) terminal

21. Which of the following irregular verbs is correct for both present and past tense?

   (A) Choose, chosen
   (B) Ring, rung
   (C) Sleep, slept
   (D) Spring, sprung

22. _____ is a word that takes the place of a noun in a sentence.

   (A) Adverb
   (B) Indirect object
   (C) Predicate
   (D) Pronoun

23. Select the sentence using a transitional word or phrase.

   (A) She thought a nice ride in the country might help him feel better unless he didn't feel up to it.
   (B) The Smith family held the town in its grasp for a quarter of a century.
   (C) We could go to the movie; on the other hand, we could go bowling.
   (D) We propose to provide shorter work days and introduce a day care center for children under six years of age.

24. Which word in the following sentence functions as an adverb?

> The performance put on by the local acting club was exceedingly well done.

(A) acting
(B) exceedingly
(C) local
(D) performance

25. Select a synonym for the italicized word in the following sentence.

> The new boss was *ungracious* to his subordinates.

(A) Affable
(B) Churlish
(C) Elegant
(D) Gracious

26. Select the best definition for the italicized word in the following sentence.

> To reduce the danger of fire damage, the roof on the new building would be made of *corrugated* steel.

(A) Convex steel
(B) Flattened steel with raised areas
(C) Steel with alternating folds and ridges
(D) Unfolded steel

27. Which of the following words is spelled incorrectly?

(A) Coronation
(B) Currency
(C) Laberinth
(D) Traitor

28. Which of the following sentences correctly uses a colon?

(A) I quote from his will: "I leave absolutely nothing to my lazy, good-for-nothing children who have bled me dry for the last forty-five years."
(B) "Ladies and Gentlemen. The Cattle Association is pleased that you have come here this evening for this fine dinner dance: and opportunity to participate in our yearly auction."
(C) The depots: along the celebrated Bailey Rail Line are Hemps Point, Marshall City, Mountain View, Dodge, Winter Haven, Bradley, Coal City, and Birmingham.
(D) The time on the clock is 0414:00.

Reading

1.	B	15.	D	29.	D	43.	B
2.	D	16.	A	30.	B	44.	B
3.	D	17.	D	31.	B	45.	C
4.	C	18.	D	32.	B	46.	A
5.	A	19.	B	33.	C	47.	D
6.	D	20.	A	34.	C	48.	C
7.	B	21.	C	35.	A	49.	C
8.	D	22.	D	36.	B	50.	C
9.	C	23.	D	37.	D	51.	D
10.	D	24.	B	38.	B	52.	B
11.	C	25.	B	39.	B	53.	A
12.	D	26.	C	40.	B		
13.	A	27.	B	41.	C		
14.	A	28.	C	42.	D		

Mathematics

1.	B	10.	C	19.	C	28.	D
2.	B	11.	C	20.	B	29.	D
3.	D	12.	D	21.	B	30.	A
4.	B	13.	B	22.	C	31.	B
5.	A	14.	B	23.	B	32.	B
6.	B	15.	D	24.	B	33.	C
7.	B	16.	B	25.	C	34.	D
8.	C	17.	B	26.	D	35.	A
9.	A	18.	D	27.	A	36.	B

ANSWER KEY
Practice Test 4

Science

1.	A	15.	C	29.	B	43.	B
2.	A	16.	C	30.	B	44.	B
3.	B	17.	B	31.	B	45.	C
4.	C	18.	D	32.	C	46.	A
5.	C	19.	C	33.	C	47.	C
6.	B	20.	A	34.	D	48.	A
7.	A	21.	A	35.	D	49.	D
8.	A	22.	D	36.	B	50.	B
9.	B	23.	D	37.	D	51.	A
10.	B	24.	A	38.	A	52.	D
11.	A	25.	C	39.	B	53.	A
12.	B	26.	B	40.	D		
13.	B	27.	A	41.	B		
14.	A	28.	C	42.	D		

English and Language Usage

1.	D	8.	D	15.	A	22.	D
2.	C	9.	A	16.	D	23.	C
3.	C	10.	D	17.	B	24.	B
4.	D	11.	D	18.	D	25.	B
5.	A	12.	B	19.	C	26.	C
6.	C	13.	C	20.	B	27.	C
7.	B	14.	A	21.	C	28.	A

ANSWER EXPLANATIONS
Reading

1. **(B)** The question asks for the heart rate. Three values are provided—HR, systolic, and diastolic. HR is the only value having any relationship with heart rate. The heart rate is 65 beats per minute. Heart rate is commonly counted in beats per minute. The remaining options are not compatible with life.

2. **(D)** The question asks for the systolic reading. The S on the monitor is the only option having to do with systolic. HR and D do not relate to the question. While the question does not require knowing anything about blood pressure and how it is written, blood pressure is written systolic over diastolic and read as 143/78. Systolic is the top number with diastolic the bottom number. The systolic number is always larger than the diastolic number.

3. **(D)** Sequencing is an ordering or a following of one thing after another. While relationship may exist, cause and effect is not an issue. The remaining options do not demonstrate anything.

4. **(C)** Student 10 is the tallest at 72 inches and the heaviest at 170 pounds. The remaining 19 students are shorter and weigh less.

5. **(A)** Students 1, 2, 3, 6, 11, 12, 13, 14, 15, and 16 weigh less than 150 pounds. The remaining students weigh 150 pounds or more.

6. **(D)** Nineteen of 20 students are 5-feet tall or taller (from 60 to 72 inches). The remaining student, at 57 inches, is less than 5-feet tall.

7. **(B)** Passages appearing in the Letters to the Editor section of a newspaper, as a rule, express opinions about an issue or issues of particular interest or concern to the writer. Such publications include both fact and opinion. In this case, the writer's intended audience is individuals who read the Letters to the Editor section of the newspaper. Individuals living in rural areas of the county, county law enforcement, and newspaper subscribers are subsets of individuals who read the Letters to the Editor section of the newspaper. More than subscribers to a newspaper actually read the paper.

8. **(D)** The word *vex* means to disturb, trouble, perplex, provoke, distress, or aggravate. The writer is clearly *vexed* about the vandalism occurring in the county. The writer is not being hostile. There is no obvious antagonism, maliciousness, or aggressiveness in the piece. *Appeasement* and *pleasantry* are closer to antonyms.

9. **(C)** Bias is opinion based on preconceived notions or ideas about a thing, person, or group of persons. In the passage, the writer is convinced that a gang of boys is responsible for the vandalism. There is nothing written to suggest this. The remaining options are facts, not opinions.

10. **(D)** The writer of the passage is attempting to persuade individuals into action. He encourages the people of the county, parents, teachers, and students to assist in solving the problem. The remaining options do not support the message of the passage.

11. **(C)** An idiom is a word or expression used instead of its usual meaning. The expression is not actually asking students to step forward or to step up onto something. The expression is asking students to take responsibility, be more active, or come forward in terms of what they may know about the vandalism. The sentence, *I heard John's uncle in Tennessee kicked the bucket last winter*, uses an idiom. The sentence does not mean the uncle literally kicked a bucket, but rather that he died. Stepping up has nothing to do with exacerbation, betrayal, or provocation.

12. **(D)** *Recalcitrant* is an adjective defined as resisting authority, disobedient, or noncompliant. The remaining options are antonyms and are not supportive of Sue Ann's suspension from school.

13. **(A)** The letters *e.g.* mean *for example*. In the sentence, all of the dog breeds in parentheses are examples of short-haired dogs.

14. **(A)** To correctly answer the question, information in the stem must be located on the chart. Randall is the second runner listed on the chart. His finishing position is the darkest horizontal bar that represents Race 1. Randall finished first in the first race.

15. **(D)** To correctly answer the question, information in the stem must be located on the chart. Tom is the fourth runner listed on the chart. Tom has the highest training hours for the second race at 42 hours per week. The remaining participants have fewer hours.

16. **(A)** The finishing position in a race is specific and usually nonmodifiable. "Training hours" is vague and nonspecific. Tom trains around 40 hours a week, while Mavis trains around 13 hours a week. Operationalizing or defining training hours would have made the study more precise. Since training is not defined, there is no way to know if the runners had professional trainers or trained on their own. There are only three 20-km races in the club's running season, and use of mixed or single gender participants may or may not have enhanced the study.

17. **(D)** Abner Johnson was married three times, first to Delphine Cadmus Walker, second to Margaret Stonehouse, and last to Hannah Marie Houeworth.

18. **(D)** Abner Johnson had a total of ten sons, five by his first wife Delphine Cadmus Walker (Aaron, George, Miner, Benjamin, and an unnamed male), four by his second wife Margaret Stonehouse (an unnamed male, Royal, Moses, and Otto), and one by his third wife Hannah Marie Houeworth (Abner).

19. **(B)** Abner Johnson's first son was born in 1779. Adeline Francis Johnson, a female, was born in 1778. Miner Orange Johnson, the third male, was born in 1782, and Abner Houeworth, the youngest son, in 1822.

20. **(A)** All of the sources are reliable except a Gaucher's disease research site selling medication to treat the disease. Research sites typically do not sell medication for treatment of a disease since the majority of treatments may be prescription-based. The remaining options are legitimate reference sources. An out-of-date medical site containing information on Gaucher's disease with a 1922 copyright would be appropriate since the scholarly paper is looking at treatment of Gaucher's disease for the last 100 years. The *Journal of the American Medical Association* was first published in 1883 and contains scholarly medical information. MedlinePlus is a health website produced by the National Library of Medicine. It made its debut in 1998.

21. **(C)** A *sucker* is an individual who is easily deceived or conned. Suckers are gullible. While the word *sucker* can mean an individual who is a laughingstock or joke, there is nothing in the passage suggestive of John being such. The fact that John is approaching his best friend about purchasing the flashlight does not suggest he is eager to please—he may see the value in his friend's counsel or he may not enjoy being chided. A solicitous individual is anxious or concerned.

22. **(D)** A hallmark of most flashlights is they have replaceable batteries and bulbs. When considering the information provided in the advertisement, John needs to think about what the ad is saying as well as what the ad is not saying. There are potential red flags in the bulleted list. The reputation of the magazine and manufacturer many be difficult to ascertain. Knowing the total cost of the purchase is not an issue since John is known for spending large amounts on purchases he knows little about. If the batteries and/or bulb are irreplaceable, the flashlight is a waste of money.

23. **(D)** *Nagged* is a synonym for *chided*. The remaining options are antonyms for *chided*.

24. **(B)** The question asks for a logical conclusion based on what you have read. Based on the passage, Angela's probability of becoming a nurse anesthetist is almost nonexistent. Course

grades are not discussed in the passage. *Probably* and *improbable* are antonyms. The passage contains enough information to reach a conclusion.

25. **(B)** The correct option is the definition of *bullheaded*. The remaining options are not supportive of the definition or of behavior demonstrated in the passage.

26. **(C)** The new word is *behave*.

    1. Secret ⇒ Becret

    2. Becret ⇒ Becrte

    3. Becrte ⇒ Behate

    4. Behate ⇒ Behave

27. **(B)** *Zetetics* is the only word found on the specified page in the dictionary. The remaining words come before *zamindari* or after *zoetrope*.

28. **(C)** The e-mail is both informational and technical. It provides information on an action the library is taking regarding library card inactivity and also tells library patrons what to do if they wish to keep their cards active. Cause and affect is illogical because *affect* is an incorrect word—it should be *effect*. The remaining options do not support the type of communication used in the e-mail.

29. **(D)** The intended audience of the e-mail is individuals who have not used their library cards for more than five years. Active library users have little or no need for the information presented in the e-mail. Library fines are not mentioned in the e-mail.

30. **(B)** *Customer* is the only word that could be a synonym for *patron*. The remaining options are not synonyms of *patron*. An advocate is a supporter of something. The probability of an individual who has not used his or her library card for five years being an advocate is low.

31. **(B)** Fact sheets are meant to inform. They are typically brief in comment and do not go into depth to explain or educate. Fact sheets can be used in virtually any setting, and can be used along with or included with other information. For example, a brochure for a specific automobile usually contains fact sheet information. The standard options on the car are usually listed without giving an explanation of what each option actually entails.

32. **(B)** Sepsis cannot occur unless an infection is present somewhere in the body. As such, it is a secondary condition with the actual infection being primary.

33. **(C)** The immune system protects again invasion of the body from foreign microbes that have the potential to cause infection. Sepsis occurs when the immune system releases chemicals into the blood to combat the infection.

34. **(C)** To correctly answer this question, you must know the definition of *hyperthermia*. The word can be broken into its parts—*hyper* meaning elevated or above and *thermia* (from *thermo*) meaning heat. The term as it relates to the human body indicates an abnormally high fever.

35. **(A)** The question requires higher-level thinking and is more complicated. A number of things must be considered to select the correct option. They are:

- What is a culture? What purpose does a culture serve? Culture is the cultivation of microorganisms. The purpose of a culture is to identify a microorganism; in this case, an infectious microorganism.

- What is an antibiotic? Why would an antibiotic be prescribed? What is the expected outcome of taking antibiotics? Antibiotics are a large group of drugs that inhibit or kill infectious microorganisms. They are used in the treatment of infections.

- How is spectrum defined? What does broad spectrum suggest in terms of antibiotics? Broad-spectrum antibiotics are a large but assorted group of antibiotics that treat infections. They act against a wide range or broad spectrum of infectious microorganisms.

■ What is the relationship between cultures and broad-spectrum antibiotics? A culture identifies a microorganism—the organism causing the infection. Once the organism is identified, an appropriate antibiotic can be administered to kill or inhibit the infectious microorganism. If the antibiotic has the power to change (by inhibiting or killing) the microorganism, then administering the antibiotic prior to drawing the cultures will alter the culture results. The broad-spectrum antibiotic is appropriate because it acts on a variety of infectious microorganisms.

36. **(B)** The bulleted statements represent *comparing and contrasting* of information. *Compare* looks at similarities, and *contrast* looks at differences.

37. **(D)** Similes show similarities between two different things as in taking a nap and nailing jelly to a tree. Alliteration uses letters of the alphabet and consonants with the same sound together. *Peter Piper picked a peck of pickled peppers* is an example of alliteration. Metaphors make implied or hidden comparisons between two unrelated things. The sentence, *Sarah's solution for any problem is a Band-Aid,* employs a metaphor. Non sequiturs are illogical or unreasonable statements, such as *All men breathe oxygenated air. Crocodiles breathe oxygenated air. Therefore, all men are crocodiles.*

38. **(B)** In this case, anthologies are collections of selected writings of an author. The anthology would contain the poetry of Kavanaugh. A poetry journal could serve as a reference but would not provide broad coverage of his poetry. Autobiographies are stories of an individual's life written by the individual and would not contain poetry. An encyclopedia would contain information about an individual but probably would not contain his written works.

39. **(B)** To correctly answer this question, a relationship must exist between information on the résumé and information from the letter of recommendation. Being a finalist for the Nobel Prize for Journalism does not does not seem to agree and stands out from the other information. It is highly doubtful that a 28-year-old individual with a 4½-year history as a reporter for a weekly newspaper serving a village of 1,200, and who has no publication history, would have the opportunity to contribute at a Nobel Prize level or be acquainted with individuals who have the ability to nominate him for a Nobel Prize. The remaining options are reasonable for an individual at this point in his career. He is interested in writing and submits his works to a local writing club contest, he participates in his community by representing his field at the local high school career day, and he is one of two reporters who take part in this monthly award competition.

40. **(B)**

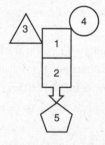

41. **(C)** Only the high amount or the estimated cost for eight weekends of painting needs to be determined. Round $780 to $800 per day and double the amount for one weekend—$1,600 per weekend. This amount times eight weekends equals $12,800 (multiply 8 × 16 = 128 and add two zeros). If the estimated cost for eight weekends is $12,800, the remaining options must be incorrect. Options (A) and (B) estimations of eight week's are too low at $6,000 and $8,500. Option (D)'s eight-weekend estimation of $14,000 is too high.

42. **(D)** Smith Bros. has the best offer. Their workmanship is guaranteed 100 percent for five years, and the owner selects the paint to be used, which means the owner determines the cost of paint. None of the other contractors make these offers. Smith Bros. also has the highest rating of the four.

43. **(B)** Jones & Walker do not do anything except paint the house. It is up to Oliver Bates, age 77, to purchase everything needed for the project, get everything to the house or have everything delivered to the house, make sure everything is available, make the needed repairs, and then clean and store everything at the end of every day with what could be six to eight weekends of painting time. Contractors typically supply everything needed for a project, and the cost is transferred to the individual. Jones & Walker are full-time college students. They paint two days a week doing five to six hours a day—this is part-time work. They may not have the resources or desire to own ladders, brushes, drop clothes, hammers, saws, and other materials needed to be regular house painters. Their satisfaction rating of one star is also a red flag.

44. **(B)** Subjective and objective data are opposites. Subjective information is what an individual says and may not be verified; objective information can be verified and seen by others. An example is body temperature. An individual says, "I am so hot. I just know I have a temperature." The statement is subjective because it is impossible to determine body temperature by observing an individual. When the temperature is actually taken by a thermometer or other heat recording device, the temperature can be verified. The actual temperature on the device can be seen by others, and if the temperature is repeated, it should be approximately the same. This is objective data. The remaining options are incorrect.

45. **(C)** Based on the information on the diagram, Fara's most appropriate action is to stay with Robin and support her. A swarm of bees is a large number of bees flying together. A swarm does not necessarily suggest danger. Attempting to scatter the bee swarm could put both girls at risk for bee stings. Leaving Robin to her own devices and going for help places Robin at an increased risk for harm or injury. Using a loud, authoritative voice will not ease her anxiety and will probably make it worse. A calm voice is most helpful to those having a panic attack.

46. **(A)** Peter and Paula are suffering from mild anxiety. Watching psychological thrillers has frightened them, and they feel there is danger in their home when there is not. They have problem solved by turning on all of the lights in the home—this shows there is no danger in the shadows. They have reasoned and taken control of their situation. Their behavior does not support the remaining types of anxiety.

47. **(D)** An outcome is a result; a positive outcome emphasizes a commendable or good result. Markus is in therapy because of anxiety which is secondary to an accident, and he is actively involved in his therapy. This is a positive outcome. For Markus to acknowledge that he has anxiety but not to be able to identify or talk about it shows little, if any, progress. To know Markus uses a coping mechanism 45 percent of the time says little because it is not known if he uses the mechanisms successfully or not. If he demonstrates coping mechanisms 45 percent of the time, it means he is unable to demonstrate coping mechanisms 55 percent of the time. Markus has received a promotion at work. While a promotion is usually good, it is not known if there is a relationship between his anxiety problems and the promotion, or if he suffers from anxiety while at work.

48. **(C)** Of the four students who interview to rent the guest house, Jini is the best prospect. Her information is positive. The remaining individuals are questionable. Annalee has difficulties handling money and solves her rent problem by moving. She is evasive about smoking and drinking and lives to party on weekends. Frannie is a smoker and drinker and states she will not smoke or drink in the house—it is doubtful she will be able to do this. She has a negative history for alcohol consumption and has shown destructive tendencies. Priscilla is the least likely to rent the guest house. She has a negative history with Mr. and Mrs. Jackson and is currently engaged to the man who kicked the door in and damaged the garage door in a fit of rage. The fact that she says they don't fight as often as they used to is a red flag.

49. **(C)** The westernmost boundary of Saudi Arabia is the Red Sea. Iraq is north of Saudi Arabia, the Persian Gulf is east, and Yemen is south.

50. **(C)** Of the options shown on the map, the Eastern Province is the largest.

51. **(D)** Jawf is closest to the West Bank at around 200 kilometers. The remaining options are greater than 200 kilometers from Jawf.

52. **(B)** While the phrase *you will see this material again* can be used in many different settings, in the teaching setting it refers to seeing the information from the lesson on a future quiz, test, or exam. The phrase has nothing to do with understanding future lessons. It is not a veiled threat, and the teacher is not joking with the class.

53. **(A)** Angela's presentation could be enhanced if she include the American system of measurement. Using the Canadian system of measurement (metric) would be appropriate if she were addressing an audience familiar with the metric system, but she is not. The class is studying transportation routes in Canada, so this is a given. Summer/winter recreation sites and the cause of winter accidents and number of deaths is illogical to include since the class focuses on geography, not social issues or information.

Mathematics

1. **(B)**

$$a^3 + 5a - 4 =$$
$$64 + 5(4) - 4 =$$
$$64 + 20 - 4 = 80$$

2. **(B)** The Pythagorean theorem is used to solve the problem. Draw a right triangle and label it if you need to visualize.

$$a = 10' \qquad b = 16'$$
$$a^2 + b^2 = c^2$$
$$16^2 + 10^2 = c^2$$
$$256 + 100 = c^2$$
$$356 = c$$
$$\sqrt{356} = c$$
$$18.87 = 19' = c$$

3. **(D)** In division, the numerator is the number above the line in a fraction, and the denominator is below the line or $\frac{n}{d}$.

$$\frac{n}{29} = 50$$
$$n = 1,450$$

4. **(B)** The rules of operation must be followed to correctly solve the equation. Parentheses have been added for clarification—the use or nonuse of parentheses does not change the answer if the order of operations is followed.

$$57 - (18 \cdot 7) - (3 \cdot 4) =$$
$$57 - 126 - 12 =$$
$$-69 - 12 = -81$$

5. **(A)** Perform the action under the square root and then determine the square root of that number.

$$\sqrt{(50)(2)} = \sqrt{100} = 10$$

6. **(B)** A number of different methods can be used to determine the answer. Ratio and proportion is used here. The total cost for summer camp is as follows:

$255 per person (cost of summer camp) = $255 × 4 = $1,020

$25 (spending money) = $25 × 4 weeks × 4 boys = $400

$200 money for family gifts

$1,020 + $400 + $200 = $1,620 (total needed) − $875 (amount saved) = $745 (amount still needed)

$$\$1,620 = 100\% :: \$745 = x\%$$
$$1,620x = 74,500$$
$$x = 45.99 = 46\%$$

7. **(B)** The decimals must be aligned to obtain the correct answer.

$$
\begin{array}{r}
879.000 \\
654.021 \\
16.420 \\
105.870 \\
+\ 10.000 \\
\hline
1,665.311
\end{array}
$$

8. **(C)** The rules of operation must be followed to solve the equation.

$x + 22(10 - 7) = 6x + 14$	$x + 22(10 - 7) = 6x + 14$
$x + 22(3) = 6x + 14$	$10.4 + 22(10 - 7) = 6(10.4) + 14$
$x + 66 = 6x + 14$	$10.4 + 66 = 62.4 + 14$
$52 = 5x$	$76.4 = 76.4$
$10.4 = x$	

9. **(A)** The following steps can be used to determine x.

STEP 1 Isolate the absolute value.

$$|2 - 3x| - 2 \geq 4$$
$$|2 - 3x| - 2 + 2 \geq 4 + 2$$
$$|2 - 3x| \geq 6$$

STEP 2 Remove the absolute value bars (|) and replace the inequality sign ($\geq$) with an equal sign (=).

$$|2 - 3x| \geq 6$$
$$2 - 3x = 6$$

STEP 3 Set up two equations (one positive and one negative) and solve for x.

$$
\begin{array}{ll}
2 - 3x = 6 & 2 - 3x = -6 \\
-3x = 4 & -3x = -8 \\
x = -1.33 & x = 2.67
\end{array}
$$
$$x \leq -1.33 \text{ or } x \geq 2.67$$

10. **(C)** The formula for percent change is used.

Original price = $5,400　　　Change amount = $6,210

Percent change (PC) = Change amount/Original price

$$PC = \frac{6,210 - 5,400}{5,400} = \frac{810}{5,400}$$

$$PC = 0.15 \text{ or } 15\%$$

11. **(C)** Walls have length, width, and height. The floor and ceiling are not counted when just the walls are to be painted. There is a total of five rooms to be painted—Rooms 1 and 5 are the same size, Rooms 3 and 4 are same size, and only one room has the dimensions of Room 2. The formula of area = 2(width × height) + 2(length × height) is used.

Rooms 1 and 5:

$$A = 2[2(w \times h) + 2(l \times h)]$$
$$A = 2[2(13 \times 12) + 2(15 \times 12)]$$
$$A = 2[312 + 360]$$
$$A = 1{,}344 \text{ sq ft}$$

Room 2:

$$A = 2(w \times h) + 2(l \times h)$$
$$A = 2(14 \times 10) + 2(12 \times 10)$$
$$A = 280 + 240$$
$$A = 520 \text{ sq ft}$$

Rooms 3 and 4:

$$A = 2[2(w \times h) + 2(l \times h)]$$
$$A = 2[2(12 \times 9) + 2(12 \times 9)]$$
$$A = 2[216 + 216]$$
$$A = 864 \text{ sq ft}$$

Rooms 1 and 5, 2, and 3 and 4 = 1,344 + 520 + 864 = 2,728 sq ft

12. **(D)**

$$A = 26 \times \$25 = \$650$$
$$B = 20 \times \$15 = \$300$$
$$C = 8 \times \$5 = \$40$$
$$\$650 + \$300 + \$40 = \$990$$

13. **(B)** The associative property of addition means that the grouping of objects added together does not matter. The question could be seen as true/false, and the correct answer can be obtained by substituting numbers for the given letters, if necessary.

$$x = 1 \qquad y = 2 \qquad z = 3$$

(A) $\quad (xy) + z = (yz) + x$
$$(1 \times 2) + 3 = (2 \times 3) + 1$$
$$2 + 3 = 6 + 1$$
$$5 \neq 7$$

(B) $\quad (x + y) + z = (x + z) + y$
$$(1 + 2) + 3 = (1 + 3) + 2$$
$$3 + 3 = 4 + 2$$
$$6 = 6$$

(C) $\quad x + x + y = z + z + x$
$$1 + 1 + 2 = 3 + 3 + 1$$
$$4 \neq 7$$

(D) $\quad x + y - z = x + z - y$
$$1 + 2 - 3 = 1 + 3 - 2$$
$$0 \neq 2$$

14. **(B)** Numbers get larger to the left of the decimal and smaller to the right of the decimal place.

1,000	100	10	1	Decimal point	$\frac{1}{10}$	$\frac{1}{100}$	$\frac{1}{1,000}$	$\frac{1}{10,000}$
4	7	5	3	.	9	8	2	1

15. **(D)** Change the sentence into an equation.

The sum of their ages is 19 years.

Samuel's age (4 times Marcy's age) = $4x$ Marcy's age = x

$$4x + x = 19$$
$$5x = 19$$
$$x = 3.8 \text{ years}$$
$$\text{Samuel} = 4x = 4 \times 3.8 = 15.2 \text{ years}$$

16. **(B)** The angles of a triangle add up to 180°. Information is then given on the three angles.

$\angle a = 56°$ $\angle b = x° + 12°$ $\angle c = x°$

$$\angle a + \angle b + \angle c = 180°$$
$$56° + x + 12° + x° = 180°$$
$$2x + 68 = 180$$
$$2x = 112$$
$$x = 56°$$

$\angle b = x + 12 = 56 + 12 = 68°$ $\angle c = x = 56°$

17. **(B)** Correctly reading the stem is paramount in answering the question. The formula for the perimeter of a rectangle is used. The question asks for the length and width of the rectangle, or the number of inches in one section of length and the number of inches in one section of width. It does not ask for the total inches in length or the total inches in width. This amount would be the perimeter or 26 inches.

$$\text{Perimeter} = \text{length} + \text{width} + \text{length} + \text{width}$$
$$\text{or}$$
$$\text{Perimeter } (P) = 2(l) + 2(w)$$

$P = 26"$ $l = x + 6$ $w = x$

$$26 = 2(x + 6) + 2x$$
$$26 = 2x + 12 + 2x$$
$$26 = 4x + 12$$
$$14 = 4x$$
$$3.5" = x$$

Length = $x + 6 = 9.5"$ Width = $x = 3.5"$

18. **(D)** To be an equal pair, $\dfrac{1}{8}$ would have to equal 0.125. The remaining options are equal pairs.

19. **(C)** The question specifically asks for four consecutive odd numbers. The simplest computations will use the lowest even numbers possible since an odd number plus an even number is odd. They are two, four, and six with x equal to the unknown.

$$x + (x + 2) + (x + 4) + (x + 6) = 344$$
$$4x + 12 = 344$$
$$4x = 332$$
$$x = 83$$
$$x + 6 = 89$$

20. **(B)** Ratio and proportion is one method for solving the problem.

$$\text{If 15 marbles} = \$22.50, \text{ then } x \text{ marbles} = \$33.00$$

$$15 = 22.5 :: x = 33$$

$$22.5x = 495$$

$$x = 22 \text{ marbles}$$

21. **(B)** The rules or orders of operation must be followed to correctly evaluate the problem.

$$15(y + 7) - 3(5 + 25 \div 5) = 100$$

$$15(y + 7) - 3\left(5 + \frac{25}{5}\right) = 100$$

$$15(y + 7) - 3(10) = 100$$

$$15y + 105 - 30 = 100$$

$$15y + 75 = 100$$

$$15y = 25$$

$$y = \frac{5}{3} \text{ or } 1.6667$$

$$15(y + 7) - 3(5 + 25 \div 5) = 100$$

$$15(1.6667 + 7) - 3\left(5 + \frac{25}{5}\right) = 100$$

$$15(8.667) - 3(10) = 100$$

$$130 - 30 = 100$$

$$100 = 100$$

22. **(C)** The decimals must be considered in order to solve the problem. The numerator has four places to the right of the decimal and the denominator has five places.

$$\frac{78.3207}{0.00715} = 10,953.94 = 10,954$$

23. **(B)** Information inside of one set of parentheses must be multiplied by the information inside of the second set of parentheses.

$$
\begin{array}{r}
5x + 2y \\
\times\, 2x + 6y \\
\hline
30xy + 12y^2 \\
+\, 10x^2 + 4xy \\
\hline
10x^2 + 34xy + 12y^2
\end{array}
$$

24. **(B)** The arithmetic average is determined by adding a series of numbers and dividing by the total of numbers in the series.

$$32 + 45 + 45 + 67 + 23 + 17 + 8 = 237 \div 7 = 33.857 = 33.86$$

25. **(C)** The problem includes both hours and minutes. A decision must be made to work in hours or minutes. The answer can be determined by either method. The following is worked in minutes, and then converted to hours.

Get up: 105 min	$325 \div 60 = 5.41\overline{6} \text{ hr}$
Breakfast: 60 min	$5 \text{ hr} \times 60 \text{ min} = 300 \text{ min}$
	$325 \text{ min} - 300 \text{ min} = 25 \text{ min}$
	5 hr 25 min
Check suitcase: 30 min	(10:00 = 9 hr 60 min)
Drive: 65 min	9 hr 60 min − 5 hr 25 min = 4:35
Check in: 45 min	Alarm time is 4:35 A.M.
+ Delay time: 20 min	
Total minutes: 325 min	

26. **(D)** Mathematical symbols are used in the options. The correct option reads *line JK is parallel to line PQ*. The remaining options are false statements. Option (B) reads *line JK is neither approximate or equal to line PQ*. Option (C) reads *line JK therefore line PQ*.

27. **(A)** Angles *c* and *b* are vertical angles and equal angles. If angle *c* is 50°, then angle *b* must be 50°. Their sum is 100°. The remaining options are incorrect.

28. **(D)** Two angles that combine to form a straight line are adjacent angles and are supplementary. The sum of two such angles is 180°. In the diagram, the following are adjacent angles: a and b, c and d, e and f, g and h, a and c, e and g, b and d, and f and h.

29. **(D)** The problem can be solved using the fraction $\left(\dfrac{4}{5}\right)$ or by changing the fraction to 0.80. Both techniques are shown below.

$\dfrac{4}{5}y - 15 + 7 = 52$	$\dfrac{4}{5}y - 15 + 7 = 52$
$\dfrac{4}{5}y - 8 = 52$	$\dfrac{4}{5}(75) - 15 + 7 = 52$
$4y - 40 = 260$	$60 - 8 = 52$
$4y = 300$	$52 = 52$
$y = 75$	
$0.8y - 15 + 7 = 52$	$0.8y - 15 + 7 = 52$
$0.8y - 8 = 52$	$0.8(75) - 8 = 52$
$0.8y = 60$	$60 - 8 = 52$
$y = 75$	$52 = 52$

30. **(A)** Hank is the oldest child and will receive the largest amount of money.

$$x + (x + 1) + (x + 2) + (x + 3) + (x + 4) = \$50$$
$$5x + 10 = 50$$
$$5x = 40$$
$$x = \$8$$

The oldest, Hank, receives $x + 4 = \$8 + \$4 = \$12$

31. **(B)** The order of operations must be followed to obtain the correct answer.

$$\frac{4(11+7)+\left(2^3 - 15\right)}{3^3 + 7} = \frac{4(18)+(8-15)}{27+7} = \frac{72-7}{34} = \frac{65}{34} = 1.91 = 1.9$$

32. **(B)**

$$\frac{34}{12} \cdot \frac{15}{7} \cdot \frac{10}{20} = \frac{5,100}{1,680} = 3.04$$

$$\frac{34}{12} \cdot \frac{15}{7} \cdot \frac{10}{20} = \frac{5,100}{1,680} = \frac{5,100 \div 2}{1,680 \div 2} = \frac{2,550}{840} = 3.04$$

$$\frac{34}{12} \cdot \frac{15}{7} \cdot \frac{10}{20} = \frac{5,100}{1,680} = \frac{5,100 \div 3}{1,680 \div 3} = \frac{1,700}{560} = 3.04$$

$$\frac{34}{12} \cdot \frac{15}{7} \cdot \frac{10}{20} = \frac{5,100}{1,680} = \frac{5,100 \div 5}{1,680 \div 5} = \frac{1,020}{336} = 3.04$$

33. **(C)**

$$\text{MDCCCXXXIX} = 1,839$$
$$\text{M} = 1,000$$
$$\text{DCCC} = 800$$
$$\text{XXX} = 30$$
$$\text{IX} = 9$$

34. **(D)** 1 in. = 2.54 cm

$$1 \text{ in.} = 2.54 \text{ cm} :: 15 \text{ in.} = x \text{ cm}$$
$$x = (2.54)(15)$$
$$x = 38.1 \text{ cm}$$

35. **(A)**

$$\text{Gasoline} = 3\% \times \$3,255 = \$97.65$$
$$\text{Insurance} = 4\% \times \$3,255 = \underline{\$130.20}$$
$$\$227.85$$

36. **(B)** The order of operations must be followed to obtain the correct answer. The mnemonic PEMDAS provides the order for solving the problem.

- P = parentheses. If parentheses are not in the problem, go to the next step. Parentheses are not necessary to indicate a function.
- E = Exponents. If exponents are not in the problem, go to the next step.
- MD = Multiplication and division. Work the equation from left to right, performing whichever function comes first.
- AS = Addition and subtraction. Work the equation from left to right, performing whichever function comes first.

The problem does not have parentheses or exponents, so the first step is to multiply 10 times 10, which equals 100. Then perform the addition of 10 + 100 + 10, which equals 120.

$$10 + 10 \times 10 + 10 =$$
$$10 + 100 + 10 = 120$$

Science

1. **(A)** Evolution is a natural process of change or transformation that occurs over time in living creatures. It is not a comparison of animals and plants. Erosion is the gradual wear down of mountain ranges. Sea creatures becoming land creatures is one example of evolution, but not the definition of the word.

2. **(A)** Baroreceptors are found in the carotid artery and aortic arch. They provide body status information to the cardiovascular system. Baroreceptors *sense* changes in pressure within the arteries. The remaining options do not support the purpose of baroreceptors.

3. **(B)** The follicle stimulating hormone (FSH) is an important part of the reproductive system in both males and females. It helps manage the menstrual cycle and follicles in females. In males, FSH and luteinizing hormone (LH) stimulate sperm production. The remaining options are not effects of FSH in males.

4. **(C)** The number of electrons in the outermost energy shell are known as valence electrons of an element. The diagram shows chloride as having an atomic number of 17. Element 17 is found in Group 17 on the Periodic Table. (The fact that both the atomic weight and group number are both 17 is coincidental. For example, sodium (Na) has an atomic number of 11 and is found in Group 1.) An atomic number of 17 places two electrons in the first energy shell, eight electrons in the second cell, and seven electrons in the third shell. Valence can, for the most part, be determined by knowing the number of valence electrons in each group. If you had problems with this question, see *www.wikihow.com/find-Valence-Electrons* and *http://dl.clackamas.edu/ch104-06/valence_electrons.htm*

5. **(C)** Antibodies are proteins that are released from lymphoid tissue by B cells. This is a basic definition of antibodies. The remaining options are incorrect.

6. **(B)** The contraction of the right ventricle pushes or forces venous blood into the pulmonary circulation. Venous blood is pumped from the ventricle into the pulmonary artery. Oxygenated blood returns from the lungs to the left atria via the pulmonary vein. The right ventricle does not prevent backflow into the right atrium, serve as a holding chamber, or stimulate filling of the left ventricle.

7. **(A)** The longitudinal fissure is the deep groove that separates the two cerebral hemispheres in the brain. A sulcus is a shallow ridge or furrow. A gyrus is an elevated ridge.

8. **(A)** The adductor magnus is located deep in the anterior thigh. The three muscles of the hamstring are located in the superficial and deep posterior thigh.

9. **(B)** Carbon dioxide is found in carbonated beverages. It produces the bubbles and fizz. The remaining options do not form carbonated water.

10. **(B)** Synovial joints have synovial or joint cavities that contain synovial fluid. These joints are diarthrotic or freely moveable and are representative of most joints in the body. Synovial fluid is a clear, yellowish, nonclotting fluid that lubricates joints.

11. **(A)** The word *adhesion* in the stem is a clue to the correct answer. Connective tissue is held together by cell adhesion proteins which are a ground substance. Proteoglycans provide ground substance firmness. Vascularity has to do with blood supply to connective tissue. Cell adhesion proteins do not support or buttress osteoblasts or osteocytes which are found in bone.

12. **(B)** Homologous pairs of chromosomes spread across the metaphase plate during metaphase I of meiosis. Chromosomes reach their respective poles during telophase I, the nuclear envelope disappears during prophase II, and the forming of daughter cells ends meiosis.

13. **(B)** The number of neutrons in an element is determined by subtracting the atomic number of the element from the atomic mass/weight of the element. Magnesium has an atomic number of 12 and atomic mass of 24.

$$\text{Atomic mass – atomic number} = 24 - 12 = 12$$

14. **(A)** A clue to the correct answer is the word *unit*. The cell is the smallest unit of life. A gland is composed of cells. A pore is a miniscule or microscopic opening. Ribosomes, found in both animal and plant cells, synthesize protein.

15. **(C)** Isotopes are atoms of the same element that have the same number of protons but a different number of neutrons. Isotopes have the same atomic number but different masses or weights.

16. **(C)** The phalanges in the foot are distal or below the metatarsals in the foot. The cuboid bone is lateral to the navicular bone. The cuneiform bone in the foot is distal to the navicular bone. The talus bone in the ankle is inferior to the malleolus of the tibia in the lower leg.

17. **(B)** The central nervous system is composed of the brain and spinal cord. The brainstem and cerebellum and cerebral hemispheres are part of the brain. Nerves branching off of the spine are part of the peripheral nervous system. The autonomic nervous system is part of the peripheral nervous system.

18. **(D)** The bones of the body are in the axial skeleton or appendicular skeleton. The axial skeleton rotates around the vertical axis of the skeleton where the appendicular skeleton is composed of the limbs that are attached to the axial skeleton. The femur is part of the appendicular skeleton.

19. **(C)** Neutrons are found within the atomic structure of an atom, but they have a neutral, not a negative charge. The remaining options are part of the atomic structure of an atom.

20. **(A)** Mixtures are amalgamations of two or more compounds, while compounds are a combination of two different elements. Compounds are held together by chemical bonds that

attract each other, and their elements are proportional in mass. They cannot be separated by physical means. Mixtures form as combinations of compounds interact, but they are not chemically bound, and substances in a mixture can be parted by physical means.

21. **(A)** Referred pain from the left ureter would manifest in the left lower quadrant. Referred pain from the right ureter would be felt in the right lower quadrant.

22. **(D)** Pain referred from the pancreas would be felt in the superior reaches of the right upper quadrant near the midline. Referred pain from the appendix would be distinct in the lower portion of the upper right quadrant near the dividing line of the upper and lower right quadrants. Referred pain from the colon would manifest in the midline of the left and right lower quadrants below the umbilicus.

23. **(D)** Peristalsis is a progressive wave of muscular action that moves digestive contents through the alimentary canal. Peristalsis is an indicator of bowel function. Activation of the reflex arc has nothing to do with peristalsis. A bowel movement cannot occur without peristalsis. Colon cells are not hyperpolarized.

24. **(A)** A key to the correct answer is breaking down the word *somatostatin*. *Somato-* is a prefix meaning body, and *statin* has to do with inhibiting. Somatotropin is a growth hormone; it inhibits, halts, or hinders growth. Somatotropin is not an amino acid derivative or an inhibitor or enhancer of dopamine.

25. **(C)** An implanted embryo secretes human chorionic gonadotropin hormone and has nothing to do with sperm production. All of the remaining options regulate sperm production.

26. **(B)** An individual with type AB blood can only donate to another individual with type AB blood. Type AB recipients can receive donor blood from any of the blood groups, but a type AB donor can only donate to a type AB recipient.

27. **(A)** There are 12 elements important in cell biology: calcium, carbon, chlorine, hydrogen, iron, magnesium, nitrogen, oxygen, phosphorus, potassium, sodium, and sulfur. Barium has many uses, but it is not required to maintain cell or human functioning. Barium is used in specific radiologic procedures.

28. **(C)** The atomic number is equal to the number of electrons present in an element. Fluorine has nine electrons, with two in the first shell and eight in the second.

29. **(B)** Organic compounds are a class of complex molecules exemplified by their use of carbon as a molecular foundation. The four types of organic compounds are carbohydrates, lipids, nucleic acids, and proteins. They are found and produced in living organisms. They are requisite for life to exist.

30. **(B)** The stem of the question provides the definition for *linkage*. Crossing over is the exchange of matching chromatid segments of homologous chromosomes with their related genes. Replication is the process of DNA making a copy of itself. Transcription is the copying of DNA segment polypeptide copied into a molecule of messenger RNA.

31. **(B)** Interferons are proteins that prevent replication of RNA viruses. After certain cells have been infected by viruses, they produce interferons which help defend against viruses. Interferons are not nonspecific skin barriers. The remaining options are nonspecific skin barriers.

32. **(C)** The origin of the nerve impulse that stimulates contraction of the diaphragm and external intercostal muscles is the medullary inspiratory center in the medulla oblongata. Located in the pons, the apneustic area stimulates the inspiratory center and prolongs the contraction of inspiratory muscles. The pneumotaxic area, also located in the pons, inhibits the inspiratory center. The Hering–Breuer reflexes are located in the bronchi and bronchioles of the respiratory tract and are activated by compression (stretching or nonstretching) of the lungs.

They assist in regulating rhythmic ventilation of the lungs and are activated when the lungs reach their physical limits.

33. **(C)** Starch is a polysaccharide composed of numerous molecules of glucose used for energy storage in plants. Common disaccharides are lactose, fructose, and sucrose. Monosaccharides are the simplest forms of carbohydrates. Trisaccharides do not exist.

34. **(D)** Passive transport is movement of ions or molecules from a higher to a lower concentration (down a gradient) and does not require energy consumption, as opposed to active transport which is movement of molecules and ions across a cellular membrane (against a gradient) from a lower to a higher concentration and requires energy consumption. Diffusion, osmosis, and dialysis are examples of passive transport. Receptor-mediated endocytosis is found in active transport.

35. **(D)** Transitional cells stretch or contract in response to body movement. These cells are epithelial in nature. The urinary bladder is an example. Columnar cells are tall and thick epithelial cells that serve to absorb and protect. Cuboidal cells are cube-shaped epithelial cells and are involved in secreting and absorbing substances. Squamous cells are flat epithelial cells and make up most of the outer layers of the skin, the passages of the digestive and respiratory tracts, and line the hollow organs.

36. **(B)** The graduated cylinder is most appropriate for measuring liquid volume. The digital and pan balances measure weight, and the hydrometer measures specific gravity.

37. **(D)** Gay-Lussac's Law shows the relationship between temperature and pressure. He determined that an increase in temperature brings about an increase in pressure when volume and mass of gas are maintained at a constant. He determined that pressure divided by temperature is a constant for gas. Since the change in pressure is directly proportional to the change in temperature, the slope of the line in the diagram is positive.

38. **(A)** The stem of the question is the definition of antigens. Neutrophils (a type of phagocyte) are white blood cells that engulf invading microorganisms. Stem cells are specialized cells that have the potential to develop into many different types of body cells.

39. **(B)** HIV is a virus that causes the collapse of the immune system. HIV destroys the CD4 helper lymphocytes in the immune system. The virus weakens the immune system and predisposes the individual to opportunistic infections which can affect any organ system. HIV and AIDS are not the same thing. HIV can lead to AIDS. AIDS is a syndrome and is the most advanced stage of HIV.

40. **(D)** The stem of the question is the description of the location of the spleen in the human body. The adrenal glands, located atop each kidney, are located in the upper left and right quadrants. The appendix is located in the right lower quadrant, and the liver is located in the right upper quadrant.

41. **(B)** A pressure wave in the arteries, known as pulse, is created when blood is pushed by the left ventricle through the arteries as the heart contracts and relaxes. The remaining options do not create a wave form referred to as the pulse.

42. **(D)** The brain is covered by the pia mater, the innermost layer, followed by the arachnoid, and, last, by the dura (outermost layer). The subarachnoid is the space under the arachnoid layer. It is not a layer.

43. **(B)** The anterior cavity of the eye contains aqueous fluid. The posterior cavity contains vitreous humor. The remaining options are components of the eye but are not cavities.

44. **(B)** The cerebrum is the largest part of the brain and is composed of the right and left hemispheres. It performs higher functions such as hearing, vision, speech, reasoning, emotions, learning, fine motor movement, and interprets touch. The temporal lobe of the cerebrum is

primarily concerned with auditory perception (hearing and selective listening). The remaining options have little or nothing to do with hearing.

45. **(C)** Endocrine glands produce two types of hormones: steroidal and nonsteroidal. Examples of steroidal hormones include aldosterone, cortisol, estrogen, and testosterone. Nonsteroidal hormones include amines (epinephrine, norepinephrine), glycoproteins (FSH, LH), peptides (oxytocin, ADH), and proteins (insulin, prolactin).

46. **(A)** An adrenal gland is located on the uppermost part of each kidney. The medulla of the adrenal gland produces the hormone adrenalin. The remaining options are not located on the kidney.

47. **(C)** The hypothesis speculating that black bearded monkeys will prefer a certain type of leaf is testable. It is specific and makes a definitive statement. The gender and tolerance hypothesis is vague and nonspecific—is gender the lumping of both male and female or is it a comparison of the two, and intolerance to what? Gender? Race? Food? "Oranges come from pear trees" is not a hypothesis since it is a fact that oranges do not come from pear trees. Interest-group contributions to a specific rescue organization is not testable since the answer can be determined by the records of contributions received by the organization as well as records kept by the various interest groups that contribute.

48. **(A)** The eight carpal bones form the wrist. They are the trapezium, trapezoid, scaphoid, lunate, triquetrum, pisiform, capitate, and hamate. The remaining options, while having to do with the hand, are not located in the circle on the diagram.

49. **(D)** The proximal phalanxes are the first finger bone segments superior to the distal and middle phalanxes, and the metacarpals are superior to the proximal phalanxes.

50. **(B)** The stem of the question describes the sciatic nerve. The common peroneal and tibial nerves are segments of the sciatic nerve as it travels down the leg. The spinal accessory nerve is the eleventh cranial nerve and has to do with turning of the head and shoulder movement.

51. **(A)** Cerebral spinal fluid is formed in the first and second or lateral ventricles in the brain. The four ventricles lie laterally in the left and right hemispheres. The lateral ventricles lie in the cerebrum of each cerebral hemisphere. The third ventricle lies in the diencephalon between the right and left thalamus, and the fourth ventricle lies between the medulla oblongata and pons. All ventricles communicate with each other.

52. **(D)** A neutralization reaction occurs when a strong base and a strong acid are combined. The end result, water and a neutral salt, does not have the characteristics of either acids or bases. The remaining options are not products of combining strong bases and strong acids.

53. **(A)** An ionic bond is created when a metallic atom allocates an electron to a nonmetal atom. A covalent bond is created when atoms of nonmetals share a pair of valence electrons.

English and Language Usage

1. **(D)** The subject of a sentence is a person, place, or thing that is *doing* or *being*. A sentence cannot be a sentence without a subject, and the subject must be a noun or pronoun. In the question, the subject *you* is implied or understood. The same is true of the following sentences. *(You) tell me the name of your brothers* and *(You) shut the window.*

2. **(C)** Correctly punctuated, the sentence reads, *The city council voted on the following measures: parking at the city zoo, repainting fire hydrants east of Baker Avenue, and increasing security at varsity home games.* The remaining options are punctuated correctly.

3. **(C)** Action verbs describe something—what a person is doing or experiencing—and allow the reader to visualize the person's activity. As verbs, participles are either past or present. The

word *swum* is an irregular past participle meaning the action occurred in the past. Present participles end in *-ing,* while past participles end in *-ed, -en, -n, -ed,* or *-t.* Two exceptions for past participles are *hung,* which ends in *-g,* and *swum,* which ends in *-m.* The remaining options use the incorrect action verb. Option (A) should be *worn,* not *wore*; option (B) should be *known,* not *knew*; and option (D) should be *drawn,* not *draw.*

4. **(D)** Interrogative pronouns are *what, which, whose, who,* and *whom,* but never *why* or *where.* Each option contains some type of pronoun, but only option (D) contains an interrogative pronoun.

5. **(A)** The word *mischievious* is spelled incorrectly in the sentence. It should be spelled *mischievous.* The words in the remaining option sentences are spelled correctly.

6. **(C)** The word *knucklehead* is a slang or informal term for a stupid or foolish person. Knuckleheads are not necessarily lazy, repulsive, or important persons. *Ethyl* is an informal term referring to tetraethyl lead that was added to gasoline to help reduce engine knocking. Leaded gasoline has not been used in the United States since the 1970s.

7. **(B)** The sentence with correct subject-verb agreement would read *None of the jokes told by the student were funny.* The phrase *told by the student* could be removed and not change the meaning or intent of the sentence. The remaining options have correct subject-verb agreement.

8. **(D)** *Excepted* is the incorrect word, and the sentence should read *The winner of the lottery graciously accepted his prize.* The word *accept* means to receive, get, or take delivery of. *Accept* is a verb. *Except* means to exclude, bar, or not include, and may be a preposition or verb. The use of *accept* or *except* in the remaining options is correct.

9. **(A)** The plural for *vita* is *vitae.* The remaining options are incorrect.

10. **(D)** Double quotation marks indicate direct speech or exactly what a speaker said. Indirect quotes do not require quotation marks since they are approximations of what a speaker said. The use of *that* signifies what follows is indirectly quoted. The remaining options demonstrate correct usage of double quotation marks.

11. **(D)** For the incorrect options, *Golden Gate Bridge* should be capitalized, *fries* should not be capitalized in *French fries,* and *monarchy* should not be capitalized.

12. **(B)** Declarative sentences make a statement or declaration and typically end with a period. Imperative sentences issue a command or a request and may end with a period or exclamation point. The remaining types of sentences are interrogative, which ask a question, and exclamatory, which express emotions and end with an exclamation point. Commas do not end sentences.

13. **(C)** *The children ran for the house, but the skunk ran ahead of them and blocked the door* is a compound sentence. The pattern for a compound sentence is [*independent clause*] [*comma*] [*coordinating conjunction*] [*followed by independent*] clause. Coordinating conjunctions are the words *and, but, for, not, or, so,* and *yet.*

14. **(A)** The incorrectly spelled words should read *happiness, pageant,* and *talcum.*

15. **(A)** Prepositions link words together and impart information to a reader. There are hundreds of prepositional words in the English language. Prepositional words cannot stand alone and are used with other words to make a prepositional phrase. For example, a prepositional phrase can be made with almost any word that has a link, connection, or correlation with the phrase *little red wagon,* such as *in the little wagon, behind the little red wagon, toward the little red wagon, to the little red wagon,* and *against the little red wagon.* The object of a preposition is the noun that follows. In the above examples, *in, behind, toward, to,* and *against* are propositions and *wagon* is the object.

16. **(D)** A direct object receives the action of a verb. Direct objects can be nouns, pronouns, phrases, or clauses. In the sentence *Marion offered a workshop on how to do origami last winter*, Marion is the subject, *offered* is the verb, and *workshop* is the direct object. To find the direct object, ask the question *what did Marion offer?* She offered a workshop. *Offered* is the sentence verb, *origami* (the art of Japanese paper folding) is a noun and specifies the type of workshop, and *winter*, a noun, provides information about time or when the workshop was offered.

17. **(B)** The subject of a sentence provides specific information and may be a word, a group of words, or a phrase. A subject can be a person, place, thing, time, or idea. In the sentence *After striking out during the championship game, Jeff threw his bat at the umpire and was ejected from the game*, Jeff is the subject, and the remainder of the sentence provides information about him—he was playing baseball during a championship game, struck out at bat, threw his bat at the umpire, and was ejected from the game. The remainder of options do not support the definition of the subject of a sentence.

18. **(D)** A simple sentence is a complete thought that stands by itself. The sentence is an independent clause followed by a period. Complex sentences are a combination of an independent clause and one or more dependent clauses. If the dependent clause comes before the independent clause, the two clauses are joined by a comma or semicolon (example: *Even though I had broken my leg, it was important for me to attend the function*). If the dependent clause comes after the independent clause, no punctuation is used between the clauses (example: *It was important for me to attend the function even though I had broken my leg*). Dependent clauses cannot stand alone and begin with a coordinating conjunction. A compound sentence is composed of two or more independent clauses joined by a coordinating conjunction (example: *Marie had never been to the city before and lost her way, but she stopped, got directions, and was only a few minutes late to her appointment*). Simple-complex sentences do not exist.

19. **(C)** *Neither . . . nor* provides correct subject-verb agreement. The word *break* (present tense) in option (A) should be *broke* (past tense). *Knowed*, in option (B), is an incorrect term and should be *knew* (past tense). *Drug*, a medication, is an incorrect word in option (D). The correct word is *dragged* (past tense).

20. **(B)** Verbs are the most important part of a sentence. For a sentence to be a sentence, it must have a verb. Verbs can be one word or more words and indicate action, circumstance, or state of being. Verbs also indicate time (past, present, or future). A single subject must have a single verb, and a plural subject must have a plural verb. There is a relationship between the subject and verb in a sentence that is more than subject-verb agreement—the verb provides information about the subject. In the sentence, Marsh discovered, and the bus departed.

21. **(C)** Irregular verbs indicating present tense are *choose, ring, sleep,* and *spring*. The words *chosen, rung,* and *sprung* are all past participles. *Slept* is past tense.

22. **(D)** The stem of the question is the definition of pronoun. The remaining options are not a definition of pronoun.

23. **(C)** Transitional words bring or link two sentences together. This provides a movement or change without jumps or breaks in thoughts or ideas. *On the other hand* is a transitional phrase. The remaining options do not contain transitional words or phrases.

24. **(B)** An adverb is a word, phrase, or clause that refashions another adverb, adjective, or clause. In the sentence, *the performance put on by the local acting club was exceedingly well done*, the word *exceedingly* changes information about the performance. The performance was not merely well done, but *exceedingly* well done. Words in the remaining option are not functioning as adverbs.

25. **(B)** An *ungracious* individual is one who is ill-mannered, unpleasant, disagreeable, or churlish. The remaining options are antonyms of *ungracious*.

26. **(C)** Corrugated steel has alternating folds and ridges and is typically used for siding or roofing of buildings. The remaining options do not support the definition of corrugated.

27. **(C)** The word should be *labyrinth*, not *laberinth*. The remaining options contain correctly spelled words.

28. **(A)** Option (B) should read *Ladies and Gentlemen: The Cattle Association is pleased that you have come here this evening for this fine dinner, dance, and opportunity to participate in our yearly auction.* A period is inappropriate after *Ladies and Gentlemen* because the phrase is not a sentence and does not contain a verb. A comma is used to separate words in a listing. Option (C) should read, *The depots along the celebrated Bailey Rail Line are: Hemps Point; Marshall City; Mountain View; Dodge; Winter Haven; Bradley; Coal City; and Birmingham.* A colon is indicated before a listing or series and introduces or presents it. Option (D) is incorrect in terms of a time format and could indicate one of two times. It could mean four o'clock in the morning, fourteen minutes and zero seconds (04:14:00), or it could mean four fourteen A.M. (04:14).

Practice Test 5

ANSWER SHEET
Practice Test 5

Reading

1. Ⓐ Ⓑ Ⓒ Ⓓ
2. Ⓐ Ⓑ Ⓒ Ⓓ
3. Ⓐ Ⓑ Ⓒ Ⓓ
4. Ⓐ Ⓑ Ⓒ Ⓓ
5. Ⓐ Ⓑ Ⓒ Ⓓ
6. Ⓐ Ⓑ Ⓒ Ⓓ
7. Ⓐ Ⓑ Ⓒ Ⓓ
8. Ⓐ Ⓑ Ⓒ Ⓓ
9. Ⓐ Ⓑ Ⓒ Ⓓ
10. Ⓐ Ⓑ Ⓒ Ⓓ
11. Ⓐ Ⓑ Ⓒ Ⓓ
12. Ⓐ Ⓑ Ⓒ Ⓓ
13. Ⓐ Ⓑ Ⓒ Ⓓ
14. Ⓐ Ⓑ Ⓒ Ⓓ

15. Ⓐ Ⓑ Ⓒ Ⓓ
16. Ⓐ Ⓑ Ⓒ Ⓓ
17. Ⓐ Ⓑ Ⓒ Ⓓ
18. Ⓐ Ⓑ Ⓒ Ⓓ
19. Ⓐ Ⓑ Ⓒ Ⓓ
20. Ⓐ Ⓑ Ⓒ Ⓓ
21. Ⓐ Ⓑ Ⓒ Ⓓ
22. Ⓐ Ⓑ Ⓒ Ⓓ
23. Ⓐ Ⓑ Ⓒ Ⓓ
24. Ⓐ Ⓑ Ⓒ Ⓓ
25. Ⓐ Ⓑ Ⓒ Ⓓ
26. Ⓐ Ⓑ Ⓒ Ⓓ
27. Ⓐ Ⓑ Ⓒ Ⓓ
28. Ⓐ Ⓑ Ⓒ Ⓓ

29. Ⓐ Ⓑ Ⓒ Ⓓ
30. Ⓐ Ⓑ Ⓒ Ⓓ
31. Ⓐ Ⓑ Ⓒ Ⓓ
32. Ⓐ Ⓑ Ⓒ Ⓓ
33. Ⓐ Ⓑ Ⓒ Ⓓ
34. Ⓐ Ⓑ Ⓒ Ⓓ
35. Ⓐ Ⓑ Ⓒ Ⓓ
36. Ⓐ Ⓑ Ⓒ Ⓓ
37. Ⓐ Ⓑ Ⓒ Ⓓ
38. Ⓐ Ⓑ Ⓒ Ⓓ
39. Ⓐ Ⓑ Ⓒ Ⓓ
40. Ⓐ Ⓑ Ⓒ Ⓓ
41. Ⓐ Ⓑ Ⓒ Ⓓ
42. Ⓐ Ⓑ Ⓒ Ⓓ

43. Ⓐ Ⓑ Ⓒ Ⓓ
44. Ⓐ Ⓑ Ⓒ Ⓓ
45. Ⓐ Ⓑ Ⓒ Ⓓ
46. Ⓐ Ⓑ Ⓒ Ⓓ
47. Ⓐ Ⓑ Ⓒ Ⓓ
48. Ⓐ Ⓑ Ⓒ Ⓓ
49. Ⓐ Ⓑ Ⓒ Ⓓ
50. Ⓐ Ⓑ Ⓒ Ⓓ
51. Ⓐ Ⓑ Ⓒ Ⓓ
52. Ⓐ Ⓑ Ⓒ Ⓓ
53. Ⓐ Ⓑ Ⓒ Ⓓ

Mathematics

1. Ⓐ Ⓑ Ⓒ Ⓓ
2. Ⓐ Ⓑ Ⓒ Ⓓ
3. Ⓐ Ⓑ Ⓒ Ⓓ
4. Ⓐ Ⓑ Ⓒ Ⓓ
5. Ⓐ Ⓑ Ⓒ Ⓓ
6. Ⓐ Ⓑ Ⓒ Ⓓ
7. Ⓐ Ⓑ Ⓒ Ⓓ
8. Ⓐ Ⓑ Ⓒ Ⓓ
9. Ⓐ Ⓑ Ⓒ Ⓓ

10. Ⓐ Ⓑ Ⓒ Ⓓ
11. Ⓐ Ⓑ Ⓒ Ⓓ
12. Ⓐ Ⓑ Ⓒ Ⓓ
13. Ⓐ Ⓑ Ⓒ Ⓓ
14. Ⓐ Ⓑ Ⓒ Ⓓ
15. Ⓐ Ⓑ Ⓒ Ⓓ
16. Ⓐ Ⓑ Ⓒ Ⓓ
17. Ⓐ Ⓑ Ⓒ Ⓓ
18. Ⓐ Ⓑ Ⓒ Ⓓ

19. Ⓐ Ⓑ Ⓒ Ⓓ
20. Ⓐ Ⓑ Ⓒ Ⓓ
21. Ⓐ Ⓑ Ⓒ Ⓓ
22. Ⓐ Ⓑ Ⓒ Ⓓ
23. Ⓐ Ⓑ Ⓒ Ⓓ
24. Ⓐ Ⓑ Ⓒ Ⓓ
25. Ⓐ Ⓑ Ⓒ Ⓓ
26. Ⓐ Ⓑ Ⓒ Ⓓ
27. Ⓐ Ⓑ Ⓒ Ⓓ

28. Ⓐ Ⓑ Ⓒ Ⓓ
29. Ⓐ Ⓑ Ⓒ Ⓓ
30. Ⓐ Ⓑ Ⓒ Ⓓ
31. Ⓐ Ⓑ Ⓒ Ⓓ
32. Ⓐ Ⓑ Ⓒ Ⓓ
33. Ⓐ Ⓑ Ⓒ Ⓓ
34. Ⓐ Ⓑ Ⓒ Ⓓ
35. Ⓐ Ⓑ Ⓒ Ⓓ
36. Ⓐ Ⓑ Ⓒ Ⓓ

ANSWER SHEET
Practice Test 5

Science

1. Ⓐ Ⓑ Ⓒ Ⓓ
2. Ⓐ Ⓑ Ⓒ Ⓓ
3. Ⓐ Ⓑ Ⓒ Ⓓ
4. Ⓐ Ⓑ Ⓒ Ⓓ
5. Ⓐ Ⓑ Ⓒ Ⓓ
6. Ⓐ Ⓑ Ⓒ Ⓓ
7. Ⓐ Ⓑ Ⓒ Ⓓ
8. Ⓐ Ⓑ Ⓒ Ⓓ
9. Ⓐ Ⓑ Ⓒ Ⓓ
10. Ⓐ Ⓑ Ⓒ Ⓓ
11. Ⓐ Ⓑ Ⓒ Ⓓ
12. Ⓐ Ⓑ Ⓒ Ⓓ
13. Ⓐ Ⓑ Ⓒ Ⓓ
14. Ⓐ Ⓑ Ⓒ Ⓓ

15. Ⓐ Ⓑ Ⓒ Ⓓ
16. Ⓐ Ⓑ Ⓒ Ⓓ
17. Ⓐ Ⓑ Ⓒ Ⓓ
18. Ⓐ Ⓑ Ⓒ Ⓓ
19. Ⓐ Ⓑ Ⓒ Ⓓ
20. Ⓐ Ⓑ Ⓒ Ⓓ
21. Ⓐ Ⓑ Ⓒ Ⓓ
22. Ⓐ Ⓑ Ⓒ Ⓓ
23. Ⓐ Ⓑ Ⓒ Ⓓ
24. Ⓐ Ⓑ Ⓒ Ⓓ
25. Ⓐ Ⓑ Ⓒ Ⓓ
26. Ⓐ Ⓑ Ⓒ Ⓓ
27. Ⓐ Ⓑ Ⓒ Ⓓ
28. Ⓐ Ⓑ Ⓒ Ⓓ

29. Ⓐ Ⓑ Ⓒ Ⓓ
30. Ⓐ Ⓑ Ⓒ Ⓓ
31. Ⓐ Ⓑ Ⓒ Ⓓ
32. Ⓐ Ⓑ Ⓒ Ⓓ
33. Ⓐ Ⓑ Ⓒ Ⓓ
34. Ⓐ Ⓑ Ⓒ Ⓓ
35. Ⓐ Ⓑ Ⓒ Ⓓ
36. Ⓐ Ⓑ Ⓒ Ⓓ
37. Ⓐ Ⓑ Ⓒ Ⓓ
38. Ⓐ Ⓑ Ⓒ Ⓓ
39. Ⓐ Ⓑ Ⓒ Ⓓ
40. Ⓐ Ⓑ Ⓒ Ⓓ
41. Ⓐ Ⓑ Ⓒ Ⓓ
42. Ⓐ Ⓑ Ⓒ Ⓓ

43. Ⓐ Ⓑ Ⓒ Ⓓ
44. Ⓐ Ⓑ Ⓒ Ⓓ
45. Ⓐ Ⓑ Ⓒ Ⓓ
46. Ⓐ Ⓑ Ⓒ Ⓓ
47. Ⓐ Ⓑ Ⓒ Ⓓ
48. Ⓐ Ⓑ Ⓒ Ⓓ
49. Ⓐ Ⓑ Ⓒ Ⓓ
50. Ⓐ Ⓑ Ⓒ Ⓓ
51. Ⓐ Ⓑ Ⓒ Ⓓ
52. Ⓐ Ⓑ Ⓒ Ⓓ
53. Ⓐ Ⓑ Ⓒ Ⓓ

English and Language Usage

1. Ⓐ Ⓑ Ⓒ Ⓓ
2. Ⓐ Ⓑ Ⓒ Ⓓ
3. Ⓐ Ⓑ Ⓒ Ⓓ
4. Ⓐ Ⓑ Ⓒ Ⓓ
5. Ⓐ Ⓑ Ⓒ Ⓓ
6. Ⓐ Ⓑ Ⓒ Ⓓ
7. Ⓐ Ⓑ Ⓒ Ⓓ

8. Ⓐ Ⓑ Ⓒ Ⓓ
9. Ⓐ Ⓑ Ⓒ Ⓓ
10. Ⓐ Ⓑ Ⓒ Ⓓ
11. Ⓐ Ⓑ Ⓒ Ⓓ
12. Ⓐ Ⓑ Ⓒ Ⓓ
13. Ⓐ Ⓑ Ⓒ Ⓓ
14. Ⓐ Ⓑ Ⓒ Ⓓ

15. Ⓐ Ⓑ Ⓒ Ⓓ
16. Ⓐ Ⓑ Ⓒ Ⓓ
17. Ⓐ Ⓑ Ⓒ Ⓓ
18. Ⓐ Ⓑ Ⓒ Ⓓ
19. Ⓐ Ⓑ Ⓒ Ⓓ
20. Ⓐ Ⓑ Ⓒ Ⓓ
21. Ⓐ Ⓑ Ⓒ Ⓓ

22. Ⓐ Ⓑ Ⓒ Ⓓ
23. Ⓐ Ⓑ Ⓒ Ⓓ
24. Ⓐ Ⓑ Ⓒ Ⓓ
25. Ⓐ Ⓑ Ⓒ Ⓓ
26. Ⓐ Ⓑ Ⓒ Ⓓ
27. Ⓐ Ⓑ Ⓒ Ⓓ
28. Ⓐ Ⓑ Ⓒ Ⓓ

READING

NUMBER OF QUESTIONS: 53

TIME LIMIT: 64 MINUTES

Instructions: Read each question thoroughly. Select the single best answer. Mark your answer (A, B, C, or D) on the answer sheet provided for Practice Test 5.

Questions 1–6 are based on the following passage.

Excerpt from Chapter Three: "Off with the Indians" from *The White Indian Boy*, an autobiography, written by Nicholas (Nick) Wilson in the early 1900s:

The night came at last when we were to leave. Just after dark I slipped away from the house and started for the bunch of willows where I was to meet the Indian. When I got there, I found two Indians waiting for me instead of one. The sight of two of them almost made me weaken and turn back, but I saw with them my little pinto pony and it gave me some courage. They had an old Indian saddle on the pony with very rough rawhide thongs for stirrup straps. At a signal from them, I jumped on my horse and away we went. Our trail led towards the north along the western shore of the Great Salt Lake.

The Indians wanted to ride fast. It was all right at first, but after a while I got very tired. My legs began to hurt me, and I wanted to stop, but they urged me along till the *peep* of day, when we stopped by some very salty springs. I was so stiff and sore that I could not get off my horse, so one of them lifted me off and stood me on the ground, but I could hardly stand up. The rawhide straps had rubbed the skin off my legs till they were raw. The Indians told me that if I would take off my trousers and jump into the salt springs it would make my legs better, but I found that I could not get them off alone; they were stuck to my legs. The Indians helped, and after some severe pain, we succeeded in getting them off. A good deal of skin came with them.

"Come now," they urged me, "jump into this water and you will be well in a little while."

Well, I jumped into the spring up to my waist. Oh, blazes! I jumped out again. Oh, my! How it did sting and smart! I jumped and kicked. I was so wild with pain that I lay on the ground and rolled around and round on the grass. After half an hour of this, I wore myself out, and oh, how I cried! The Indians put down a buffalo robe, and rolled me onto it and spread a blanket over me. I lay there and cried myself to sleep.

1. *The White Indian Boy* is an example of a

   (A) mixed primary and secondary source.
   (B) primary source.
   (C) secondary source.
   (D) tertiary source.

2. The style of writing used in the passage is

   (A) argumentative.
   (B) exposition.
   (C) narrative.
   (D) persuasive.

3. The italicized word *peep* in the passage suggests Nick and the Indians rode

(A) through the night and did not stop until the break of day.
(B) through the night in anticipation of hearing the songs of the night birds.
(C) until Nick tired and started to softly cry.
(D) until the horses were tired.

4. Which of the following is implied in the passage about Nick's first hours with the Indians?

(A) Nick had been fooled by the Indians.
(B) The hours were exciting and filled with adventure.
(C) The Indians and Nick rode throughout the night in fear of being discovered.
(D) What started out as adventure ended with misadventure.

5. Nick's adventures with the Indians started in

(A) the Great Plains.
(B) the mountains of the West.
(C) what is now the state of Utah.
(D) The geographical location cannot be established.

6. What was the primary cause of Nick's agony when he jumped into the salt spring?

(A) He was a novice rider.
(B) Keeping his legs tensed to keep from falling off of the horse
(C) Riding on a saddle he was not used to
(D) Rough rawhide stirrup straps

---

7. Which of the following states does not belong in the list?

Alabama	Louisiana
Florida	Mississippi
Georgia	Texas

(A) Alabama
(B) Georgia
(C) Louisiana
(D) Mississippi

8. What is the best definition of the italicized word in the following passage?

John's mother had given him $500 to buy school clothes for the upcoming year. This, coupled with what he had saved over the summer, would allow him to purchase everything he needed and wanted—including a pair of bright red *speedos*.

(A) A pair of men's tight-fitting swimming trunks
(B) A pair of men's warm-up pants
(C) An Italian winter jacket with detachable sleeves
(D) Long-distance running shoes

Questions 9–12 are based on the following passage.

Mountain Pass State Park closed for the season on October 22 following a record two-day snowfall of 17 feet in the lower elevations. The park will not be open again until late spring or early summer of next year. Thirty-three late-season campers ignored the park ranger's warnings to leave the park after 2 feet of snow had fallen and had to be rescued by helicopter.

Looking back on the season, many feared the increase in usage fees two years ago would lower the number of individuals visiting the park. However, improvement in parkwide services is credited for making this season's attendance record the highest in the past 15 years. A breakdown of visitors by state saw a 25 percent increase in out-of-state visitors, with a 40 percent increase of in-state visitors. Throughout the park, campsite reservations ran at 80–90 percent for all areas, and the majority of campsites are 95 percent booked for next season. Businesses within the park saw a 65 percent increase in sales, and gasoline sales increased by 28 percent.

The mayor of Parkside, the village nearest the park entrance, said village businesses had experienced a 55 percent increase in *revenue*, and lodging facilities had run at nearly 100 percent all season. He anticipates a good season next year.

9. Which of the following would be appropriate for publication of the passage?

(A) *Mountain Pass State Park Monthly*
(B) *Ranger Troop 54 Quarterly Happenings*
(C) *The Parkside Tribune*
(D) *Travel Journey magazine*

10. What is implied in the passage about Mountain Pass State Park's revenue for the season?

(A) Revenue increased because of an increase in visitors to the park.
(B) Revenue increased because Mountain Pass State Park is the closest area with mountains and camping facilities.
(C) Revenue stayed the same because the cost of living is higher.
(D) Revenue stayed the same to make up for the shortfall of previous years.

11. What was the writer's intent for writing this passage?

(A) To challenge the reader
(B) To inform the reader
(C) To make a political statement
(D) To warn of impending misuse of nature by increasing numbers of visitors

12. What is a synonym for the italicized word *revenue* in the last paragraph?

(A) Cash flow
(B) Duty
(C) Fluid assets
(D) Salary

13. What is the meaning of the italicized word in the following sentence?

Many young people of today seem to *adulate* wealth and living the good life more than being productive, law-abiding citizens.

(A) Believing good things will come to those who work hard

(B) Living above your means and placing your financial future in jeopardy

(C) Showing uncritical praise, devotion, or admiration of someone or something

(D) Wanting, desiring, or longing for something that may be out of reach without permanent or temporary concessions

Questions 14–17 are based on the following chart.

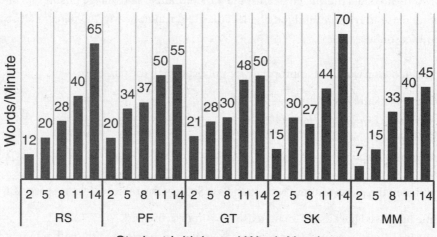

Typing Words/Minute by Week

14. How many students are included in the chart?

(A) 2

(B) 3

(C) 4

(D) 5

15. Which student had the second-lowest typing words/minute in Week 8?

(A) GT

(B) PF

(C) RS

(D) SK

10. Which student had the greatest improvement in typing words per minute during the 14-week period?

(A) GT

(B) MM

(C) RS

(D) SK

17. What does analysis of the chart data suggest?

    (A) Gender influences typing speed.
    (B) There is too much variability to make a determination.
    (C) Typing speed increases over time.
    (D) Typing speed remains static over time.

Questions 18–23 are based on the following passage.

Frank had been an assistant to the scoutmaster for two years and had accompanied him on fourteen camping trips with troops of eight- to eleven-year-old mountain scouts. Frank enjoyed telling scary stories to the groups. It was his favorite activity after teaching hiking skills, and he was known for his scary, *keep-you-awake-at-night* stories. Frank made sure he never told the same story twice and searched the Internet for new ideas on a regular basis.

Tonight's story had been one of his best, and the weather had been his ally. He called the story "The Lullaby Whistler." It was the story of a *maniacal* escapee from a prison farm who whistled lullabies as he stalked and dismembered his young victims. The weather added suspense to the story. The wind periodically whistled through the pines and carried usually ignored sounds into the camp. Frank was sure there were a lot more imaginary things going "bump in the night" than there usually were.

Making sure the scouts were tucked in for the night took longer than usual. Many were still somewhat spooked by the story and the weather, but Frank assured them that "The Lullaby Whistler" was just a story and night winds were the norm for this time of year. As expected, the majority of the scouts elected to leave lamps on in their tents.

Frank completed his evening rounds and was preparing for bed when he thought he heard a new sound that almost sounded like a whistled lullaby in the wind. He ignored the sound because there were always new sounds to be heard in the forest, and besides, the wind in the pines always made strange reverberations. He'd been in his sleeping bag for a short time when he heard the whistling again. This time the sound seemed to be moving against the wind. He was certain he'd heard sounds like something moving in the bushes outside of his tent. Frank was beginning to feel a little unnerved. Suddenly something hit his tent, and the whistling sound of a lullaby filled the air. Frank didn't wait to see what was going to happen next. He bolted out of his sleeping bag and nearly took the tent down. As he scrambled out of the tent he tripped, screamed, and fell into a crowd of laughing and shrieking mountain scouts who had finally procured their revenge.

18. Which of the following writing styles is used in the passage?

    (A) Compare/contrast
    (B) Narrative
    (C) Problem/solution
    (D) Sequencing

19. What does the italicized phrase *keep-you-awake-at-night* imply?

    (A) Anticipation about the next day's activities
    (B) The scouts ate sugary snacks while listening to scary stories, and they were not ready to settle down and go to sleep.
    (C) "The Lullaby Whistler" coupled with the wind provoked uncertainty and trepidation that negatively influenced sleep.
    (D) The wind blowing in the pines

20. What does the passage suggest about Frank?

   (A) He gets some satisfaction from frightening the young scouts with his scary stories.
   (B) He tells scary stories because they are an expectation of the camping experience.
   (C) He uses the scary stories as teaching moments to help the young scouts learn.
   (D) His telling of scary stories gives the scoutmaster solitary time to plan for the next day's activities.

21. What is an antonym for the italicized word *maniacal* in the passage?

   (A) Compos mentis
   (B) Deranged
   (C) Meshugge
   (D) Psychotic

22. What frightened or unnerved Frank when he was in his tent?

   (A) His imagination got the better of him.
   (B) Males' response to fear is different than females' response.
   (C) Fear is transmissible.
   (D) Camping in an unfamiliar environment

23. Which of the following writing styles is used in the passage?

   (A) A mixture of formal and informal
   (B) Exposition
   (C) Formal
   (D) Informal

24. What is your first action in solving the following equation?

$$\frac{17+3\times7+4(7-13)}{40} =$$

   (A) Adding 17 + 3
   (B) Dividing by 40
   (C) Multiplying 3 × 7
   (D) Subtracting 7 − 13

25. The information guides at the top of a page in a dictionary are *Capitalization 2.734* and *Capitalization 2.980*. Which of the following will be found on this page?

   (A) Capitalization 2.568
   (B) Capitalization 2.733
   (C) Capitalization 2.789
   (D) Capitalization 2.981

26. The speaker at the seminar told the audience that there were numerous etiologies for small-business failures. What does his statement suggest?

   (A) A lack of management skills leads to numerous small-business failures.
   (B) Formal courses in business management will reduce small-business etiologies.
   (C) Small-business failures are caused by many different phenomena.
   (D) Small businesses constantly fail because of lack of support from local and federal agencies.

Questions 27–29 are based on the following table of contents from a geometry review book.

27. In which of the following chapters would you expect to find information on the basics of triangles?

(A) Chapter 3
(B) Chapter 4
(C) Chapter 7
(D) Chapter 8

28. A student missed a post-test question on the amount of fluid a cylinder will hold. Which of the following chapters should the student review?

(A) Chapter 1
(B) Chapter 3
(C) Chapter 5
(D) Chapter 9

29. Prior to taking the post-test, a student wants to double check the formula for the surface area of a cube. Which of the following chapters contains this information?

(A) Chapter 2
(B) Chapter 5
(C) Chapter 8
(D) Chapter 10

Questions 30–34 are based on the following passage on pain.

Pain is unique to the individual. This means that pain is subjective and exists whenever and wherever the individual says it does. An individual's pain may be *demonstrative* or inexpressive. How pain is expressed often has a cultural basis. Pain is never a diagnosis, but a symptom of a problem that can range from a headache brought on by stress, overworking a muscle, a broken bone, or an indication of organ failure. Pain can range from a mild annoyance to debilitation. A pain scale is often used to aid in determining the intensity of pain. The scale ranges from one to ten, with one indicating no pain or pain free and ten indicating the worst pain possible.

Pain has three basic components—a stimulus, a sensation of pain, and a reaction. The acknowledgment of pain requires a functioning nervous system. The stimulus may be external and in the environment or internal and originate in the body. A realization of pain involves the nervous system, as the stimulus is transmitted and responded to. The reaction to pain can involve any body system and typically has a psychological component.

While it may seem odd, pain is beneficial. Pain can serve as an early warning system and can give indications that things are not going as they should.

30. The purpose of the passage is to

   (A) encourage use of home remedies to treat pain.
   (B) encourage visits to health-care providers.
   (C) inform.
   (D) persuade.

31. Pain can be said to be

   (A) detrimental.
   (B) expected.
   (C) idiosyncratic.
   (D) objective.

32. The mother said her three-year-old son's pain is *demonstrative*. What is the best explanation of *demonstrative*?

   (A) Only the health-care provider has the skill to determine how the child expresses his pain.
   (B) Only the mother can describe her son's pain.
   (C) The child must be questioned to understand his pain.
   (D) The child's pain is readily observable.

33. A man visits his health-care provider because of stomach pain that he develops after eating and in the middle of the night. This is an example of pain serving as a(n)

   (A) early warning system.
   (B) indication the man needs to change his diet.
   (C) indication the problem will worsen if not treated.
   (D) indication of a potential problem in the nervous system.

34. What does the use of a pain scale to determine an individual's pain level insinuate?

   (A) Different pain scales can be used for young and old.
   (B) Greater amounts of information can be gathered from more complex pain scales.
   (C) Health-care providers can use a pain scale to get a more tangible sense of an individual's pain.
   (D) Verbal pain scales are more accurate than numerical ones.

---

35. Follow the instructions to change the word *question* to a new word.

   1. Move the *t* to before the *q*.
   2. Drop *on* and replace with *ch*.
   3. Drop *ues* and replace with *om*.
   4. Reverse the order of *t* and *q*.
   5. Drop *i* and replace with *a*.
   6. Drop *q* and replace with *s*.

The new word is

   (A) sequel.
   (B) stoma.
   (C) stomach.
   (D) stomich.

36. What is your first action in solving the following equation?

$$25 + 20 \div 5 - 20 + 5 =$$

(A) Add 25 + 20
(B) Cancel +20 and –20
(C) Divide 20 by 5
(D) Subtract 5 from –20

Questions 37–39 are based on the following café menu in a ranching/farming community of 7,500.

THE MAGNOLIA CAFÉ

(Est. 1972)

Wednesday Specials

10:30 A.M. – 8:00 P.M.

All specials served with choice of salad bar/dinner salad, three vegetables, bread, dessert, and never-ending drink refills.

Additional 15% discount at checkout for 60–74 years

Over 75 years always eat free of charge

Call ahead—Carry out welcome

Papa's Favorite
Chicken Fried Steak with Cream Gravy
Gents—$8.75 (reg. $11.50)
Ladies—$7.50 (reg. $9.50)
Kids—$4.00 (reg. $6.00)

Pirate's Feast
Hamburger/Cheeseburger
Gents—$9.00 (reg. $10.50)
Ladies—$7.95 (reg. $9.50)
Kids—$4.00 (reg. $6.50)

Mama's Favorite
Chicken and Dumplings
Gents—$8.50 (reg. $10.00)
Ladies—$6.50 (reg. $8.50)
Kids—$3.95 (reg. $5.50)

Cook's Favorite
Smoked Brisket
Gents—$12.00 (reg. $15.00)
Ladies—$10.50 (reg. $12.50)
Kids—$4.75 (reg. $7.50)

Southern Delight
Fried Chicken
Gents—$8.95 (reg. $12.00)
Ladies—$7.50 (reg. $10.00)
Kids—$4.75 (reg. $6.95)

Grannie's Favorite
Salad Bar & Vegetable Plate
Gents—$7.50 (reg. $8.59)
Ladies—$5.00 (reg. $6.50)
Kids—$3.00 (reg. $4.50)

37. How many beef specials are offered?

(A) 1
(B) 3
(C) 4
(D) 5

38. Excluding Grannie's Favorite, what is the most economical special for ladies less than 50 years of age?

(A) Mama's Favorite
(B) Papa's Favorite
(C) Pirate's Feast
(D) Southern Delight

39. Which of the following options is the least economical special for gents less than 50 years of age?

(A) Cook's Favorite
(B) Grannie's Favorite
(C) Mama's Favorite
(D) Pirate's Feast

---

40. "I know you consider Ken a friend, but I'd watch what you say around him. He's nothing but a big *blabbermouth*."

Select the best alternative for the word *blabbermouth*.

(A) Ken can't keep his mouth shut.
(B) Ken is a stupid person.
(C) Ken is flirtatious.
(D) Ken thinks he knows it all.

41. A chapter in a book entitled *Roses Around the World* has the following subheadings: (a) History of Roses; (b) Growing Roses in Various *Climes*; (c) Varieties of Roses; and (d) Year-round Care of Roses. What is a synonym for *climes*?

(A) Countries
(B) Elevations
(C) Soil types
(D) Weather zones

42. All of the organs in the human body work in concert to sustain life. The heart is one of the most important organs. Life is impossible without an effectively working heart. The arterial system allows the heart to transport oxygenated blood to the body and the venous system works to carry deoxygenated blood from the body back to the heart. Like all organs, the heart is susceptible to damage and/or death from an insufficient blood supply resulting in a lack of tissue oxygenation. In medical or technical terms, the condition is referred to as a myocardial infarction (MI). Defining this term indicates primary damage to

(A) heart chambers.
(B) heart electrical conduction.
(C) heart muscle.
(D) heart valves.

Questions 43–47 are based on the following communication.

MEMORANDUM

TO: Randall Watson, Analyst 2nd class, Division IV
FROM: Mike Abercrombee, Division IV Supervisor
Date: November 15
Subject: Theft of secure documents and subsequent actions

This memo is to serve as an overview of our meeting last week, and the findings of the Disciplinary Committee regarding charges brought against you.

On November 2, you were removed from your position until a formal hearing could be held to address the charges of theft and sale of secure documents brought against you. Computer access to the public and private company website was also terminated.

On November 7, you met with the Disciplinary Committee regarding the formal charges of theft and exchange of classified information for personal gain. After presentation of *irrefutable* evidence, you admitted your guilt in this matter and expressed regret for your actions.

In coming to a decision, the Disciplinary Committee reviewed disciplinary action taken against you two years ago for the same problem. At that time, you were suspended from employment without pay and benefits for a period of six months, reduced from Analyst 6th class to Analyst 2nd class which reduced your clearance status to Primary, and placed on probation for 18 months after returning to work.

Little committee discussion was necessary since learning did not take place after the first incident. The Disciplinary Committee recommends immediate termination. Their decision has been forwarded to Audie Johnson, Company Chairman, for signature.

Within the next 24 hours, you will receive a formal letter via registered mail officially terminating your employment. During this same time frame, officials from Legal Services will be meeting with the Princeton County Attorney to pursue criminal charges against you.

[Based on Policy 42.92.3a–42.95.8 of the Employee Handbook, Security has hand delivered this memo to you, and will escort you from the building to your car where you will be escorted from company parking to a public street. As per policy, all of your personal belongings (excluding company identification and other company property) will be returned to you following the results of legal actions taken against you. Failure to comply with the above-referenced policies will result in your immediate arrest.]

43. Is the information in the memo delineated?

   (A) No, the information is illogical.
   (B) No, the information is imprecise.
   (C) Yes, the information is clearly and precisely presented.
   (D) Yes, the information is sketchy.

44. Which of the following correctly identifies the type of writing?

   (A) Expository
   (B) Narrative
   (C) Persuasive
   (D) Technical

45. What is an appropriate synonym for the word *irrefutable*?

(A) Assailable

(B) Controversial

(C) Overwhelming

(D) Questionable

46. What is the logical conclusion of the memo?

(A) Randall will appeal the Disciplinary Committee's decision and keep his job.

(B) Randall will be able to find a similar job in another state.

(C) The memo is a threat.

(D) The probability is high that Randall will serve prison time.

47. What is the nature of the information presented in the memo?

(A) Conjecture

(B) Explicit

(C) Guesswork

(D) Threat

Questions 48–51 are based on the following chart.

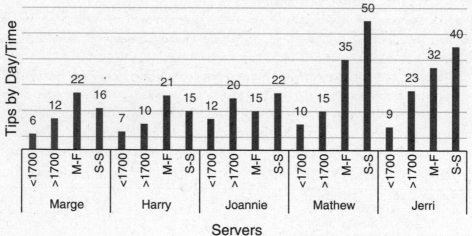

48. What server has the lowest number of tips before 1700 (before 5:00 P.M.)?

(A) Harry

(B) Jerri

(C) Marge

(D) Mathew

49. Which server had the highest number of tips after 1700 (after 5:00 P.M.)?

    (A) Jerri
    (B) Joannie
    (C) Marge
    (D) Mathew

50. Estimate the number of tips Jerri received Monday through Friday and Saturday and Sunday?

    (A) Approximately 40
    (B) Approximately 50
    (C) Approximately 60
    (D) Approximately 70

51. Were the number of tips higher during the week or on weekends? (Estimate your answer.)

    (A) This cannot be determined since there are more days during the week than on weekends.
    (B) The number of tips was highest during the week.
    (C) The number of tips was highest during weekends.
    (D) The number of tips for each is basically the same.

Questions 52–53 are related to the Dewey decimal system.

    070 News media, journalism & publishing
    071 Newspapers in North America
    072 Newspapers in British Isles; in England
    073 Newspapers in central Europe; in Germany
    074 Newspapers in France & Monaco
    075 Newspapers in Italy & adjacent islands
    076 Newspapers in Iberian Peninsula & adjacent islands
    077 Newspapers in eastern Europe; in Russia
    078 Newspapers in Scandinavia
    079 Newspapers in other geographic areas

52. A daily newspaper in Norway publishes a weekly edition in English. In what section of the Dewey decimal system would you find this edition?

    (A) 071 Newspapers in North America
    (B) 075 Newspapers in Italy & adjacent islands
    (C) 078 Newspapers in Scandinavia
    (D) 079 Newspapers in other geographical areas

53. Samuel is majoring in Spanish and has an assignment to locate and translate a newspaper article from a newspaper published in a Spanish-speaking country. In what section would he find a newspaper written in Spanish?

    (A) 076 Newspapers in Iberian Peninsula & adjacent islands
    (B) 074 Newspapers in France & Monaco
    (C) 070 News media, journalism & publishing
    (D) 079 Newspapers in other geographical areas

MATHEMATICS

NUMBER OF QUESTIONS: 36

TIME LIMIT: 54 MINUTES

> **Instructions:** Read each question thoroughly. Select the single best answer. Mark your answer (A, B, C, or D) on the answer sheet provided for Practice Test 5.

1. Solve the following equation. Round your answer to the nearest hundredth.

   $15x + 7x - 28 - (-2) = 0$

   (A) 1.08
   (B) 1.18
   (C) 1.25
   (D) 1.36

2. The instructions on a prescription label read: Take 5 milliliters every 6 hours followed by 8 ounces of water. How many teaspoons of medication will you take in a 24-hour period?

   (A) 2 tsp
   (B) 4 tsp
   (C) 6 tsp
   (D) 8 tsp

3. A man tells his grandchildren that he is 22,567 days old. How old is he in years? Round your answer to the nearest tenth.

   (A) 59.7
   (B) 61.8
   (C) 66.0
   (D) 73.4

4. Add the following. Round your answer to the nearest whole number.

   $616.78 + 8.3411 + 55.214 + 22.5088 =$

   (A) 701
   (B) 702
   (C) 703
   (D) 704

5. Sylvie is planning on spending $75 to buy her best friend a gift. Her mother finds out and tells Sylvie she must spend the money on buying gifts for her three sisters and best friend since all four individuals helped her with her project. Sylvie decides that she will spend 40 percent on her best friend and 20 percent on each of her sisters. What amount of money will be spent on Sylvie's best friend and each of her sisters?

   (A) $15 on the best friend and $20 on each sister
   (B) $20 on the best friend and $18 on each sister
   (C) $30 on the best friend and $15 on each sister
   (D) $35 on the best friend and $13 on each sister

6. Sam is building a new chicken coop and decides to attach one long side of the coop to the south side of his barn facing the garage. Measurements for the chicken coop sides are 22 feet long by 15 feet high and 15 feet wide by 15 feet high. He decides to purchase chicken wire available in rolls of 40 feet long by 5 feet wide. How many rolls of chicken wire does he need to purchase?

   (A) 2.5 rolls
   (B) 4 rolls
   (C) 5.5 rolls
   (D) 6 rolls

7. Solve for x in the following problem.

   $$17x - 22 + 7x - 7 = 61$$

   (A) 3.75
   (B) 2.54
   (C) 3.21
   (D) 7.7

8. Simplify the following expression.

   $$\frac{7}{8} \div 50\% =$$

   (A) 0.4375
   (B) $\dfrac{7}{40}$
   (C) 1.75
   (D) $4\dfrac{3}{8}$

9. Polly wants to know her current grade going into the final exam in her history class. According to the syllabus, each exam is worth 20 percent, the history project 20 percent, presentation 10 percent, and the final exam 30 percent. What is her grade going into the final exam? Her grades are below:

   Test 1—75

   Test 2—89

   History Project—85

   Presentation—80

   (A) 66%
   (B) 80%
   (C) 83%
   (D) 94%

10. Phil needs to weigh between 68.0 and 72.57 kilograms for his wrestling weight class. He currently weighs 139 pounds. His goal is to weigh 155 pounds by the beginning of the fall semester. How many kilograms does Phil need to gain?

   (A) 7.27 kg
   (B) 8.43 kg
   (C) 10.53 kg
   (D) 12 kg

11. Evaluate the following expression if $a = 15$, $b = 5$, and $c = 10$.

$$\frac{b+c}{a} + \frac{8}{a-c} =$$

(A) $-\dfrac{42}{5}$

(B) $\dfrac{13}{5}$

(C) $\dfrac{42}{5}$

(D) $\dfrac{8}{15}$

12. Multiply the following.

$$(4a + b)(4a + 5b) =$$

(A) $8a^2 + 6b^3$

(B) $16a^2 + 24ab + 5b^2$

(C) $18a + 5a^2b + 5b^2$

(D) $80a^2b^2$

13. Simplify the following fraction.

$$\frac{119}{68} =$$

(A) 0.75

(B) 1.74

(C) 1.75

(D) 2.75

14. Add the following fractions. Present your answer in a decimal format. Round your answer to the nearest hundredth.

$$\frac{6}{21} + \frac{13}{15} =$$

(A) 0.53

(B) 0.68

(C) 1.15

(D) 1.62

15. Select the unequal pair from the following.

(A) $\dfrac{3}{4}$, 0.75

(B) 1.68, $1\dfrac{34}{50}$

(C) 5, $\dfrac{40}{7}$

(D) $\dfrac{250}{50}$, 5

16. One angle in a triangle measures 105°, and the second angle measures 20°. What is the measurement in degrees of the third angle?

(A) 55°
(B) 120°
(C) 235°
(D) The answer is impossible to determine without knowing the type of triangle.

17. The sum of four consecutive odd numbers is 200. What is the largest of the four consecutive numbers?

(A) 45
(B) 47
(C) 51
(D) 53

18. Sarah and Abigail are first cousins. Sarah is four times as old as Abigail. How old is Abigail if the difference between their ages is 15 years?

(A) 3
(B) 5
(C) 11
(D) 19

19. A prop for the school play calls for a 5-foot cube to be painted green. A pint of paint will cover 100 square feet. How many pints of paint will be purchased if two coats of paint are needed?

(A) 2
(B) 3
(C) 4
(D) 5

20. Denver, Colorado, is often referred to as the Mile-High City. How many yards above sea level is the city?

(A) 1,760
(B) 2,250
(C) 5,280
(D) 6,000

21. A right triangle measures 6.5 inches on one side and 8.75 inches on another side. What is the length in inches of the hypotenuse?

(A) 9.4 in.
(B) 10.9 in.
(C) 11 in.
(D) 12.3 in.

22. Simplify the following expression.

$$\frac{6 - \dfrac{7}{8}}{4 + \dfrac{2}{3}}$$

(A) 1.1
(B) 1.5
(C) 2.0
(D) 3.2

23. Solve for x in the following equation.

$$3(14x - 14) + (3x + 4) - 13 = 39$$

(A) 1.38
(B) 1.42
(C) 2.00
(D) 2.18

24. Simplify the following expression.

$$4\frac{4}{5} - 2\frac{7}{8} =$$

(A) $1\dfrac{3}{40}$

(B) $1\dfrac{37}{40}$

(C) $2\dfrac{1}{3}$

(D) $2\dfrac{1}{8}$

25. Solve the following equation.

$$\frac{4x}{5} + 10 = 20$$

(A) 1.5
(B) 3.5
(C) 7.5
(D) 12.5

26. A cylinder has a diameter of 8 inches and a height of 50 inches. What is its volume?

(A) 1,553 cu in.
(B) 1,553 gal
(C) 2,512 cu in.
(D) 2,512 gal

27. Mary is a poor typist, and her term project is due in a week. According to the word count, the paper is approximately 53 pages in length. She enlists the help of Winnie and Susan. Mary can type one page in one hour, Winnie can type seven pages in three hours, and Susan can type five pages in 30 minutes. How many days will it take to type the term project if they can type a total of four hours each day? (Round your answer to the nearest whole number.)

(A) 4 days
(B) 5 days
(C) 6 days
(D) 7 days

28. Simplify the following equation.

$$5x + 15 = 50 - x$$

(A) $5.83\overline{3}$
(B) 12.501
(C) 14.823
(D) 15.243

29. Evaluate the following expression if $c = 7$ and $d = 10$.

$$\frac{c}{4d} + \frac{c+d^2}{c} =$$

(A) 0.857
(B) 2.43
(C) 10.5
(D) 15.46

30. Harley and Bob are investing in a business venture. They need a total of $5,495. Harley is contributing 62 percent of the needed money. What amount will Bob be contributing?

(A) $1,892.34
(B) $2,088.10
(C) $2,199.00
(D) $2,348.33

31. A store manager wants to know his store's sales average for the past six days. The sales are as follows:

$785 $1,150 $980 $772 $1,300 $842

What is the average sales for the past six days?

(A) $799.38
(B) $884.25
(C) $971.50
(D) $1,341.44

32. Stanley's next baseball game is in the suburb of a city he has never been to. He consults a map and determines that the distance is 3.5 inches from his house to his destination. How many miles is he from his destination if the map scale is 0.5 inches is equal to 0.5 mile?

(A) 1 mile
(B) 2.5 miles
(C) 3.0 miles
(D) 3.5 miles

33. The cost of a medication has risen 85 percent in the last year. What is the present cost of the medication if the original price was $325?

(A) $587.33
(B) $601.25
(C) $650.00
(D) $750.42

34. Cliff's mother has given him $2 to spend at the school bazaar. He purchases six cookies for $0.50 a piece, two peanut bars at $0.20 apiece, and a carton of milk for $0.60. He also wants to buy a glitter pencil for $0.55. Does Cliff have enough money to buy the glitter pencil?

(A) Cliff does not have enough money to buy the glitter pencil.
(B) Cliff has enough money to buy the glitter pencil and another peanut bar.
(C) Cliff has exactly enough money to buy the glitter pencil.
(D) Cliff has more than enough money to buy the glitter pencil.

35. A going-out-of-business sale claims tremendous markdowns on all items. One ad advertises a 54 percent markdown of a top-of-the-line television at checkout. What is the cost of the item at checkout if the original price was $2,250.99?

(A) $1,035.46
(B) $1,125.50
(C) $1,215.53
(D) $1,301.77

36. Find the area of $\triangle ABC$.

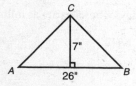

(A) 20.59 sq. in.
(B) 91.00 sq. in.
(C) 157.34 sq. in.
(D) 182 sq. in.

SCIENCE

NUMBER OF QUESTIONS: 53

TIME LIMIT: 63 MINUTES

> **Instructions:** Read each question thoroughly. Select the single best answer. Mark your answer (A, B, C, or D) on the answer sheet provided for Practice Test 5.

1. Based on the Periodic Table of Elements (page 53), what is the atomic number of potassium (K) if it has 19 protons?

    (A) 12
    (B) 17
    (C) 19
    (D) 20

2. Enzymes

    (A) are organic catalysts.
    (B) are expended in chemical processes.
    (C) inhibit chemical processes.
    (D) release hydroxyl ions in cellular solutions.

3. The _____ hormone(s) produced by the _____ function to _____.

    (A) androgens and estrogens, adrenal cortex, promote absorption to the kidneys
    (B) epinephrine and norepinephrine, adrenal medulla, stimulate the fight-or-flight response
    (C) insulin, posterior pituitary, promote glycogenesis
    (D) thyroid stimulating, pancreas, raise blood sugar

4. All of the following are clues that a chemical reaction has occurred EXCEPT

    (A) a new element is formed.
    (B) gas is created.
    (C) heat is taken in or given off.
    (D) something new has been produced and can be seen.

5. An individual has problems with visual perception after falling and hitting the back of his head. What lobe of the brain controls visual perception?

    (A) Brainstem
    (B) Frontal lobe
    (C) Occipital lobe
    (D) Parietal lobe

6. The thoracic cavity is found in the

    (A) dorsal cavity.
    (B) frontal plane.
    (C) transverse plane.
    (D) ventral cavity.

7. _____ are nonprotein molecules that aid enzymes.

   (A) Atoms
   (B) Cilia
   (C) Cofactors
   (D) Filaments

8. Duplication of DNA occurs during which of the following stages of the cell cycle?

   (A) Cytokinesis
   (B) Interphase
   (C) Mitosis
   (D) Prophase

9. The molecular formula or mass of NaCl is

   (A) 31.4309 g/mol.
   (B) 35.4609 g/mol.
   (C) 58.4428 g/mol.
   (D) 64.0128 g/mol.

10. All of the following are categories of tissue EXCEPT

    (A) cardiac.
    (B) connective.
    (C) epithelial.
    (D) nervous.

11. The periosteum

    (A) arises from fibrous membranes and hyaline cartilage during embryonic development.
    (B) covers the outer layer of compact bone tissue.
    (C) encases the diploë during bone growth.
    (D) is sandwiched between layers of spongy bone tissue.

12. All of the following are movable, flexible regions of the vertebral column EXCEPT

    (A) cervical.
    (B) coccyx.
    (C) lumbar.
    (D) thoracic.

13. Which of the following is an example of a synarthrotic joint?

    (A) It is between the axis and atlas vertebrae.
    (B) It is between the humerus and ulna.
    (C) It is between the metacarpals and phalanges.
    (D) It is between the sockets and teeth.

14. Which of the following becomes engorged with blood during an erection?

   (A) Corpus cavernosa
   (B) Ejaculatory ducts
   (C) Testes
   (D) Vas deferens

15. Which of the following contributes to muscle fatigue?

   (A) Decreased accumulation of lactic acid
   (B) Inadequate amounts of ATP
   (C) Increased muscle contraction
   (D) Lack of muscle activity

16. All of the following are dimensions of volume EXCEPT

   (A) height.
   (B) length.
   (C) mass.
   (D) width.

17. _____ are responsible for removing foreign material from the lungs.

   (A) Alveolar tissues
   (B) Capillaries
   (C) Cilia
   (D) Microphages

Questions 18–19 are based on the following image.

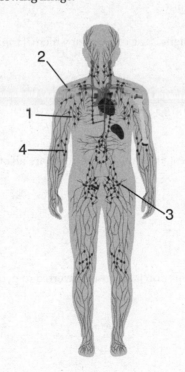

18. Number 3 represents which of the following lymph nodes?

    (A) Inguinal
    (B) Peritoneal
    (C) Submaxillary
    (D) Supratrochlear

19. Number 2 represents which of the following lymph nodes?

    (A) Cervical
    (B) Deltopectoral
    (C) Submental
    (D) Superficial cubital

20. The _____ protects the openings of the urethra and vagina.

    (A) hymen
    (B) labia majora
    (C) labia minora
    (D) perineum

21. Which of the following determines an individual's basic skin color by controlling the amount of melanin synthesized and deposited in the epidermis?

    (A) Exposure to the sun
    (B) Genes
    (C) Melanocytes
    (D) Volume of blood in the capillaries

22. In environmental chemistry, sunlight is the catalyst for which of the following?

    (A) Acid rain
    (B) Industrial pollution
    (C) Ocean acidification
    (D) Smog

23. The elements present in the greatest amounts in living cells are all of the following EXCEPT

    (A) calcium.
    (B) hydrogen.
    (C) nitrogen.
    (D) oxygen.

24. During which type of cellular respiration is glucose converted to pyruvic acid?

    (A) Aerobic
    (B) Anaerobic
    (C) Glucogenesis
    (D) Krebs citric acid cycle

25. A neuron is said to be (at) _____ when it is not carrying an impulse.

(A) action potential

(B) contracting

(C) depolarized

(D) resting potential

26. The Islets of Langerhans in the pancreas

(A) controls the release of sugar in the pancreas.

(B) inhibits reabsorption of sodium.

(C) regulates glycogen storage in the liver.

(D) stimulates reabsorption of sodium.

27. Adenosine triphosphate (ATP) molecules function to

(A) conserve lipids.

(B) inhibit carbohydrates.

(C) join with other enzymes to catalyze chemical reactions.

(D) store energy.

28. Humans belong to the order named

(A) Homo sapiens.

(B) Mammalia.

(C) Primates.

(D) Vertebrata.

29. The foremost purpose of the vertebral column is to

(A) prevent flexion of the back.

(B) protect the spinal cord.

(C) provide stability for sensory and motor neurons.

(D) provide the ventral aspect of the thorax.

30. During the clotting process, fibrinogen is converted to

(A) degradation products.

(B) factor XIII.

(C) fibrin.

(D) thrombin.

31. The process of breaking down waste products and excessive proteins to produce urea is called

(A) convolution.

(B) deamination.

(C) differentiation.

(D) parturition.

32. _____ are the only sources of fiber for the human body.

(A) Fat soluble vitamins

(B) Plant sources

(C) Red meats

(D) Water soluble vitamins

33. In the research process, data collection has four main steps. All of the following are steps of data collection EXCEPT

    (A) analysis.
    (B) measurement.
    (C) observation.
    (D) samples.

34. A patient presents with tetany (acute recurrent tonic contractions and muscle pain). The health-care provider suspects the patient is deficient in

    (A) calcium.
    (B) iron.
    (C) manganese.
    (D) sodium.

35. Digestion of fats is assisted by

    (A) bile.
    (B) chyme.
    (C) pancreatic enzymes.
    (D) proteolytic enzymes.

36. Select the testable hypothesis.

    (A) A nurse's perception of health-care institution bureaucracy will vary with his or her level of educational preparation.
    (B) Pre-election polls are strong indicators of election success.
    (C) The majority of elementary school children bring their lunch to school.
    (D) Winter snow at higher elevations is a predictor of snow at lower elevations.

37. Where is an occipital injury found?

    (A) Between the hemispheres in the frontal lobe
    (B) In front of the cranium
    (C) On top of the head
    (D) The back of the head

38. What is absolute zero?

    (A) An arbitrary number dependent upon the temperature scale in use
    (B) The constant temperature needed to keep ice frozen
    (C) The highest level at which gas will evaporate
    (D) The lowest temperature a gas can achieve

39. Which of the following contains some of the strongest muscles in the body?

    (A) Cervix
    (B) Uterus
    (C) Vagina
    (D) Vulva

40. Oxygen enters the cell by which of the following processes?

   (A) Active transport
   (B) Diffusion
   (C) Osmosis
   (D) Vesicular transport

41. Transmission across a synapse cannot occur without the release of which of the following?

   (A) Myelinated Schwann cells
   (B) Neuronal impulses
   (C) Neurotransmitters
   (D) Stable membrane potentials

42. An individual with known heart disease is prescribed an aspirin a day to prevent

   (A) blood thinning.
   (B) cardiac pain.
   (C) plaque proliferation.
   (D) platelet agglutination.

43. How many neutrons does an atom of krypton (Kr) have?

   (A) 48
   (B) 35
   (C) 84
   (D) 120

44. Which of the following contains an ionic bond?

   (A) $CaCl_2$
   (B) CO_2
   (C) H_2
   (D) H_2O

45. The larynx is _____ to the esophagus.

   (A) inferior
   (B) intermediate
   (C) proximal
   (D) superior

46. A diuretic is a medication that increases the volume of urine by pulling water and sodium from the body. Select the component that fulfills this function.

   (A) Cortex
   (B) Hilum
   (C) Nephron
   (D) Ureters

47. Which of the following is the pumping chamber for systemic circulation?

    (A) Left atrium
    (B) Left ventricle
    (C) Right atrium
    (D) Right ventricle

48. The _____ is an opening across the interatrial septum that closes at birth.

    (A) ductus arteriosus
    (B) foramen ovale
    (C) mitral stenosis
    (D) truncus arteriosis

49. Ventricular filling begins when which of the following valves open and allow blood to fill the ventricles?

    (A) Aortic bicuspid valves
    (B) Atrioventricular valves
    (C) Fossa ovalis valves
    (D) Semilunar valves

50. What occurs after data collection in the research process?

    (A) Analysis
    (B) Hypothesis development
    (C) Problem identification
    (D) Question asking

51. _____ is the process of gas exchange between the atmosphere and the tissues of the body.

    (A) External respiration
    (B) Inspiration and expiration
    (C) Internal respiration
    (D) Pulmonary-cardiac ventilation

52. Which of the following systems is responsible for gas transport?

    (A) Cardiovascular
    (B) Nervous system
    (C) Pulmonary system
    (D) Renal system

53. A nerve tract is a bundle of _____ in the central nervous system.

    (A) bipolar nerve fibers
    (B) dealienated nerve fibers
    (C) multipolar nerve fibers
    (D) myelinated nerve fibers

ENGLISH AND LANGUAGE USAGE

NUMBER OF QUESTIONS: 28

TIME LIMIT: 28 MINUTES

> **Instructions:** Read each question thoroughly. Select the single best answer. Mark your answer (A, B, C, or D) on the answer sheet provided for Practice Test 5.

1. Select the compound sentence with a coordinating conjunction.

   (A) After they stopped and ate hamburgers and fries for supper, Tom remembered they were supposed to eat with his parents.
   (B) He did not study for the exam because he preferred being with his friends.
   (C) Johnathan cannot dribble a basketball, and he cannot score a basket.
   (D) Mary arrived early for the first day of class.

2. Select the correctly spelled word.

   (A) Accomodate
   (B) Paraphernalia
   (C) Questionaire
   (D) Withold

3. Which of the following contains punctuation errors?

   (A) "Did you see that?" said Abe. "I hope he does it again."
   (B) Families spent evenings listening to the radio prior to the advent of television.
   (C) He was angry and screamed at his mother until he started to cry.
   (D) "When will you leave for the train," asked Monica. "Probably not for another hour," said Mary.

4. Which of the following indicates an unexpected alteration in thought, explanation, or definition and breaks the continuity of a sentence?

   (A) Apostrophe (')
   (B) Colon (:)
   (C) Dash (—)
   (D) Quotation marks (". . .")

5. Select the sentence containing an indirect object.

   (A) Martin Jones, whose son won the scholastic award, will be the speaker.
   (B) The religious sect did not believe women should work outside of the home.
   (C) The parents bought their children new cars when they turned 18.
   (D) Do you understand what I am saying?

6. Which of the following is representative of nominative pronouns demonstrating first-, second-, and third-person plural?

   (A) I, you, he/she/it
   (B) Our/ours, your/yours, their/theirs
   (C) Us, you, them
   (D) We, you, they

7. Which of the following is a simple sentence?

   (A) Andrew mowed the lawn and pulled weeds in the garden.
   (B) The group could not decide where to go for dinner, and finally split into three groups and ate at different places.
   (C) The tornado alarm sounded and the students stood and quietly got under their desks.
   (D) When the moon is full.

8. Select the direct object in the following sentence.

   Frank Hamilton, a music instructor at the local junior college, offers a free class in beginning guitar.

   (A) Class
   (B) Guitar
   (C) Instructor
   (D) Offers

9. Select the sentence that uses the italicized word correctly.

   (A) His constant banging on that drum *aggravates* me.
   (B) Most agreed that Watcher's Bend was the most beautiful *site* in the county.
   (C) The air conditioner runs almost *continuously* during the month of August.
   (D) The *alter* in the small church contained culturally relevant objects.

10. Which of the following suffixes means "kill"?

    (A) –cide
    (B) –ee
    (C) –pnea
    (D) –sophy

11. Select the sentence using coordinating conjunctions.

    (A) Ryan and his friends had planned on hiking the river on Saturday, but Sam and Mary decided to go fishing instead.
    (B) Rather than stand in line for hours in the hot sun, Peter decided to purchase his admission packet online.
    (C) John ran from the sound of the explosion, whereas, I ran toward it.
    (D) Dwight returned the birthday gift to the store.

12. What do the italicized words in the following sentence indicate?

The pottery course required *pre- and post-tests* on pottery painting and firing.

(A) Pre- and post-testing will always demonstrate a difference in abilities.
(B) Pre- and post-testing will add to the basic cost of the course.
(C) Testing on pottery painting and firing is required before the beginning of the course and at the end of the course.
(D) Testing on pottery painting and firing is required midway through the course and at the end of the course.

13. Which of the following sentences follows the rules of capitalization?

(A) "Marsha," said her father, "Pay attention when I'm talking to you."
(B) By the time Henry reached the registration table, algebra 1542 was closed.
(C) Many believe the victorian era permanently stained American culture.
(D) The new President told the crowd he looked forward to flying on Air Force One.

14. What do the italicized words in the following sentence suggest?

The climb had been more difficult than most of the climbers expected, and the guide told them they needed to *cowboy up* in order to reach the climber's cabin before nightfall.

(A) Be ecologically responsible
(B) Face a formidable task
(C) Help others
(D) Think clearly

15. Which of the following parts of speech is necessary to have a complete sentence?

(A) Adverb
(B) Gerund
(C) Preposition
(D) Verb

16. Select the most meaningful passage incorporating the following four sentences.

■ Flying in a bush plane would be the last part of their journey to reach their destination.
■ The couple had saved their money for two years to take a trip to Alaska.
■ They would fly from Dallas to Olympia and then to Anchorage.
■ They'd been told they were going at the best time of year to see wildlife.

(A) The couple had saved their money for two years to take a trip to Alaska. They'd been told they were going at the best time of year to see wildlife. They would fly from Dallas to Olympia and then to Anchorage. Flying in a bush plane would be the last part of their journey to reach their destination.
(B) They would fly from Dallas to Olympia and then to Anchorage. They'd been told they were going at the best time of year to see wildlife. Flying in a bush plane would be the last part of their journey to reach their destination. The couple had saved their money for two years to take a trip to Alaska.
(C) Flying in a bush plane would be the last part of their journey to reach their destination. They would fly from Dallas to Olympia and then to Anchorage. They'd been told they were going at the best time of year to see wildlife. The couple had saved their money for two years to take a trip to Alaska.
(D) They'd been told they were going at the best time of year to see wildlife. Flying in a bush plane would be the last part of their journey to reach their destination. The couple had saved their money for two years to take a trip to Alaska. They would fly from Dallas to Olympia and then to Anchorage.

17. Select the compound sentence.

    (A) The team had struggled all season to win just one game; however, in their last game against the number one team in the conference, they finally won.
    (B) The children and their parents celebrated by eating at their favorite restaurant and seeing a movie.
    (C) The chess club met every Saturday afternoon at one o'clock.
    (D) If I were young again, I would live my life differently and try to be a better parent to my children.

18. Gabe wants to research Civil War battles that took place in what is now Texas. Which of the following would be his best source of information?

    (A) A historical dictionary
    (B) A thesaurus
    (C) An encyclopedia of the Civil War in America
    (D) A biography of commanders of brigades from Texas during the Civil War

19. Select the sentence that contains an error in word usage.

    (A) When the elementary school principal stated that contact sports were inappropriate for elementary school children, he inferred that the school's football program should be eliminated.
    (B) After years of running competitively, John felt he could speak for numerous long-distance runners who would support an additional race each season.
    (C) The family wished to remain anonymous donors and did not want their financial contribution to be publically acknowledged.
    (D) That old junker of a car that Mike loves is in need of repair.

20. Which of the following is often served as the final course of a meal?

    (A) Daserrt
    (B) Dassert
    (C) Desert
    (D) Dessert

21. Select the sentence lacking style and clarity.

    (A) Apples, pears, peaches, and bananas were on sale at the market every Saturday afternoon.
    (B) Beth longed for a new computer, but she could only afford a refurbished one.
    (C) Since the football team lost in the Super Bowl, we went ahead and bought season tickets for next year.
    (D) John and I listened respectfully as the elderly gentleman gave the history behind the World War I monument.

22. Select the second-person singular possessive pronouns.

    (A) Her, hers, his, its
    (B) Mine, my
    (C) Our, ours
    (D) Your, yours

23. Deduce the meaning of the italicized word based upon clues given in the sentence.

> Most agreed the man was *obtuse* because he always had to have directions repeated three or four times.

(A) Astute
(B) Not paying attention
(C) Sensitive
(D) Slow to understand

24. Which of the following demonstrates correct capitalization?

(A) "I've always had fond memories of my High School days."
(B) Do you know if our Uncle Henry gathered enough wood for the smoker?
(C) My favorite winter activity is ice skating.
(D) The Gods have favored us once again.

25. Which of the following is a synonym for *demagogue*?

(A) Conformist
(B) Conventionalist
(C) Rabble-rouser
(D) Supporter

26. What are the descriptive words in the following sentence?

> The last game of the season was canceled because of freezing rain.

(A) Game, rain
(B) Last, freezing
(C) Of the season, of freezing rain
(D) Season, because

27. Select the phrase that correctly completes the following sentence.

> Marge Swanson is not only an excellent teacher but _____.

(A) also is a strong student advocate
(B) is also a strong student advocate
(C) she is a strong student advocate also
(D) she is a strong student advocate

28. Which of the following sentences misuses or adds unnecessary words or phrases?

(A) "Is it really true that George Washington chopped down a cherry tree?" asked the student.
(B) The assignment requested students to write five sentences using different meanings of the word "pass."
(C) The couple loved to walk in the forest when it snowed.
(D) The only reason I came here tonight was that I thought someone might listen to my opinion.

WANT MORE PRACTICE?

Visit *barronsbooks.com/tp/TEAS/* for access to an additional online practice test. Conveniently accessible on your computer, smartphone, or tablet.

ANSWER KEY
Practice Test 5

Reading

1.	B	15.	C	29.	D	43.	C
2.	C	16.	D	30.	C	44.	A
3.	A	17.	C	31.	C	45.	C
4.	D	18.	B	32.	D	46.	D
5.	C	19.	C	33.	A	47.	B
6.	D	20.	A	34.	C	48.	C
7.	B	21.	A	35.	C	49.	A
8.	A	22.	A	36.	C	50.	D
9.	C	23.	D	37.	B	51.	C
10.	A	24.	D	38.	D	52.	C
11.	B	25.	C	39.	A	53.	A
12.	A	26.	C	40.	A		
13.	C	27.	B	41.	D		
14.	D	28.	D	42.	C		

Mathematics

1.	B	10.	A	19.	B	28.	A
2.	B	11.	B	20.	A	29.	D
3.	B	12.	B	21.	B	30.	B
4.	C	13.	C	22.	A	31.	C
5.	C	14.	C	23.	C	32.	D
6.	B	15.	C	24.	B	33.	B
7.	A	16.	A	25.	D	34.	A
8.	C	17.	D	26.	C	35.	A
9.	C	18.	B	27.	A	36.	B

ANSWER KEY
Practice Test 5

Science

1.	C	15.	B	29.	B	43.	A
2.	A	16.	C	30.	C	44.	A
3.	B	17.	D	31.	B	45.	D
4.	A	18.	A	32.	B	46.	C
5.	C	19.	B	33.	A	47.	B
6.	D	20.	C	34.	A	48.	B
7.	C	21.	B	35.	A	49.	B
8.	B	22.	D	36.	A	50.	A
9.	C	23.	A	37.	D	51.	A
10.	A	24.	B	38.	D	52.	A
11.	B	25.	D	39.	B	53.	D
12.	B	26.	C	40.	B		
13.	D	27.	D	41.	C		
14.	A	28.	C	42.	D		

English and Language Usage

1.	C	8.	A	15.	D	22.	D
2.	B	9.	C	16.	A	23.	D
3.	D	10.	A	17.	A	24.	C
4.	C	11.	A	18.	C	25.	C
5.	C	12.	C	19.	A	26.	B
6.	D	13.	D	20.	D	27.	B
7.	A	14.	B	21.	C	28.	D

ANSWER EXPLANATIONS
Reading

1. **(B)** *The White Indian Boy* is the story of Nick Wilson's autobiographical account of his growing up in the late 1800s. Autobiographies are considered primary sources. The remaining options do not meet the criteria for autobiographical works.

2. **(C)** *The White Indian Boy* is written in a narrative style. It tells a story and is entertaining. It also includes facts, opinions, and biases. Expository writing explains and provides facts and figures without opinions. Persuasive writing is opinionated, bias filled, and may or may not be factual. Its purpose is to persuade or convince you of something. Argumentative writing styles investigate a specific topic, and require the reader to consider and evaluate evidence and, perhaps, form an opinion.

3. **(A)** *Day peep* or *peep of day* is the dawn or beginning of a new day. The passage provides clues for the word *peep* used in the phrase *peep of day*. Nick's journey with the Indians began at night, and they rode until the *peep of day*, suggesting they rode throughout the night and did not stop until daybreak. *Peep* does not have any relationship with the remaining options.

4. **(D)** Nick's first night with the Indians quickly becomes unpleasant. His journey with the Indians begins with trepidation when he finds two Indians waiting for him instead of one, but he decides to accompany them when he sees his pinto pony. The journey has no problems at first, but the Indians want to ride fast and Nick tires, his legs hurt, and he wants to stop. There is no stopping, and after riding long enough for Nick's legs to stiffen and for the rough thongs to rub his thighs raw, they stop. Nick is urged to jump into a salt spring to help his legs. After assistance with removing his trousers, he jumps into the spring and experiences excruciating pain. He ends up crying himself to sleep. The passage provides no evidence of Nick being fooled by the Indians, having an exciting adventure, or of being fearful of being discovered.

5. **(C)** The passage states Nick and the Indians rode along the western shore of the Great Salt Lake, which is in present day Utah. Nick and the Indians are west of the Great Plains and east of the Rocky Mountains.

6. **(D)** The rough rawhide stirrup straps rubbed Nick's inner thighs raw. Putting salt into a wound causes extreme pain. There is no evidence in the passage about Nick's riding ability, if he was in danger of falling off of his pony, or if he was riding on a saddle he was not used to. If stiff legs from prolonged riding were his only problem, jumping into the salt spring would not have been painful.

7. **(B)** Each of the listed states, except Georgia, borders or has a portion of its border on the Gulf of Mexico. Georgia's eastern border is on the Atlantic Ocean.

8. **(A)** The correct option is the definition of *speedos*. The remaining options do not satisfy the definition.

9. **(C)** The local newspaper, *The Parkside Tribune*, is the most appropriate publication for the passage—it's local information that has interest to those in the area. The *Mountain Pass State Park Monthly* would focus on happenings inside the park, not on happenings outside of the park. A youth organization quarterly, like the park publication, would have an inward focus, not outward. While a travel magazine might feature the park in an article, the majority of information in the passage would not be of interest to magazine readers.

10. **(A)** Revenue increased because of the increase in visitors to the park. Simply put, an increase in visitors increases revenue because visitors spend money for gasoline, food, lodging, and entertainment. The passage does not provide information about the park in relation to other mountain areas with camping facilities, the cost of living, or shortfall in previous years.

11. **(B)** The author's intent for writing the passage is to inform readers of happenings in the area. There is nothing challenging in the passage, it is not political in nature, and it does not suggest misuse of the environment brought about by an increased number of visitors to the area.

12. **(A)** All of the options are synonyms for *revenue*. However, *revenue* must be defined in terms of context. In the passage, revenue has to do with *cash flow*—the increase in money coming into the area from visitors to the area. *Duty* is a tax on foreign goods, *fluid assets* have to do with cash reserve, and *salary* is money paid for work performed.

13. **(C)** The correct option is the definition of *adulate*. The remaining options are incorrect definitions of the word.

14. **(D)** Chart data are from five students: RS, PF, GT, SK, and MM.

15. **(C)** RS had the second-lowest typing time in Week 8 with 28 words per minute. SK had the lowest time in Week 8 with 27 words per minute.

16. **(D)** The answer to the problem can be estimated. GT and MM can be eliminated because their highest scores are 20+ points lower than RS and SK. There is a three-point difference between RS and SK's lowest scores and a five-point difference between their highest scores suggesting SK has shown the greatest improvement in typing words per minute.

17. **(C)** The chart suggests that typing speed increases over time. The chart shows a definite trend of improvement over time. The five students are typing more words per minute from Week 2 to Week 14. Their rate of increase is not the same, but an increase is shown. The gender of the five students is not given. Variability is not an issue, and typing speed did not remain static; it was dynamic.

18. **(B)** The passage is a narrative that tells a story and is meant to entertain. The passage does not compare or contrast, does not identify a problem or solution, and is not an example of sequencing.

19. **(C)** The phrase *keeps-you-awake-at-night* indicates something that prevents you from sleeping at night. The condition can be caused by numerous things such as worry, illness, and an unfamiliar environment. Based on the passage, "The Lullaby Whistler" and wind were the problem. Words and phrases must always be evaluated in terms of context. Consider the word *pass*, for example. There is a difference based on context in the following three phrases: *the quarterback threw a Hail Mary pass to his best receiver*; *the mountain pass presented difficulties for the novice climbers*; and *the student wanted to pass the exam*. Without knowing the context, it is impossible to understand the meaning of *pass*.

20. **(A)** The use of the word *enjoyed* in the passage is important—Frank enjoys telling scary stories to children. Individuals invest time and energy into activities they enjoy because they get something out of it. Enjoyed activities are satisfying. Options (B) and (C) are false statements. While it's common to hear about camping and scary stories, they are not necessarily an expectation of camping. There is nothing to suggest that Frank uses his scary stories as teaching moments. The passage gives no information on the scoutmaster's activities when Frank is storytelling.

21. **(A)** A *compos mentis* individual has a sound mind, an intact memory, and the ability to understand. It is an antonym for *maniacal*, which suggests madness and uncontrolled reasoning, excitement, or frenzy. The remaining options are synonyms of *maniacal*.

22. **(A)** Being able to define *imagination* is a key to correctly answering the question. In the passage, imagination is the ability to form mental concepts or images of things that are not real or determined by the senses. While Frank saw the wind as an element that enhanced his story, it also affected him and played a part in his undoing. Frank's imagination turned noises into elements of the scary story he'd told the mountain scouts. Unknown to Frank was the

mountains scouts' involvement, which heightened his anxiety/fear, and ultimately brought about actions that made him the brunt of the mountain scouts' prank. The passage does not indicate the gender of the mountain scouts. Fear is not transmissible, and the passage gives no indication of Frank's level of familiarity with the environment.

23. **(D)** The focus of informal writing is to communicate information that is meaningful and easily understood. Informal writing may contain characteristics of everyday spoken conversation and incorporate slang words/phrases and contractions. Feelings may also be presented or evident in informal writing. The writing style is not exposition or a mix of formal and informal.

24. **(D)** The order of operations must be used to obtain the correct answer. Based on this, the first action is to perform the function inside of the parentheses (7 − 13). While computation is not required, it is shown below.

$$\frac{17+3\times7+4(7-13)}{40}=$$

$$\frac{17+3\times7+4(-6)}{40}=$$

$$\frac{17+21+(-24)}{40}=$$

$$\frac{17+21-24}{40}=$$

$$\frac{14}{40}=\frac{7}{20}=0.35$$

25. **(C)** Capitalization 2.789 is found between Capitalization 2.734 and Capitalization 2.980. The remaining options are found either before Capitalization 2.734 or after Capitalization 2.980.

26. **(C)** The word *etiologies* must be correctly defined to answer the question. *Etiology* means cause or causation. There are many causes for small-business failure. Option (A) is incorrect because the stem states numerous causes, and lack of management skills is only one cause. Option (B) is an illogical sentence. Option (D) is an incorrect statement—the word *constantly* is a synonym of *always*. The use of the word *always* is highly suggestive of an incorrect statement.

27. **(B)** A triangle is a geometric shape. Information on triangles would be found in Chapter 4. Chapter 9 would not include information on triangles. Options (C) and (D) would contain information on specific aspects of triangles such as the perimeter and area of a triangle, not basic information.

28. **(D)** Volume is the amount, mass, or quantity an object or substance occupies. Chapter 9 addresses volume. The remaining options do not deal with volume.

29. **(D)** Surface area is the sum of all the areas of all the spaces that cover the surface of a solid object. Information on the surface area of a cube would be found in Chapter 10. The remaining options do not address surface area.

30. **(C)** The purpose or intent of the passage is to inform. The passage provides informal, simple information about the nature of pain. The passage does not encourage visits to a health-care provider, encourage the use of home remedies, or attempt to persuade the reader.

31. **(C)** The first two sentences of the passage state that pain is unique to the individual, is subjective, and exists whenever and wherever the individual says it does. *Idiosyncratic*, meaning unique to the individual, is the only option that supports this. Pain is not always detrimental, is not always an expectation, and is not objective. Subjective information is what the patient or individual says; objective information is what a health-care provider or another individual sees or observes.

32. **(D)** Something *demonstrative* is characterized by or involves demonstration—it is observable. The mother is saying her son presents certain observable behavior when he is in pain. *Demonstrative* and *description* are not synonymous. Three-year-olds typically do not have the ability to explain pain. Option (C) is a false statement.

33. **(A)** Pain presenting in specific areas at distinct times indicates an abnormality in function. Option (A) is the only logical answer. The remaining options are speculation since the cause of the problem is not known.

34. **(C)** Pain scales focus on the intensity or amount of an individual's pain. The scale allows the individual, not the health-care provider, to determine the intensity. The stem questions the use of a pain scale, not the type of pain scale used. Options (B) and (D) are false statements. Verbal pain scales are less accurate than numerical ones because words may be defined or interpreted differently by each individual. More complicated pain scales are more difficult to use and interpret.

35. **(C)** The new word is *stomach*.
    1. Move the *t* to before the *q* (tquesion).
    2. Drop *on* and replace with *ch* (tquesich).
    3. Drop *ues* and replace with *om* (tqomsich).
    4. Reverse the order of *t* and *q* (qtomich).
    5. Drop *i* and replace with *a* (qtomach).
    6. Drop *q* and replace with *s* (stomach).

36. **(C)** The order of operations must be used to obtain the correct answer. Based on this, the first action is to perform the division of 20 by 5 since there are no exponents, brackets, or parentheses. While computation is not required, it is shown below.

$$25 + 20 \div 5 - 20 + 5 =$$
$$25 + \frac{20}{5} - 20 + 5 =$$
$$25 + 4 - 20 + 5 = 34 - 20 = 14$$

37. **(B)** Three Specials with beef are offered—Papa's Favorite, Pirate's Feast, and Cook's Favorite.

38. **(D)** Southern Delight is the most economical for ladies with $2.50 off of the regular price of $10.00. The remaining specials offer between $1.55 and $2.00 off of the regular price. The answer can be estimated.

39. **(A)** Cook's Favorite is the least economical. Of all the items for gents, it is the most expensive at regular or Wednesday Special pricing.

40. **(A)** *Blabbermouth* is a slang term for an individual who cannot keep his or her mouth shut or someone who can't keep confidences or secrets. Blabbermouths are typically not stupid, flirtatious, or know-it-alls.

41. **(D)** *Climes* is a synonym for *weather zones*. The remaining options are not synonyms for *clime*.

42. **(C)** Knowledge and correct application of word parts is necessary to correctly answer this question.
    - *My* or *myo* = muscle
    - *Cardi* = heart
    - *Infarction* (from the Latin, *infarcire*) = to plug or cram, usually in terms of an artery.

    A myocardial infarction is commonly called a *heart attack*. It consists of heart muscle damage and/or death from obstruction of arterial blood flow. Myocardial infarctions are medical emergencies and may be fatal even with medical treatment.

43. **(C)** The information in the memo is clearly delineated. It provides who, where, what, why, and when of the incident in a logical, precise, thorough fashion.

44. **(A)** The writing type in the memo is expository. Its purpose is to explain, inform, and/or describe. The memo is not a narrative, does not attempt to persuade, and is not technical in nature.

45. **(C)** *Irrefutable* can be defined as something that cannot be disproven. Evidence presented at Randall's disciplinary hearing could not be invalidated, contradicted, or challenged. *Overwhelming* is a synonym for *irrefutable*.

46. **(D)** Based on information presented in the memo, it is logical to conclude that Randall's behavior places him at high risk for serving time in prison for theft and sale of classified documents. His risk is heightened because the current incident is his second offense. Randall's response to the memo is not known, it is questionable he will find out-of-state employment in a similar position, and the memo is not a threat.

47. **(B)** Explicit information is exact and to the point. The information is not speculative, assumptive, or guesswork, and the memo is not a threat.

48. **(C)** Marge has the lowest number of tips before 5:00 P.M. with six tips. The remaining servers have from seven to twelve tips for the same time frame.

49. **(A)** Jerri had the highest number of tips after 1700 (after 5:00 P.M.) with 23 tips. The remaining servers had tips ranging from 10 to 20.

50. **(D)** Jerri's tips for Monday through Friday and Saturday and Sunday are approximately 70 (lower 32 to 30, and 40=40)—her actual number is 72.

51. **(C)** Estimation can be used to answer the question since an actual number is not asked for. An estimation of Saturday and Sunday was 150 tips (actual number 143) with Monday through Friday 130 tips (actual 125). The stem does not ask if the number of tips for Monday through Friday and Saturday and Sunday is approximate.

52. **(C)** The Scandinavian region is in northern Europe and is comprised of Denmark, Finland, Iceland, Norway, and Sweden.

53. **(A)** The Iberian Peninsula is found in southwestern Europe. The countries of Spain, Portugal, and portions of Gibraltar comprise the Iberian Peninsula.

Mathematics

1. **(B)**

$$15x + 7x - 28 - (-2) = 0 \qquad 15x + 7x - 28 - (-2) = 0$$
$$15x + 7x - 28 + 2 = 0 \qquad 22(1.1818) - 28 + 2 = 0$$
$$22x - 26 = 0 \qquad 25.996 - 26 = 0$$
$$22x = 26 \qquad 26 - 26 = 0$$
$$x = 1.1818 \qquad 0 = 0$$

2. **(B)** Ratio and proportion can be used to solve the problem.

$$1 \text{ tsp} = 5 \text{ ml} \qquad 5 \text{ ml} \times 4 \text{ doses} = 20 \text{ ml}$$
$$1 \text{ tsp} = 5 \text{ ml} :: x \text{ tsp} = 20 \text{ ml}$$
$$5x = 20 \text{ ml}$$
$$x = 4 \text{ tsp}$$

3. **(B)** Ratio and proportion can be used to solve the problem.

$$1 \text{ year} = 365 \text{ days}$$

$$365 \text{ days} = 1 \text{ year} :: 22{,}567 \text{ days} = x \text{ years}$$

$$365x = 22{,}567$$

$$x = 61.827 = 61.8 \text{ years}$$

4. **(C)** The decimals must be aligned when adding the numbers.

$$
\begin{array}{r}
616.7800 \\
8.3411 \\
55.2140 \\
+\ 22.5088 \\
\hline
702.8439 = 703
\end{array}
$$

5. **(C)** The answer to this problem can be determined by a number of methods.

$$\$75 \times 40\% = \$30 \text{ (best friend)} \qquad \$75 - \frac{\$30}{3} = \$15 \text{ (each sister)}$$

or

$$40\%(x) + 3[20\%(x)] = \$75$$

$$40x + 60x = 75$$

$$100x = 75$$

$$x = 0.75$$

$$40\% \times 0.75 = \$30 \text{ (best friend)} \qquad 20\% \times 0.75 = \$15 \text{ (each sister)}$$

6. **(B)** Drawing a diagram will make this easier to visualize. One long side of the chicken coop will be attached to the barn leaving the one long side and two short sides to be fenced.

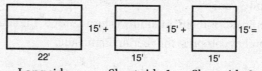

Long side   Short side 1   Short side 2

One roll of chicken wire is 40 feet long by 5 feet wide. This means that each side of the coop needs a total of three strips of chicken wire to equal 15 feet in height.

$$\text{Long side} = 22' \times 3 \text{ strips} = 66' \qquad \text{Short side} = 2(15' \times 3 \text{ strips}) = 90'$$

$$66' + 90' = 156' \div 40' = 3.9 = 4 \text{ rolls of chicken wire}$$

7. **(A)**

$$17x - 22 + 7x - 7 = 61$$
$$24x - 29 = 61$$
$$24x = 90$$
$$x = 3.75$$

$$17x - 22 + 7x - 7 = 61$$
$$17(3.75) - 22 + 7(3.75) - 7 = 61$$
$$63.75 - 22 + 26.25 - 7 = 61$$
$$90 - 29 = 61$$
$$61 = 61$$

8. **(C)** The problem can be solved using fractions or decimals.

$$\frac{7}{8} \div 50\% = 0.875 \div 0.5 = 1.75$$

or

$$\frac{7}{8} \div 50\% = \frac{7}{8} \div \frac{1}{2} = \frac{7}{8} \times \frac{2}{1} = \frac{14}{8} = 1\frac{3}{4}$$

9. **(C)** Polly has 70% of her course grades, only the final exam at 30% is unknown. Her grades calculated by weight are below.

$$\text{Test 1} - 75 \times 20\% = 15.0$$
$$\text{Test 2} - 89 \times 20\% = 17.8$$
$$\text{History Project} - 85 \times 20\% = 17.0$$
$$\text{Presentation} - 80 \times 10\% = 8.0$$
$$\text{Test 1} + \text{Test 2} + \text{History Project} + \text{Presentation} = 70\%$$
$$15 + 17.8 + 17 + 8 = 70\%$$
$$57.8 = 70\%$$
$$\text{If } 57.8 = 70\% \text{ then } x = 100\%$$
$$57.8 = 70\% \therefore x = 100\%$$
$$70x = 5{,}780$$
$$x = 82.57 = 83\%$$

An estimate of Polly's course grade before the final exam is in the 80s. If Polly's grade seems illogical, consider a student who made 100 on each of the four graded components. His or her current grade before the final exam would be 100. This can be calculated using the steps used to calculate Polly's grade.

$$\text{Test 1} - 100 \times 20\% = 20$$
$$\text{Test 2} - 100 \times 20\% = 20$$
$$\text{History Project} - 100 \times 20\% = 20$$
$$\text{Presentation} - 100 \times 10\% = 10$$
$$\text{Test 1} + \text{Test 2} + \text{History Project} + \text{Presentation} = 70\%$$
$$20 + 20 + 20 + 10 = 70$$
$$70 = 70\%$$
$$\text{If } 70\% = 70 \text{ then } 100\% = x$$
$$70 = 70 \therefore 100 = x$$
$$70x = 7{,}000$$
$$x = 100\%$$

10. **(A)** Weight needs to be in kilograms. One kilogram = 2.2 pounds.

$$\frac{115 \text{ lb}}{2.2 \text{ lb}} - \frac{139}{2.2} = \text{kg}$$

$$70.45 \text{ kg} - 63.18 \text{ kg} = 7.27 \text{ kg}$$

11. **(B)**

$$a = 15 \qquad b = 5 \qquad c = 10$$

$$\frac{b+c}{a} + \frac{8}{a-c} = \frac{5+10}{15} + \frac{8}{15-10} = \frac{15}{15} + \frac{8}{5} = 1 + \frac{8}{5} = 1\frac{8}{5} = \frac{13}{5}$$

12. **(B)**

$$4a + b$$
$$\underline{\times \ 4a + 5b}$$
$$20ab + 5b^2$$
$$\underline{+ \ 16a^2 + 4ab}$$
$$16a^2 + 24ab + 5b^2$$

13. **(C)** The problem can be simplified using two techniques. You can simply divide 68 into 119, or you can reduce the fraction to its lowest term by dividing both the numerator and dominator by the largest number that will divide evenly into both.

$$\frac{119}{68} = 1.75$$

or

$$\frac{119}{68} = \frac{119 \div 17}{68 \div 17} = \frac{7}{4} = 1.75$$

14. **(C)** A number of techniques can be used to simplify the problem. The third technique adds an additional step.

$$\frac{6}{21} + \frac{13}{15} = \frac{6 \times 5}{21 \times 5} + \frac{13 \times 7}{15 \times 7} = \frac{30}{105} + \frac{91}{105} = \frac{121}{105} = 1.15$$

or

$$\frac{6}{21} + \frac{13}{15} = \frac{6 \times 15}{21 \times 15} + \frac{13 \times 21}{15 \times 21} = \frac{90}{315} + \frac{273}{315} = \frac{363}{315} = 1.15$$

or

$$\frac{6}{21} + \frac{13}{15} = \frac{6 \div 3}{21 \div 3} + \frac{13}{15} = \frac{2}{7} + \frac{13}{15} = \frac{2 \times 15}{7 \times 15} + \frac{13 \times 7}{15 \times 7} = \frac{30+91}{105} = \frac{121}{105} = 1.15$$

15. **(C)**

$$\frac{40}{7} = 5\frac{5}{7} = 5.71$$

$$5 \neq 5.71$$

16. **(A)** A triangle has three angles totaling 180°. Two of the three angles total 125° leaving a third angle of 55°.

17. **(D)** The stem indicates that there are four consecutive odd numbers and their total is 200. Let x equal the original and increase each additional x by 2.

$$x + (x + 2) + (x + 4) + (x + 6) = 200 \qquad\qquad x + (x + 2) + (x + 4) + (x + 6) = 200$$
$$4x + 12 = 200 \qquad\qquad\qquad 47 + 49 + 51 + 53 = 200$$
$$4x = 188 \qquad\qquad\qquad\qquad 200 = 200$$
$$x = 47$$
$$x + 6 = 47 + 6 = 53$$

18. **(B)** Change the sentence into an equation. Let x equal Abigail's age, so Sarah's age would be equal to $4x$. Their age difference is 15 years. The words *age difference* indicates that subtracting their ages is equal to 15.

$$4x - x = 15$$
$$3x = 15$$
$$x = 5$$
$$\text{Abigail} = x = 5 \text{ years}$$

19. **(B)** A cube is a geometric shape having six equal faces or sides. The square footage of the surface area of a cube is the sum of the area of all of its sides.

$$\text{Area} = \text{length} \times \text{width} = 5 \text{ ft} \times 5 \text{ ft} = 25 \text{ sq ft}$$
$$6 \text{ sides} \times 25 \text{ sq ft} = 150 \text{ sq ft}$$
$$150 \text{ sq ft} \times 2 \text{ coats} = 300 \text{ sq ft} = 3 \text{ pints of paint}$$

20. **(A)**

$$1 \text{ mile} = 5{,}280 \text{ feet} = 1{,}760 \text{ yards}$$

21. **(B)** A right triangle has one angle of 90°. The hypotenuse is the side opposite the right angle. The Pythagorean theorem is used to determine the length of the hypotenuse. Draw and label a right triangle if visualization is needed.

$$a - 6.5'' \qquad b - 8.75'' \qquad c = \text{unknown}$$
$$a^2 + b^2 = c^2$$
$$6.5^2 + 8.75^2 = c^2$$
$$42.25 + 76.56 = c^2$$
$$118.81 = c^2$$
$$\sqrt{118.81} = c$$
$$10.9'' = c$$

22. **(A)**

$$\frac{6 - \dfrac{7}{8}}{4 + \dfrac{2}{3}} = \frac{5\dfrac{1}{8}}{4\dfrac{2}{3}} = \frac{\dfrac{41}{8}}{\dfrac{14}{3}} = \frac{41}{8} \div \frac{14}{3} = \frac{41 \times 3}{8 \times 14} = \frac{123}{112} = 1.098 = 1.1$$

23. **(C)**

$$3(14x - 14) + (3x + 4) - 13 = 39$$
$$42x - 42 + 3x - 9 = 39$$
$$45x - 51 = 39$$
$$45x = 90$$
$$x = 2$$

$$3(14x - 14) + (3x + 4) - 13 = 39$$
$$3(14 \cdot 2 - 14) + (3 \cdot 2 + 4) - 13 = 39$$
$$3[(14 \cdot 2) - 14] + [(3 \cdot 2) + 4] - 13 = 39$$
$$3(28 - 14) + (6 + 4) - 13 = 39$$
$$3(14) + 10 - 13 = 39$$
$$42 + 10 - 13 = 39$$
$$39 = 39$$

24. **(B)**

$$4\frac{4}{5} - 2\frac{7}{8} = 4\frac{4 \times 8}{40} - 2\frac{7 \times 5}{40} = 4\frac{32}{40} - 2\frac{35}{40} = 3\frac{72}{40} - 2\frac{35}{40} = 1\frac{37}{40}$$

or

$$4\frac{4}{5} - 2\frac{7}{8} = \frac{24}{5} - \frac{23}{8} = \frac{24 \times 6}{5 \times 8} - \frac{23 \times 5}{8 \times 5} = \frac{192}{40} - \frac{115}{40} = 1\frac{37}{40}$$

25. **(D)**

$$\frac{4x}{5} + 10 = 20$$
$$\left(\frac{5}{4}\right)\left(\frac{4}{5}\right)x = 10\left(\frac{5}{4}\right)$$
$$x = \frac{50}{4}$$
$$x = 12.5$$

$$\frac{4x}{5} + 10 = 20$$
$$\left(\frac{4}{5}\right)(12.5) + 10 = 20$$
$$\frac{50}{5} + 10 = 20$$
$$10 + 10 = 20$$
$$20 = 20$$

26. **(C)** The formula for the volume of a cylinder is $V = (\pi r^2)h$. The volume of a cylinder is measured in cubic inches (cu. in.).

$$\pi = 3.14 \qquad r = 4 \text{ in} \left(\frac{1}{2} \text{ of diameter of 8 in.}\right) \qquad h = 50 \text{ in.}$$
$$V = (\pi r^2)h$$
$$V = (3.14 \times 4^2)50$$
$$V = (3.14 \times 16)50$$
$$V = (50.25)50$$
$$V = 2,512 \text{ cu. in.}$$

27. **(A)**

$$\text{Mary} = 1 \text{ pg/hr} \qquad \text{Winnie} = 7 \text{ pg/3 hr} \qquad \text{Susan} = 10 \text{ pg/1 hr}$$
$$18 \text{ pg} - 5 \text{ hr} :: 53 \text{ pg} - x \text{ hr}$$
$$18x = 265$$
$$x = 14.7 \text{ hr} \div 4 \text{ hrs/day} = 3.68 = 4 \text{ days}$$

28. (A)

$$5x + 15 = 50 - x$$
$$6x + 15 = 50$$
$$6x = 35$$
$$x = 5.83\overline{3}$$

$$5x + 15 = 50 - x$$
$$5(5.83\overline{3}) + 15 = 50 - 5.833$$
$$29.167 + 15 = 44.167$$
$$44.167 = 44.167$$
$$44.2 = 44.2$$

29. (D)

$$c = 7 \qquad d = 10$$

$$\frac{c}{4d} + \frac{c+d^2}{c} = \frac{7}{4 \times 10} + \frac{7+10^2}{7} = \frac{7}{40} + \frac{107}{7} = \frac{49}{280} + \frac{4{,}280}{280} = \frac{4{,}329}{280} = 15.46$$

30. (B)

$$\text{Harley} = 62\% \qquad \text{Bob} = 38\% \qquad \text{Total needed } \$5{,}495$$

$$\$54{,}965 \cdot 62\% = 5{,}495 \cdot 0.62 = \mathbf{\$3{,}406.90}\ (\text{Harley})$$

$$\$5{,}495 \cdot 38\% = 5{,}495 \cdot 0.38 = \mathbf{\$2{,}088.10}\ (\text{Bob})$$

$$\$3{,}406.90 + \$2{,}088.10 = \$5{,}495$$

$$\$5{,}495 = \$5{,}495$$

31. (C) An average or mean is determined by totaling a number of items, and then dividing by the number of items.

$$\frac{\$785 + \$1{,}150 + \$980 + \$772 + \$1{,}300 + \$842}{6} = \frac{\$5{,}829}{6} = \$971.50$$

32. (D) A number of methods can be used to solve the problem. Ratio and proportion are used below.

$$\text{Scale: } 0.5 \text{ in.} = 0.5 \text{ mile} \qquad \text{Distance} = 3.5 \text{ in.}$$
$$\text{If } 0.5 \text{ in.} = 0.5 \text{ mile, then } 3.5 \text{ in.} = x \text{ miles}$$
$$0.5 = 0.5 :: 3.5 = x$$
$$0.5x = 1.75$$
$$x = 3.5 \text{ miles}$$

33. (B) A number of methods can be used to solve the problem. The formula for percent change is used below.

$$\text{Starting point} = \$325 \qquad \text{Increase} = 85\% \qquad x = \text{Present cost}$$

$$100\% + \text{Percent rise} = \text{Present cost/Starting point}$$

$$85\% = \frac{x}{\$325}$$

$$0.85 = \frac{x}{\$325}$$

$$x = \$601.25$$

34. (A) Cliff has spent $1.50 on cookies, peanut bars, and milk. The glitter pencil costs five cents more than what he has.

$$\text{Cookies} = (2 \times 0.25) = \$0.50 \quad \text{P-bars} = (2 \times 0.20) = \$0.40 \quad \text{Milk} = \$0.60 \quad \text{Pencil} = \$0.55$$
$$\$0.50 + \$0.40 + \$0.60 = \$1.50 \text{ spent} \qquad \$1.50 + 0.55 = \$2.05$$

35. **(A)** The stem of the question provides the advertised cost of the television ($2,250.99) and the amount of markdown (54%). The cost of the television at check-out needs to be determined.

$$\text{Starting point} = \$2,250.99 \qquad \text{Percentage markdown} = 54\%$$
$$\text{If } 100\% = \$2,250.99 \text{ then } 54\% = \$x$$
$$1.00 = 2,250.99 :: 0.54 = x$$
$$x = (2,250.99)(0.54)$$
$$x = \$1,215.53$$
$$\$2,250.99 - 1,215.53 = \$1,035.46$$

36. **(B)** The formula for determining the area of a triangle must be used.

$$base = 26 \text{ in.} \qquad height = 7 \text{ in.}$$
$$\text{Area } (A) = 0.5(b)(h)$$
$$A = 0.5(26)(7)$$
$$A = 0.5(182)$$
$$A = 91 \text{ sq in.}$$

Science

1. **(C)** The number of protons is equal to the atomic number. Potassium has an atomic number of 19 and a total of 19 protons.

2. **(A)** Catalysts are proteins capable of producing chemical reactions or changes in organic substances. Catalysts are not depleted in this process. Enzymes control the rate of chemical reaction but do not inhibit it. Bases release hydroxyl ions in solutions.

3. **(B)** One adrenal gland is located on the top of each kidney. Hormones from the adrenal gland assist with (1) blood sugar control, (2) protein and fat consumption, (3) stress response, and (4) blood pressure regulation. Androgens (substances that produce male characteristics) and estrogens (substances that produce female characteristics) are produced primarily in the gonads (testes in the male and ovaries in the female) and promote secondary sex characteristics. Insulin is produced in the pancreas and lowers blood sugar. The thyroid stimulating hormone, produced in the anterior pituitary, stimulates the thyroid.

4. **(A)** New elements are formed during nuclear reactions, not chemical reactions. The remaining options are indicators that a chemical reaction has occurred.

5. **(C)** The occipital lobe located on the back of the head is responsible for processing visual stimuli from the eyes. Individuals injuring the occipital lobe may have problems recognizing familiar objects. The remaining structures of the brain do not have this ability.

6. **(D)** Also called the anterior cavity, the ventral cavity contains the thoracic cavity that encases the heart and lungs. The posterior or dorsal cavity includes the cranial and vertebral cavities. The frontal or coronal plane divides the body into anterior and posterior sections. The transverse or horizontal plane divides the body into superior and inferior sections.

7. **(C)** A cofactor is a nonprotein component of enzymes. Cofactors help enzymes function. Organic cofactors are referred to as coenzymes. Examples are biotin and pyridoxal phosphate. Examples of inorganic cofactors are cobalt, copper, and magnesium. The remaining options do have this function.

8. **(B)** Interphase is the nondividing but metabolically active period of the cell cycle. Cytokinesis is the process of producing two daughter cells and follows the mitotic or meiotic division of the nucleus. Prophase is the first step of meiosis and mitosis.

9. **(C)** The terms *molecular weight* and *molecular mass* may be used interchangeably in chemistry although they are not the same thing. Mass is the amount of matter in an object and weight is the pull or acceleration of gravity of an object's mass. The molecular formula or mass is the number of atoms in a molecule or compound. The number of molecules are added together to obtain the molecular formula or mass. Molecular mass = atomic weight of element $\times$ the number of molecules present.

NaCl has one molecule of sodium and one molecule of chlorine and could be written as $Na_1Cl_1 = 22.98976928 + 35.453 = 58.4428$ g.

As an example, H_2SO_4 or $H_2S_1O_4$ has two atoms of hydrogen, one atom of sulfur, and four atoms of oxygen $= 2(1.008) + 32.065 + 4(15.9994) = 2.016 + 32.065 + 63.9976 = 98.0786 = 98$ g.

10. **(A)** The human body has four types of tissues: connective, epithelial, muscle, and nervous. Muscle tissue is composed of cardiac muscle, skeletal muscle, and smooth muscle.

11. **(B)** The periosteum is the dense, fibrous outer layer of compact bone that muscles attach to. Spongy bone tissue is called diploë. It is sandwiched between two layers of compact bone. The skeleton develops from fibrous membranes and hyaline cartilage during early development.

12. **(B)** The vertebral column is composed of 33 vertebrae. The seven cervical vertebrae, 12 thoracic vertebrae, and 5 lumbar vertebrae compose the 24 presacral vertebrae which are followed by the sacrum (5 fused sacral vertebrae) and 4 fused coccygeal vertebrae. The 24 presacral vertebrae allow flexion and movement of the vertebral column; the coccyx does not.

13. **(D)** Joints are classified according to their structure and function. Synarthrotic articulations or joints are immovable or fixed. They may be fibrous or cartilaginous in nature. Gomphosis occurs between the teeth and their sockets where the two are connected by periodontal ligaments. They are considered peg and socket joints. Their functional class is synarthrosis (immovable) and structural class is fibrous. The remaining options are examples of diarthrotic or movable joints.

14. **(A)** There are three cylindrical masses in the penis that serve as erectile bodies. These are the two corpora cavernosa and the corpus spongiosum. The remaining options do not become engorged with blood during an erection.

15. **(B)** It is important to differentiate between weakness and fatigue. Weakness is the lack of physical or muscle strength. Fatigue is a feeling of tiredness, exhaustion, or a need to rest because of decreased energy or strength. Muscle fatigue is a decrease in the capability of muscles to generate force. The majority of muscle fatigue is exercise induced. Muscle cells need a constant supply of energy for metabolic reactions. Adenosine triphosphate (ATP) is the source of the chemical energy needed for cells to perform their tasks. Inadequate amounts of ATP leads to muscle fatigue. Inadequate amounts of oxygen, glucose, and ATP, and buildup of lactic acid result in muscle fatigue. An increase in lactic acid levels and decrease in muscle contractions are seen in muscle fatigue. A lack of muscle activity will not cause muscle fatigue.

16. **(C)** Volume is the amount of space a substance occupies. It is measured in terms of height, length, and width. The volume of both regular and irregular substances can be measured. Mass is the amount of matter in a substance or object.

17. **(D)** Macrophages are one form of white blood cells that get rid of unwanted foreign bodies or particles. They are formed via monocyte differentiation. As part of the immune system, macrophages use phagocytosis to engulf and destroy these unwanted particles. Macrophages have the ability to differentiate between particles that belong and those that do not.

18. **(A)** Lymph nodes are bean-shaped bodies located along the lymphatic system. Lymph nodes have the functions of defense via filtration and phagocytosis and hemopoiesis. The inguinal nodes are found in the left and right groin. Lymph from the legs and external genitalia flow through these. The remaining are lymph nodes found in other areas of the body.

19. **(B)** The deltopectoral or infraclavicular lymph nodes filter lymphatic fluid from the upper arm and breast. The remaining options are lymph nodes in other parts of the body.

20. **(C)** The labia minora are cutaneous folds that form part of the external female genitalia. Their purpose to protect the clitoris, urinary meatus, and vagina. The remaining options are components of the female anatomy.

21. **(B)** Genes exercise primary control over melanocytes' production of melanin that determines the quantity of melanin deposited in the epidermis which governs skin color. Lengthy exposure to the sun increases melanocyte synthesis. The volume of blood in the *skin* capillaries modifies skin color—the option is vague and nonspecific because the location of the capillaries is not stated.

22. **(D)** Smog forms when pollution from motor vehicles and factory smokestacks becomes trapped and concentrated. The sun's energy is the catalyst that leads to smog formation. Acid rain is created when atmospheric water reacts with sulfur dioxide and nitrogen oxides creating a pH of less than 5.6. Industrial pollution is nonspecific. It does specify the type of pollution—water, air, soil, and so on. Ocean acidification is created when atmospheric carbon dioxide enters the ocean and overcomes the natural carbon cycling of ocean systems.

23. **(A)** The elements carbon, hydrogen, nitrogen, and oxygen are found in the greatest quantities in living cells. The elements calcium, chlorine, iodine, iron, magnesium, potassium, phosphorus, sodium, and sulfur are found in smaller quantities.

24. **(B)** Oxygen is not required for anaerobic respiration that takes place in the cytoplasm of cells. Glucose, activated by ATP, is converted to pyruvic acid during this process. Aerobic respiration, also called the Krebs citric acid cycle, takes place in the mitochondria of cells and requires oxygen. Pyruvic acid is key in both the anaerobic and aerobic processes. Glycogenesis is the synthesis of glycogen from glucose.

25. **(D)** Resting potential occurs when a polarized neuron is not carrying an impulse. The neuron has action potential when carrying an impulse. The remaining options do not satisfy the stem.

26. **(C)** Glycogen storage in the liver is regulated by the Islets of Langerhans in the pancreas. Another function is accelerating oxidation of sugar in the cells.

27. **(D)** ATP (adenosine triphosphate) is a coenzyme that fuels life. It carries energy to cells. ATP does not conserve lipids, inhibit carbohydrates, or act as a catalyst.

28. **(C)** The classification of humans is as follows:

    Kingdom (Animalia) → Phylum (Chordata) → Subphylum (Vertebrata) → Class (Mammalia) → Order (Primates) → Family (Hominidae) → Genus (*Homo*) → Species (*Homo sapiens*)

29. **(B)** The vertebral column, or backbone, is composed of individual vertebrae running from the base of the skull to the coccyx. The foremost function of the vertebral column is to protect the spinal cord. Nerves diverging from the spinal cord branch out to all parts of the body. Other functions include bolstering the head and trunk and serving as joining points for muscles and ribs. The vertebral column allows for flexion. It does not provide neuronal stability. It provides for the dorsal aspect of the thorax.

30. **(C)** Hemostasis is accomplished via three steps: (1) vasoconstriction of damaged vessel; (2) formation of platelet plug; and (3) coagulation in which factor X and prothrombinase is formed, prothrombin is converted to thrombin, and fibrinogen is converted to fibrin.

31. **(B)** The stem is the definition of *deamination*. The remaining options do not meet the criteria for deamination.

32. **(B)** Plant sources are the only source for fiber in the human body. Fiber is not a nutrient. It enhances the elimination of waste products. Fiber adds bulk and water and softens the stool. The remaining options are not sources of fiber.

33. **(A)** Analysis follows data collection. The substeps of data collection are observing, measuring, sampling, and organizing.

34. **(A)** Calcium is the most abundant mineral in the human body and is required for tooth and bone formation, blood clotting, and nerve and muscle activity. Sufficient body calcium is needed to prevent tetany. Iron, manganese, and sodium are not factors in tetany. Knowing the definition of *tetany* provides clues for calcium as the correct response.

35. **(A)** Bile, an alkaline, yellow, brown, or greenish fluid, is produced and secreted by the liver and is stored in the gallbladder where it is concentrated. Bile travels through the common bile duct to the duodenum where it aids in the absorption and digestion of fats and the absorption of fat soluble vitamins (A, D, and K). Bile is composed of bile acids, salts, and cholesterol. The remaining options do not aid in the digestion of fats.

36. **(A)** *A nurse's perception of health-care institution bureaucracy will vary with his or her level of educational preparation* is a testable hypothesis because it can be determined experientially whether the hypothesis is likely to be false or more likely to be true. The remaining hypotheses are not testable. Pre-election polls are not reliable and are predominantly biased. For example, if people from a county who have never elected a Democratic official are asked who they forecast the next governor of the state will be, in all likelihood, they will say the next governor will be the Republican candidate. The hypothesis regarding elementary school children bringing their lunches to school is not a hypothesis. The question does not need scientific inquiry; the answer can be determined by counting the number of elementary students who bring their lunch to school. Snow at a higher elevation is not a valid predictor of snow at a lower elevation. Higher elevations typically receive more snow than lower elevations. A good example is the location of winter ski areas.

37. **(D)** The occipital area is the back of the head. The remaining cerebral areas are found in other areas.

38. **(D)** The lowest temperature a gas can achieve is the definition of absolute zero. The remaining options do not satisfy the definition of absolute zero.

39. **(B)** The cervix, uterus, vagina, and vulva are components of the female reproductive system. The uterus is a hollow muscular organ composed of three layers: the endometrium or reproductive layer; the myometrium or middle layer which composes the muscular wall of the uterus and plays a key role in the childbirth process; and the outer layer or perimetrium, a thin layer of epithelial cells that covers the uterus. The cervix and vulva are not muscular in nature, and while the vagina does have a muscle layer and becomes an enlarging passageway during childbirth, it does not have the strength of the uterus.

40. **(B)** Oxygen enters the cells by way of diffusion. Diffusion is a means of passive transport that basically means spreading or scattering. The process does not require energy. Movement of substances through cell membranes is classified as passive or active processes. Diffusion and osmosis are passive mechanisms, and active transport, phagocytosis, and pinocytosis

are active mechanisms. Transcytosis, or vesicular transport, is a mechanism of transcellular transport across a cell and is not involved in the process of diffusion.

41. **(C)** Neurotransmitters are chemicals that relay signals between neurons. Acetylcholine, epinephrine, norepinephrine, dopamine, gamma aminobutyric acid (GABA), glutamine, and serotonin are examples of neurotransmitters. The remaining options are not involved in this process.

42. **(D)** Aspirin, or acetylsalicylic acid (ASA), is used as an anti-inflammatory, analgesic, and antipyretic. Aspirin also prevents platelet agglutination or platelet clumping. Platelet agglutination is part of the sequence of events leading to thrombus (clot) formation which is seen in heart attacks and strokes. Aspirin does not prevent blood thinning, cardiac pain, or platelet proliferation.

43. **(A)** A neutron is a neutral particle in the nucleus of an atom that has a mass of 1 amu. The number of neutrons in an element can be determined by subtracting the atomic number of the element from the atomic mass (weight) of the element.

$$\text{Krypton: Atomic number} = 36 \qquad \text{Atomic mass} = 83.798$$

$$\text{Atomic mass} - \text{Atomic number} = \text{Number of Neutrons}$$

$$83.798 - 36 = 47.798 = 48 \text{ Neutrons}$$

44. **(A)** Calcium chloride contains an ionic bond. Calcium is an alkaline earth metal and chlorine is a halogen, a nonmetal. Bonds are valence electrons that connect the atoms or molecules and compounds together. Ionic bonds are formed between nonmetal and metal elements and require the transfer of a valence electron from the metal element to the nonmetal element. Ionic compounds are held together by ionic bonds. An ionic bond generates two oppositely charged ions. The following contain ionic bonds: KCl, MgO, $FeSe$, and $CaCl_2$. Covalent bonds are formed between nonmetal elements, and a valence electron is shared. Covalent bonds can be polar or nonpolar. Examples containing covalent bonds are H_2O, H_2, and CO_2.

45. **(D)** The larynx is above or superior to the esophagus. It is not inferior, intermediate, or proximal to the esophagus.

46. **(C)** The key to correctly determining the answer to this question is knowing how and where water is pulled from the body. Nephrons are filtering elements within the kidneys. They are the basic structural and functional units of the kidney. The nephron's primary purpose is to control water and other soluble substances by blood filtration. The nephron reabsorbs what is needed and excretes the rest as urine.

47. **(B)** The left ventricle is larger than the right ventricle and has thicker more muscular walls. The left ventricle pumps blood into the systemic circulation which carries oxygenated blood away from the heart and into the body. It includes the arterial and venous systems and culminates with blood returning to the heart via the vena cava veins. The left atrium is a holding chamber. The right ventricle is concerned with venous blood getting to the lungs.

48. **(B)** The foramen ovale, an opening in the interatrial septum, allows circulation to bypass the pulmonary system prior to birth when the fetal lungs are still developing. This opening normally closes at birth. The remaining options are congenital cardiac conditions except for mitral stenosis that usually results from disease.

49. **(B)** The heart has two atrioventricular valves: the tricuspid valve between the right atrium and right ventricle, and the bicuspid valve between the left atrium and left ventricle. Ventricular filling occurs when these two valves open. The fossa ovalis is located in the right atrium. The semilunar valve is an aortic valve. Breaking the word *atrioventricular* into its parts provides a clue to the answer.

50. **(A)** Analysis follows data collection in the research process. The remaining options take place prior to analysis.

51. **(A)** The stem is the definition of *external respiration*. Inspiration and expiration is the process of breathing. Internal respiration occurs within the body. Pulmonary-cardiac ventilation occurs during cardiopulmonary resuscitation.

52. **(A)** Transportation and distribution of oxygen throughout the body and collecting carbon dioxide and returning it to the lungs is the responsibility of the cardiovascular system. The remaining systems are not involved with transportation and distribution.

53. **(D)** Bundles of myelinated nerve fibers comprise nerve tracts in the central nervous system. Neurons are unipolar, bipolar, or multipolar. There is no such thing as a dealienated nerve fiber.

English and Language Usage

1. **(C)** Compound sentences are composed of two independent clauses. They are connected or linked together using a coordinating conjunction. Coordinating conjunctions can be remembered by using the acronym FANBOYS (For-And-Nor-But-Or-Yet-So). Coordinating conjunctions usually require the use of a comma to separate the independent clauses. The remaining options do not contain coordinating conjunctions. Option (A) is a complex sentence; option (B) is a complex sentence. The word *because* is a subordinating conjunction. Option (D) is a simple sentence.

2. **(B)** *Paraphernalia* is spelled correctly. The correct spelling for the remaining options is *accommodate, questionnaire,* and *withhold*.

3. **(D)** A question mark is needed after Monica's question, not a comma. The remaining options are punctuated correctly.

4. **(C)** The stem identifies the use of a dash. An apostrophe can indicate an exclusion of letters in a word, show plurals in numerals, and show possession. A colon is used to introduce or start a series or list and also comes before a statement. Quotation marks indicate direct speech or the exact words spoken by an individual. They are also used before and after titles.

5. **(C)** An indirect object identifies *to* or *for whom*, and *to what* and *for what* action the verb performs. In the sentence, *The parents bought their children new cars when they turned 18,* the verb is *bought,* the who is the *parents,* the what is *cars,* and the for whom is *children.* The remainder of the options do not contain indirect objects in the sentences.

6. **(D)** Nominative pronouns are the subject in a sentence. *We, you,* and *they* are nominative first-, second-, and third-person plural. *I, you, he/she/it* are nominative first-, second-, and third-person singular. Objective pronouns are objects in a sentence. *Us, you,* and *them* are objective first-, second-, and third-person plural. Possessive pronouns show possession, control, ownership, or rights. *Our/ours, your/yours,* and *their/theirs* are first-, second-, and third-person plural.

7. **(A)** Simple sentences or independent clauses are complete thoughts. They contain a single or compound subject and a single or compound verb. Option (B) is a compound-complex sentence. Option (C) is a compound sentence. Option (D) is a dependent clause and is not a sentence.

8. **(A)** A direct object is the receiver or recipient of action in a sentence. In the sentence, *Frank Hamilton, a music instructor at the local junior college, offers a free class in beginning guitar, Frank Hamilton* is the subject, *a music instructor . . .* is a dependent clause that further identifies or defines Frank Hamilton, *offers* is the verb, and *class* is the direct object.

9. **(C)** *Continuously* is the correct word and means constantly, endlessly, or nonstop. Option (A) should use the word *annoy* instead of *aggravate*. An annoyance is something that bothers or gets on your nerves; aggravation is something that worsens or exacerbates. Option (B) should use the word *sight* instead of *site*. *Sight* is something seen with the eyes, something that is viewed or noticed. *Site* is a location or place. Option (D) should use the word *altar* instead of *alter*. An altar is an elevated place or structure where religious rites are performed. *Alter* means to change.

10. **(A)** The suffix *-cide* means kill or the act of killing. Examples are *homicide*, *herbicide*, and *bacteriocidal*. The suffix *-ee* means receiver or performer. Examples are *employee*, and *volunteer*. *Apnea* and *orthopnea* are examples of the suffix *-pnea*, and *philosophy* is an example of the suffix *-sophy*.

11. **(A)** Coordinating conjunctions can be remembered by using the acronym FANBOYS (For-And-Nor-But-Or-Yet-So). Coordinating conjunctions usually require the use of a comma to separate the independent clauses. Options (B) and (C) use the subordinating conjunctions *rather than* and *whereas*. Option (D) does not use a conjunction.

12. **(C)** The question asks what the italicized words indicate. *Pre-* and *post-tests* are given to assess knowledge before and after information is given—often in a formally structured way. Option (A) is automatically incorrect because of the words *will always*, and pre- and post-tests may not test abilities as they only test knowledge. Cost of pre- and post-testing is added into the cost of a course, if necessary. Option (D) is illogical.

13. **(D)** *President* is always capitalized when referring to the President of the United States. Air Force One is the traffic control sign for any U.S. Air Force aircraft carrying the President of the United States. It is always capitalized since it is a particular object. Option (A) is an example of interrupted direct speech; the word *pay* should not be capitalized. In option (B), the title of the algebra course should be capitalized and should read *Algebra 1542. The Victorian Era* in option (C) requires capitalization since it is a name applied to a recognized historic, cultural era.

14. **(B)** *Cowboy up* is a slang term. It means facing a formidable task, not bowing to adversity of hardship, or not giving up. The remaining options are not supportive of the term.

15. **(D)** Verbs are a category of words that normally express an action or occurrence, a state of being, or a relationship between things. It is impossible to have a sentence without a verb. Verbs are classified as action (*run, threw, climbed*) and nonaction (*dislike, believe, have, taste*). Sentences may or may not have adverbs, gerunds, and/or prepositions.

16. **(A)** The four sentences can be randomly grouped in any fashion to present the information. However, random ordering of the sentences produces a jumbled array of thoughts that have no order or specific meaning for the reader. The stem asks for the most meaningful passage. This suggests order and reasonable thought. Option (A) provides this. The remaining options appear haphazardly thrown together.

17. **(A)** Compound sentences are composed of two independent clauses (complete sentences). The sentences are connected using a coordinating conjunction which is typically followed by a comma. The word *however* is the coordinating conjunction. Options (B) and (C) are simple sentences, and option (D) is a complex sentence that uses the subordinating conjunction *if*.

18. **(C)** An encyclopedia is a resource containing topics in alphabetical order. They can be general (*Encyclopedia Britannica*) or specific (an encyclopedia of the Civil War in America). The remaining options would not provide the information Gabe wants to research.

19. **(A)** The correct word in the sentence should be *implied,* not *inferred.* To *imply* is to suggest or hint without actually saying what is meant. In the sentence, the principal makes the statement that contact sports are inappropriate in the elementary grades. He does not say that the football program should be eliminated, but he suggests that it should be. To infer is to deduce or make a conjecture. An individual could infer that red lights at intersections mean little to drivers if the majority of drivers ignore red lights. The remaining options contain correct word usage.

20. **(D)** Of the four options, (A) and (B) are fabricated words. Depending on how the word is pronounced and used, a desert is an arid geographical region or abandonment without intending to return. *Dessert* satisfies the definition given in the stem and is spelled correctly.

21. **(C)** As written, the sentence suggests that season tickets were purchased because the team lost in the Super Bowl. This is a confusing statement—use of the word *since* is ambiguous. Use of a word such as *although* would clarify and add meaning to the sentence. The remaining options have both style and clarity.

22. **(D)** Second-person singular possessive pronouns are *your* and *yours*. The words are also second-person plural possessive. *Her, hers, his,* and *its* are third-person singular possessive, *my* and *mine* are first-person singular possessive, and *our* and *ours* are first-person plural possessive pronouns. You may have noticed that option (A) has four pronouns and the remaining options have three pronouns. If you selected option (A) because you were guessing, you most likely selected the option because it contains four pronouns where the remainder contains three. Selecting an option because it is the longest or has the longest listing is a myth and demonstrates poor guessing.

23. **(D)** *Obtuse* means simpleminded, thickheaded, slow, or dull. Astute and sensitive are antonyms for *obtuse*. Based on the sentence, the man is slow to understand. The sentence does not suggest that the man is not paying attention.

24. **(C)** The words *winter* and *ice skating* are not capitalized in the correct option. The remaining options contain capitalization errors. *High school* is not capitalized since it is preceded by a possessive word (*my*); it is also nonspecific. *Uncle* before Henry is not capitalized since is it preceded by a possessive (our), and *gods* is not capitalized because the sentence speaks of gods in general.

25. **(C)** A *demagogue* is an individual, usually a political leader or speaker, who acquires power and recognition by provoking passions and intolerances of people. *Rabble-rouser* is a synonym for *demagogue*. The remaining options are antonyms of *demagogue*.

26. **(B)** The words *last* and *freezing* are descriptive words. Both words add meaning to the sentence. It was not just any game, but the last game of the season, and cancellation was not just because of rain, but because of freezing rain. The remaining options are not descriptive words in the sentence.

27. **(B)** Marge Swanson is two things—an excellent teacher and a strong student advocate. *Not only* precedes *excellent teacher* and *but* precedes *strong student advocate*. The sentence is balanced. In this case, the descriptions are presented in the same form. The remaining options are not correctly or effectively written and are not balanced.

28. **(D)** The sentence contains additional words or phrases that are unnecessary and misuses words. Correctly written, the sentence reads, *I came here tonight because I thought someone might listen to my opinion*. The remaining options are correctly written.

NOTES

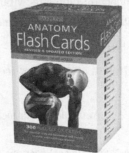
 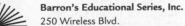

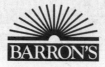
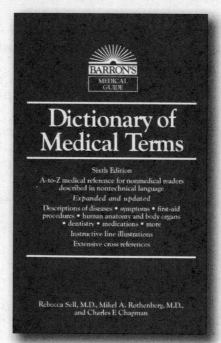

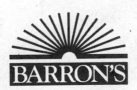

WE SALUTE THEIR HISTORICAL ACHIEVEMENTS!
From Nightingale to Nursing in the Twenty-first Century

Celebrating Nurses
A Visual History

Dr. Christine Hallett; U.S. Consultant Joan E. Lynaugh, R.N., M.S.N., Ph.D., F.A.A.N.

This refreshing narrative history of nursing marks an exception to standard, often dry academic descriptions of the nursing profession. It presents dramatic, highly readable illustrated stories of nursing's pioneering, often heroic leaders. Following an account of early nineteenth-century nursing practice during the Napoleonic Wars, the book goes on to highlight the life and work of Florence Nightingale who, in the 1850s, elevated nursing to a respected branch of medicine when she served on the Crimean War's battlefields. Also chronicled are the contributions to nursing by Clara Barton, founder of the American Red Cross, and the poet Walt Whitman during the American Civil War. Surgical nursing first became important in the late nineteenth century, following discoveries by Robert Koch in Germany and Louis Pasteur in France of germ theory and infection control. Early twentieth-century accounts chronicle the origin of public health services, and include the story of Adelaide Nutting, the world's first professor of nursing at Columbia Teacher's College in New York. Here too is the story of Edith Cavell, who was executed for helping Allied soldiers escape from German-occupied Belgium during World War I. Nursing's contributions during World War II, as well as in the Korean and Vietnam wars are also described in several vivid accounts. A concluding chapter explains how twenty-first-century nursing has expanded to cover many duties that were once the responsibility of junior doctors. The book's absorbing text is complemented with approximately 200 illustrations and photos.

Hardcover w/jacket, 192 pp., 8 ¹/₂" x 10 ¹/₂"
ISBN-13: 978-0-7641-6286-2, ISBN-10: 0-7641-6286-1
$24.99, Can$29.99

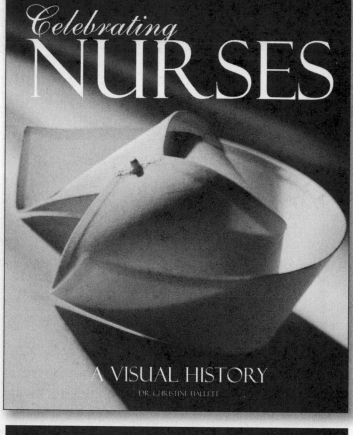

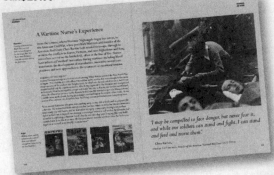

Dr. Christine Hallett, Ph.D. is a Registered Nurse and the Director of the Center for the History of Nursing and Midwifery at the University of Manchester, U.K. She also holds fellowships with the Royal Society of Medicine and the Royal Society for the Arts, U.K.

Joan E. Lynaugh, Ph.D., R.N., is Professor Emerita of the School of Nursing at the University of Pennsylvania and the Barbara Bates Center for the Study of the History of Nursing.

Highlights from Celebrating Nurses

- Early Military Nursing in the Napoleonic wars and Florence Nightingale in the Crimean War
- What is a Nurse? How the nursing vocation evolved into a highly respected profession
- Surgical Nursing and the emergence of nurses in the operating room
- The Establishment of Nursing Schools, starting in 1907 when Adelaide Nutting at Columbia Teachers College in New York became the world's first nursing professor

Barron's Celebrates National Nurses Week

National Nurses Week is celebrated annually from May 6th, also known as National Nurses Day, through May 12th, the birthday of Florence Nightingale, the founder of modern nursing.

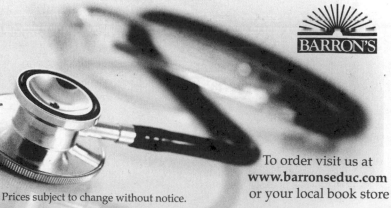

BARRON'S

Barron's Educational Series, Inc.
250 Wireless Blvd.
Hauppauge, N.Y. 11788
Call toll-free: 1-800-645-3476

(#190) R 4/10

In Canada:
Georgetown Book Warehouse
34 Armstrong Ave.
Georgetown, Ontario L7G 4R9
Call toll-free: 1-800-247-7160

To order visit us at
www.barronseduc.com
or your local book store

Prices subject to change without notice.